SPRINGER SERIES IN NEUROPSYCHOLOGY

Harry A. Whitaker, Series Editor

## Springer Series in Neuropsychology

Harry A. Whitaker, Series Editor

---

*Phonological Processes and Brain Mechanisms*
H.A. Whitaker (Ed.)

*Contemporary Reviews in Neuropsychology*
H.A. Whitaker (Ed.)

*Neuropsychological Studies of Nonfocal Brain Damage: Dementia and Trauma*
H.A. Whitaker (Ed.)

*Linguistic Analyses of Aphasic Language*
W.U. Dressler and J.A. Stark (Eds.)

*Synesthesia: A Union of the Senses*
R.E. Cytowic

*Discourse Ability and Brain Damage: Theoretical and Empirical Perspectives*
Y. Joanette and H.H. Brownell (Eds.)

*Morphology, Phonology, and Aphasia*
J.-L. Nespoulous and P. Villiard (Eds.)

*Cognitive Microgenesis: A Neuropsychological Perspective*
R.E. Hanlon (Ed.)

*Neuropsychology and the Law*
J. Dywan, R.D. Kaplan, and F.J. Pirozzolo (Eds.)

Robert E. Hanlon
Editor

# Cognitive Microgenesis

## A Neuropsychological Perspective

Foreword by Anne Harrington

With 29 Illustrations

Springer-Verlag
New York Berlin Heidelberg London
Paris Tokyo Hong Kong Barcelona

Robert E. Hanlon
Departments of Rehabilitation
and Neuropsychology
University of California at Los Angeles
300 U.C.L.A. Medical Plaza, B100
Los Angeles, CA 90024
USA

Library of Congress Cataloging-in-Publication Data
Cognitive microgenesis: a neuropsychological perspective / Robert E. Hanlon, editor.
p. cm. — (Springer series in neuropsychology)
Includes bibliographical references.
ISBN-13:978-1-4612-7778-1 e-ISBN-13:978-1-4612-3056-4
DOI: 10.1007/978-1-4612-3056-4
1. Brain—Evolution. 2. Brain—Growth. 3. Neuropsychology.
4. Cognitive science. I. Hanlon, Robert E. II. Series.
[DNLM: 1. Cognition. 2. Neuropsychology. WL 103 C676]
QP376.C58 1991
612.8'2—dc20 90-10408

Printed on acid-free paper.



Typeset by Best-set Typesetters, Ltd., Chai Wan, Hong Kong.

9 8 7 6 5 4 3 2 1

ISBN-13:978-1-4612-7778-1

# Foreword

If scientific research traditions can be awarded philosophical epitaphs, perhaps an appropriately suggestive one for microgenesis would be Heraclitus's classic statement: "We step and we do not step into the same river, we are and we are not." For this is the heart, it seems to me, of the challenge microgenesis aims to confront: In what sense is the brain as an object of scientific inquiry the same object from moment to moment and in what sense is it eternally harnessed to the unidirectional laws of time and process and change? Philosophically, the microgenetic enterprise has been all about mediating this tension between the imperatives of stable identity and those of transmutation and process. Scientifically, the challenge that has faced microgenesis historically has been the profound one of symbolically and pictorially capturing on a three-dimensional printed page the deep truth that the brain is a four-dimensional object.

The earliest and still most enduring metaphor used to convey the microgenetic principle of four-dimensionality drew on images of hierarchy, one of 19th-century evolution's conceptual legacies to psychological and neurological theorizing. The hierarchy metaphor—first formulated into a form practical for brain science research by the British neurologist John Hughlings Jackson—was made all the more compelling for the insight it seemed to offer into the *nature* of the change one could expect to see in mind–brain processes as they passed through progressively more complex levels of the system. In this sense, microgenesis and Freudian psychoanalysis are two results of a broad fin de siècle attempt to reformulate static, surface-oriented models of mind–brain using the Darwinian and Haeckelian legacy of a truncated replaying of past history in the present moment.

Historically, a case for intriguing family resemblances between the original ambitions of dynamic psychiatry (including but not limited to the work of Freud) and the past and present ambitions of the microgenetic program in neurology can be expounded still further. In each case, we are concerned with a research program to recover the normally hidden processes leading to the final (mental) product, pathology is seen as an important window onto a normally subterranean terrain of not-yet-actualized experience, and the untidy world of affect and motivation (whether we choose to use the language of *ids* or that of limbic processes) is drawn into a necessary partnership with the unfolding processes of perceptual and cognitive formation. The German experimental psychologist, Friedrich Sander, who coined the German term *Aktualgenesis*, was fascinated by the powerful emotionality associated with early (normally preconscious) stages of perception, as well as the powerful pull of something one might want to call "will" toward final consolidation of the image (Hermann, 1976, p. 600).

More broadly, microgenesis may be considered an enduring neurological legacy of a general reorientation in philosophy which began around the turn of the century and that, in various ways, would begin to stress the radical historicity of fundamental reality. Keynote contributions in this process of questioning and recasting of problems have ranged from the concept of creatively unfolding time (*durée réelle*) in the work of Henri Bergson to the "process philosophy" of Alfred North Whitehead.

At the same time, the speculative potentialities of microgenesis have necessarily been disciplined by the pragmatic challenges it faces from laboratory and clinical data. For this reason, it has slowly, over the course of this century, arrived at a point where it can now aspire to become something that "process philosophy" never could or would be: a research paradigm with sufficient explanatory scope and predictive power to guide and integrate multidisciplinary investigations into cognitive processes and neuropsychological functioning. If microgenesis succeeds in its quest to be integrated into the mainstream of cutting-edge neuropsychology, this will not be solely because it was always more "true" than other, more static paradigms. It will have succeeded because it persisted in the hard work of transforming its deep truths into the practical insights and technologies required of every productive science.

## Reference

Hermann, T. (1976). Ganzheitspsychologie und Gestalttheorie. In: *Die Psychologie des 20. Jahrhunderts*: *Vol. 1. Die europäische Tradition* (pp. 573–658). Kindler Verlag, Zürich.

Department of the History of Science
Harvard University
Cambridge, MA

ANNE HARRINGTON, PHD

# Contents

# Contributors

TALIS BACHMANN, PHD Department of Psychology, University of Tartu, Tartu, Estonia, USSR

JASON W. BROWN, MD Department of Neurology, New York University Medical Center, New York, NY 10016, USA

HUGH W. BUCKINGHAM, PHD Interdepartmental Linguistics Program, Louisiana State University, Baton Rouge, LA 70803, USA

INGEGERD CARLSSON, PHD Department of Psychology, Lund University, S-223 50 Lund, Sweden

JOHN A. CEGALIS, PHD 9 Trafalgar Square, Nashua, NH 03063, USA

JURIS G. DRAGUNS, PHD Department of Psychology, Pennsylvania State University, University Park, PA 16802, USA

GARY GOLDBERG, MD Electrodiagnostic and Stroke Centers, Moss Rehabilitation Hospital and Departments of Physiology and Physical Medicine and Rehabilitation, Temple University School of Medicine, Philadelphia, PA 19141, USA

ROBERT E. HANLON, PHD Departments of Rehabilitation and Neuropsychology, University of California at Los Angeles, Los Angeles, CA 90024, USA

UWE HENTSCHEL, PHD Department of Psychology, University of Leiden, 2300RA Leiden, The Netherlands

RALPH E. HOFFMAN, MD Yale Psychiatric Institute, Yale University School of Medicine, New Haven, CT 06520, USA

Arn Hosemann, PhD Department of Psychology, University of Leiden, 2300RA Leiden, The Netherlands

Aki M. Johanson, PhD Department of Psychology, Lund University, S-223 50 Lund, Sweden

Manfred Kießling, PhD Department of Psychology, University of Leiden, 2300RA Leiden, The Netherlands

George Kurian, PhD Institute for Yoga and Consciousness, Vijayanagaram Palace, Andhra University, Visăkhapatnam 530 023, India

Åsa Lilja, PhD Department of Psychology, Lund University, S-223 50, Lund, Sweden

Paul D. MacLean, MD National Institute of Mental Health, Poolesville, MD 20837, USA

Avraham Schweiger, PhD Department of Psychology, University of California at Los Angeles, Los Angeles, CA 90024, USA

Gudmund J.W. Smith, PhD Department of Psychology, Lund University, S-223 50, Lund, Sweden

# Introduction

Microgenesis represents a process model of cognitive formation in which the structural development of mental phenomena is considered to evolve through qualitatively different stages, ultimately emerging in consciousness and behavioral expression. The fundamental assumption of microgenesis is that all mental representations, including ideas, perceptions, words, actions, and affects, result from a formative process that is responsible for their emergent structure. This process involves a progressive unfolding in microtime, spanning milliseconds or seconds, that ultimately achieves conscious awareness. Awareness of mental events in consciousness represents the end point of multiple preconscious stages through which a cognition is formed. Conscious events, such as volitional movement, veridical object perception, articulate speech, and mental images are the end stage of the cognitive process and the surface level of cognitive structure. They are the outcome of a microdevelopmental process that is reiterated in the occurrence of every representation.

The primary focus of microgenesis is on the stages through which a mental representation unfolds. This approach examines the processing stages underlying representations through experimental methods designed to elicit preliminary stages of the cognitive progression and/or through the process-oriented assessment and interpretation of the symptoms and errors emitted by patients with brain lesions. According to Froehlich (1984), microprocesses to be assessed are conceptualized as an ordered sequence of events that occurs in the temporal period between the presentation of a stimulus and the formation of a single, stabilized cognitive response.

A fundamental principle, conceived by Werner (1948, 1957) and elaborated by Arieti (1962), is that microgeny recapitulates, but does not repeat, phylogeny and ontogeny. The idea that phylogenetic and ontogenetic patterns are retraced in microgeny implies that this process may be conceptualized as a natural developmental progression that unfolds over the temporal period of milliseconds or seconds and recapitulates evolutionary and maturational processes, psychologically and biologically.

A basic element in microgenetic theory is the idea that preliminary or premature stages that precede conscious representations are an integral part of the structure of the representation, a concept identical to that in evolutionary theory. The microdevelopmental progression may be considered a type of instantaneous evolution. Like evolution and maturation, it is assumed to proceed in a forward direction. Draguns (1983) speculates that the adaptive nature of microgenesis is based on the properties of dissonance, incongruity, and conflict, which guide the formative process toward the completion of its course.

The microprocessing approach incorporates the principle of hierarchical organization within the stage model of cognitive formation. However, there are distinct differences between microgenetic theory and Jacksonian concepts. In Jackson's view (1932), cognition is hierarchically ordered as a function of development and damage to the later superficial levels in the hierarchy of neuropsychological function releases normally inhibited archaic systems. Conversely, the microgenetic approach holds that preliminary stages are not released or disinhibited from above but exhibit a form of cognition consistent with a certain level of derivation (Brown, 1988b). The structure of cognition arises from the transformation of early processing stages into subsequent stages, rather than higher, more volitional stages controlling lower, automatic ones. In microgenesis, the direction of processing is not descending control by higher centers over lower output levels but an emergent process from depth to surface.

The microgenetic conceptualization of a symptom is crucial to an understanding of the model. In contrast to the traditional view in which symptoms are viewed as deficits brought about by damage to underlying mechanisms, on the microgenetic approach, according to Brown (1977, 1988b), symptoms reflect normal subsurface processing mediated by the damaged region. An important point is that symptoms are not attenuations but submerged levels, which are normally transformed in cognitive formation. Pathology disrupts the microgenetic progression at a subsurface stage and exposes the normal processing at the disrupted point in the structuration process. Symptoms reflect a particular moment in microgeny, the variability of which is determined by the level achieved as the normal process unfolds. Focal lesions induce a circumscribed disruption in the formative process, but the processing mediated by the damaged area still occurs as the exposed point evolves through successive stages in a normal manner. The argument is that in brain pathology the symptom reflects the stage of cognitive formation where the normal structural progression is derailed, as the result of a lesion.

There are two important implications of this perspective for neuropsychology. First, it postulates that the neurodynamic states underlying cognitive functions are generated as wave fronts (Bernstein, 1967) or fields (Braak, 1980; Sanides, 1970), rather than centers or modules. Clearly, this view requires a shift in thinking from conventional static center, modular, and connectionistic models to one in which transformations underlying behavior unfold over coupled neural and cognitive processing stages. Second, the concept of pathology as a disruption or derailment, rather than as a deficit or loss implies that, with the exception of cases of massive brain damage, functions are not destroyed or eliminated from the repertoire of behavior but persist in an altered form and have the potential to be retrieved. Theoretically, this means that recovery of cognitive function following brain damage as well as the remediation of dysfunctional cognitive systems are possible.

## History

With this introduction to the principles of microgenetic theory, a brief overview of the historical development of the model may help to resolve misconceptions of this hierarchically organized stage model of cognitive processing (see also Brown, 1972; Flavell & Draguns, 1957; Hanlon & Brown, 1989). Originating from assumptions on the structural development of thought, the early experimental psychologists of Würzburg and Leipzig, despite the methodological drawbacks of the introspective approach, produced the conceptual precursors of microgenesis. Though crude, these experiments led to the description of a nonsensory or imageless event or state of consciousness immediately following the presentation of a stimulus, a stage that corresponded to the birth of a thought. The model of meaning that emerged from this work was important in that it represented an attempt to describe the microstructure of the cognitive process, based on the idea of a microtemporal transition underlying thought.

Following the proposals of the early Würzburg psychologists on the transitional stages of thought formation, Arnold Pick (1913) presented a hierarchical model of language organization, based on his observations and analyses of the utterances of aphasic patients. Pick described four hierarchical stages through which thought develops in the process of language production. He believed that this microtemporal sequence originated in a prelinguistic stage consisting of the initial formulation of the thought as a loose structural assembly of components, followed by stages of predication, development of the utterance pattern, and word choice and articulation, respectively. In 1920, following a series of case studies involving detailed clinical observations, Liepmann proposed a theory of apraxia, which divided the apraxias into three major forms, according to the point in the physiological and temporal organization of movement at which the process was disrupted. He held that the different types of apraxia (i.e., limb-kinetic, ideomotor, ideational) represent moments in the action development (see Brown, 1988a).

Until this time, studies and theories based on the process perspective had focused on the formation of thought, language, and action. Influenced by the Gestalt movement, however, Sander (1928/1962) and his group in Leipzig initiated the experimental study of the temporal development of percepts. Sander proposed a theory of perception in which the process of object formation, referred to as *Aktualgenese*, evolved through several phases of perceptual microdevelopment. He maintained that the process of perception developed from an initial stage of a diffuse percept through progressive differentiation and discrimination to a distinct configuration.

Sander (1928/1962) was responsible for the development of experimental paradigms and techniques, designed explicitly to demonstrate microgenetic phenomena. These paradigms involved presentation of stimuli in obscured or fragmented conditions, including poor illumination, peripheral location, and tachistoscopic exposure (see Froehlich, 1984). Following the initial presentation, a series of presentations were completed that were characterized by successive increases in distinctiveness and clarity. Based on his belief that the perceptual process is composed of a series of distinct stages of which we are consciously unaware, by restricting the normal perceptual progression experimentally, these stages could be delineated and analyzed.

In cases of perceptual disorder resulting from brain damage, such as agnosia, Pötzl (1928, 1960) noted the intrusive recurrence of unreported elements in subsequent object descriptions. For example, a green asparagus stalk that was not reported on one task recurred a few moments later in the description of a person as having a green tie (see Brown, 1988a). He then confirmed this effect in normal subjects. Following the tachistoscopic presentation of scenes, he found that unreported fragments were integrated into dreams and were recalled in morning dream reports. These findings, which were subsequently confirmed by Fisher (1960), sparked great interest in subliminal perception. Furthermore, the implication that subconscious residues are linked to early stages in object formation and that the symptoms of perceptual dysfunction can be reproduced through experiments in percept formation was influential in later studies of perceptgenesis.

Building on the findings of Sander and the concept of *Aktualgenese*, Conrad (1947) presented a microgenetic interpretation of aphasia. He described four levels of disorder in the word formation process, which may occur in aphasia, corresponding to Sander's (1928/1962) four-stage progression in perceptual microdevelopment. Conrad believed that cognitive formation depends on the simultaneous processes of differentiation and integration, and either one or both of these components are disrupted in aphasia.

At about the same time, Yakovlev (1948) published a seminal paper on the evolution of motility in which the different forms of motility and action systems were mapped to structural levels in the evolution of the forebrain. He differentiated behavior into three spheres of movements: visceral motility, such as respiration; motility of the outward expression of internal states, as in the facial expression, vocalizations, and postures associated with pain, fear, pleasure, and so on; and motility of effectuation, such as locomotion, manual manipulation, and tool use. Yakovlev, however, did not believe that these three spheres of motility represented independent categories of behavior. Rather, he insisted that "every movement and posture is an integral part of the total behavior which evolves and proceeds as a unity in time" (1948, p. 315). He elaborated on the action systems derived from these spheres of motility and proposed a hierarchical model of the neural structures that mediate the evolution of behaviors from visceral to expressive to effective.

Perhaps the most creative and expansive microgenetic theory of thought formation was proposed by Schilder (1951). Schilder viewed thought disorders as "abortive formations produced in the course of the differentiation-process of thought" (p. 514). The fundamental premise to Schilder's model is that mental contents or "presentations" are progressively incorporated within the developing thought structure. On this view, thought originates in a diffuse concept of the direction that its structural development will take, based on the goal established at the moment of conception. Subsequently, the thought evolves through a series of preliminary stages, which constitutes the preparatory phase, during which mental contents progressively influence the formative process. The passage to consciousness is governed by the dual processes of similarity and contiguity, resulting in the emergence of object-directed, reality-oriented thought.

On the view that schizophrenic thought disorders reflect abortive formations in the differentiation process that ordinarily evolves to reality-oriented and rational thought, Schilder proposed similar descriptions of disorders of language and perception. The symptoms of aphasia and agnosia were thought to reflect the coming-to-the-fore of earlier stages in their microgeny. A fundamental idea in Schilder's theory is that the process of thought development recapitulates the phylo-ontogeny of cognition. Additionally, and in keeping with the Jacksonian idea of hierarchical organization, he concluded that this developmental progression occurs through the psychic exchanges between the neural levels in the hierarchy (Schilder, 1953).

The developmental theorist Heinz Werner was responsible for introducing the methodological techniques used by Sander (1928/1962) to demonstrate perceptual microgenesis to English-speaking countries. Werner (1956), in fact, is credited with coining the term *microgenesis* in translation of the German word *Aktualgenese* in a paper on the microgenetic analysis of aphasia (see Flavell & Draguns, 1957). Werner (1956) put forth two basic assumptions:

> First, the functions underlying abnormal behavior are in their essence not different from those underlying normal behavior. Second, any human activity such as perceiving, thinking, acting, etc. is an unfolding process, and this unfolding of

microgenesis, whether it takes seconds or hours or days, occurs in developmental sequence. (p. 347)

Werner stressed that the unfolding of cognition retraces levels or stages in evolution and ontogeny. Drawing from the work of Pick, Sander, and Conrad, as well as his own experiments on the comparative developmental theory (1948), Werner described the semantic spheres through which linguistic processes develop in microgenetic progression. Catán (1986) provided a detailed review of the contributions of Werner, Vygotsky, and Luria to microgenetic theory, particularly from a developmental perspective.

Following the decline of behaviorism in the 1950s, there was renewed interest in information processing and mediational activity, which resulted in a resurgence of microgenetic research (Draguns, 1984). Much of the experimental work on the microgenetic model has been conducted in Europe, particularly at Lund University by Gudmund Smith and his colleagues, through their extensive research on percept-genesis. Founded on the classic microgenetic methods originally employed by Sander, two tachistoscopic procedures—the Meta-Contrast Technique (Kragh & Smith 1970) and the Defense Mechanism Test (Kragh, 1969; Westerlundh, 1976), in which incongruent and/or threatening stimuli are successively presented to evoke anxiety—have been used to examine normal and psychopathological personality organization.

Microgenetic methods and constructs have also been used in the experimental analysis and interpretation of subliminal perception (Dixon, 1981; Hentschel, Smith, & Draguns, 1986). Froehlich (1984), following Sander (1928/1962), has differentiated two types of microgenetic experimental procedures: (1) merogenetic techniques, which entail progressive stimulus presentations from degraded fragmentation to uniform configuration, which elicits imaginal activity and hypothesizing based on sequential comparisons, and (2) hologenetic techniques, which are based on a progressive change in the energy level of presentation of a structurally intact stimulus (i.e., luminosity, clarity, etc.), which reveal the stages of meaning assessment through progressive figure–ground discriminations.

Brown (1977, 1988b) has proposed a microgenetic interpretation of the symptoms of brain damage, which holds that the symptoms of neuropathology represent a premature exposure of preliminary levels in the microstructure of cognition that are normally transformed. Others who have presented microgenetic interpretations of the manifestations of neurological and neuropsychiatric conditions include Goldberg (1985, 1987) and Hoffman and Sledge (1984). More recently, Hanlon, Brown, and Gerstman (1990) have applied microgenetic principles in the development of a therapeutic intervention with brain-damaged patients.

The two historical tracts in work based on microgenetic principles, the clinical-theoretical and the experimental, continued relatively independently through the 1970s. However, with the advances in the neurosciences and the increased sophistication of methods employed in the study of neurocognitive processes, the 1980s saw the merging of these two tracts, primarily through the work and influence of individuals such as Smith, Brown, and Froehlich. Although insufficiently integrated into the mainstream of both neuropsychology and cognitive psychology, this work represents an intriguing, "alternative" approach to the study of cognitive processes and the manifestations of neuropathology.

## Overview

The present volume was conceived to bring together a number of notable neurologists, neuropsychologists, and cognitive psychologists who have expressed views, developed models, or conducted experimental work based on microgenetic theory. The division of this collection of chapters into the two sections of (I) clinical and theoretical views and (II) experimental approaches to cognitive processing and personality not only represents a practical separation based on the conceptual nature of the chapter but also reflects the two different but interrelated veins that have emerged in work on microgenesis. This book is an attempt to unify these two veins in a collaborative project with the singular objective of understanding cognitive process and neuropsychological function.

In Chapter 1, Paul MacLean discusses the role of the cerebellum, through interconnections with the prefrontal cortex and thalamus, in highly complex cognitive operations, such as planning, mathematical functions, and prediction. With intriguing evidence based on the triune structure of the forebrain and the fractal aspects of microgenesis, he elaborates on the neofrontocerebellar mechanisms that may be implicated in computation and prediction.

Gary Goldberg stresses the need for a sound theoretical foundation for neurorehabilitation, in Chapter 2. Following a detailed analysis of the microgenetic process from the dynamical systems perspective, he proposes that the dual premotor systems hypothesis, a model of action formation based on microgenetic principles, may serve as a heuristic framework for interpreting the performance errors of brain-damaged subjects and developing strategic rehabilitation programs.

In Chapter 3, Jason Brown describes the dynamic structure of mental states and the concept of a stratified cognition. He elaborates on the neuroanatomical framework of cognition, based on extensive work on the microgenetic model, and speculates on the formative nature of consciousness. George Kurian, in Chapter 4, presents a cogent analysis of the recent findings on semantic processing and hemispheric asymmetry and argues that such findings are consistent with, and indeed, may be explained by microgenetic theory.

In Chapter 5, Avraham Schweiger elucidates some of the difficulties with traditional cognitive and neuropsychological approaches that have stressed the functional separation of perception and action. Based on the Piagetian approach to cognitive development, which stresses the integration of perception and action, he argues that action and perception emerge through progressive stages in a unified microgenetic process. John Cegalis provides an extensive and detailed review of the work of a number of cognitive theorists who have focused on perceptual microgenesis, in Chapter 6, and constrasts the microgenetic perspective with that of information processing approaches. He outlines the conditions considered to be necessary and sufficient for perceptual microgenesis and cautions as to the limitations of the model.

Ralph Hoffman presents a compelling interpretation of schizophrenic language production from the microgenetic perspective in Chapter 7. With numerous examples of schizophrenic speech and evidence from previous studies, Hoffman suggests that errors generated by schizophrenics reveal distinct stages in the microgenetic progression of language production. In Chapter 8, Hugh W. Buckingham provides a comparative analysis of the psycholinguistic model of sentence production proposed by Merrill Garrett and the microgenesis of language formation developed by Jason Brown. Based on the common elements of hierarchical organization and parallel processing, Buckingham succeeds in mapping Garrett's functional model to Brown's microgenetic theory, arriving at an integrated neuropsychological interpretation of language production and paraphasic errors. In closing the section on theoretical interpretations and clinical applications, Hanlon discusses some of the shortcomings of the cognitive rehabilitation movement, and following Goldberg, stresses the need for a theory of neurorehabilitation. This is followed by a description of studies involving language rehabilitation, particularly the facilitation of language production, which have been based on microgenetic theory.

Gudmund Smith opens the section on experimental work with a cogent and convincing thesis on the importance of reconsidering methods employed in the study of perception and the need to incorporate microgenetic approaches that may examine various aspects of cognitive processing and structuration. As co-founder of the Lund school of percept-genesis, Smith calls for the shift to a process perspective in the analysis of both cognition and personality, to more fully explain neuropsychological function. In Chapter 11, Carlsson, Lilja, Smith, and Johanson describe the methods used to assess cognitive processing and personality variables, based on the percept-genetic model outlined by Smith, and present the findings of two studies that incorporated these methods.

Talis Bachmann (Chapter 12) reviews recent findings on visuoperceptual processing derived from work in experimental cognition, using various visual information-processing paradigms. He concludes that the results of studies involving visual masking, binocular rivalry, and global/local visual processing support the main postulates of cognitive microgenesis. In Chapter 13, Hentschel, Kießling, and Hosemann present a study that incorporated microgenetic methodology and resulted in illuminating findings regarding the influence of anxiety on attentional mechanisms and the apparent interaction of specific defense mechanisms and anxiety on attentional regulation. Juris Draguns concludes the volume with an informed and insightful overview of experimental work conducted from the microgenetic perspective and directed toward the assessment of personality. Draguns surveys the techniques that have been employed to date and proposes that the percept-genetic techniques hold great promise as established methods for future research on cognitive processes.

Current work on this theoretical perspective is rather sparse. However, as a result of the seemingly growing dissatisfaction with conventional center, modular, and componential theories of neurocognition, interest in microgenesis is increasing. The degree to which the theoretical principles, clinical interpretations, and experimental techniques of the microgenetic model will be incorporated within neuropsychology remains to be seen. The current movement within cognitive psychology and the neurosciences, involving the analysis of cognitive processes, rather than the products of cognitive formation, is encouraging. Furthermore, this refocusing on process-oriented approaches to the study of cognition suggests that the time has come to seriously consider this perspective.

## *References*


Arieti, S. (1962). The microgeny of thought and perception. *Archives of General Psychiatry, 6,* 76–90.

Bernstein, N. (1967). *The coordination and regulation of movements.* Oxford, UK: Pergamon.

Braak, H. (1980). *Architectonics of the human telencephalic cortex.* Berlin: Springer-Verlag.

Brown, J.W. (1972). *Aphasia, apraxia, and agnosia.* Springfield, IL: Charles C. Thomas.

Brown, J.W. (1977). *Mind, brain, and consciousness.* New York: Academic Press.

Brown, J.W. (1988a). *Classics in neuropsychology: Selected papers on agnosia and apraxia.* Hillsdale, NJ: Erlbaum.

Brown, J.W. (1988b). *The life of the mind.* Hillsdale, NJ: Lawrence Erlbaum.

Catán, L. (1986). The dynamic display of process: Historical development and contemporary uses of the microgenetic method. *Human Development, 29,* 252–263.

Conrad, K. (1947). Über den Begriff der Vorgestalt und seine Bedeutung für die Hirnpathologie. *Nervenarzt, 18,* 289–293.

Dixon, N. F. (1981). *Preconscious processing.* Chichester: Wiley.

Draguns, J.G. (1983). Why microgenesis? An inquiry on the motivational sources of going beyond the information given. *Archives of Psychology, 135,* 5–16.

Draguns, J.G. (1984). Microgenesis by any other name . . . . In W. Froehlich, G. Smith, J. Draguns, & U. Hentschel (Eds.), *Psychological processes in cognition and personality.* Washington, DC: Hemisphere.

Fisher, C. (1960). Introduction: Preconscious stimulation in dreams, associations, and images. *Psychological Issues, 2,* 1–40.

Flavell, J.H., & Draguns, J. (1957). A microgenetic approach to perception and thought. *Psychological Bulletin, 54,* 197–217.

Froehlich, W.D. (1984). Microgenesis as a functional approach to information processing through search. In W. Froehlich, G. Smith, J. Draguns, & U. Hentschel (Eds.), *Psychological processes in cognition and personality* (pp. 19–52). Washington, DC: Hemisphere.

Goldberg, G. (1985). Supplementary motor area structure and function: Review and hypotheses. *The Behavioral and Brain Sciences, 8,* 567–616.

Goldberg, G. (1987). From intent to action: Evolution and function of the premotor systems of the frontal lobe. In E. Perecman (Ed.), *The frontal lobes revisited* (pp. 273–306). New York: IRBN Press.

Hanlon, R., & Brown, J.W. (1989). Microgenesis: Historical review and current studies. In A. Ardila & F. Ostrosky-Solis (Eds.), *Brain organization of language and cognitive processes* (pp. 3–15). New York: Plenum.

Hanlon, R.E., Brown, J.W., & Gerstman, L. (1990). Enhancement of naming in nonfluent aphasia through gesture. *Brain and Language, 38,* 298–314.

Hentschel, U., Smith, G., & Draguns, J. (Eds.) (1986). *The roots of perception.* Amsterdam: Elsevier North-Holland.

Hoffman R., & Sledge, W. (1984). A microgenetic model of paragrammatisms produced by a schizophrenic speaker. *Brain and Language, 21,* 147–173.

Jackson, J.H. (1932). In J. Taylor (Ed.), *Selected writings of John Hughlings Jackson: Vol. 2.* London: Hodder & Stoughton.

Kragh, U. (1969). *DMT-defense mechanism test.* Stockholm: Skandinaviska Testforlaget.

Kragh, U., & Smith, G.J.W. (Eds.) (1970). *Percept-genetic analysis.* Lund, Sweden: Gleerup.

Liepmann, H. (1920). Apraxie. *Ergebnisse der gesamten Medizin, 1,* 516–543.

Pick, A. (1913). *Die agrammatischen Sprachstörungen.* Berlin: Springer-Verlag.

Pötzl, O. (1928). *Die optisch-agnostischen Störungen.* Leipzig, Germany: Deutiche.

Pötzl, O. (1960). The relationship between experimentally induced dream images and indirect vision. *Psychological Issues, 2,* 41–120. (original work published 1917)

Sander, F. (1962). Experimentelle Ergebnisse der Gestaltpsychologie. In F. Sander & H. Volkelt (Eds.), *Ganzheitspsychologie.* Munich, Germany: Beck. (Reprinted from E. Becher (Ed.), *10 Kongreß bericht experimentelle Psychologie*, 1928. Jena: Fischer)

Sanides, F. (1970). Functional architecture of motor and sensory cortices in primates in light of a new concept of neocortex evolution. In C. Noback & W. Montagna (Eds.), *Advances in primatology* Vol. 2, pp. 137–208. New York: Appleton-Century-Crofts.

Schilder, P. (1951). On the development of thoughts. In D. Rapaport (Ed.), *Organization and pathology of thought* (pp. 497–518). New York: Columbia University Press.

Schilder, P. (1953). *Medical psychology.* New York: International Universities Press.

Werner, H. (1948). *Comparative psychology of mental development.* New York: International Universities Press.

Werner, H. (1956). Microgenesis and aphasia. *Journal of Abnormal Social Psychology, 52,* 347–353.

Werner, H. (1957). The concept of development from a comparative and organismic point of view. In D.B. Harris (Ed.), *The concept of development* (pp. 125–148). Minneapolis: University of Minnesota Press.

Westerlundh, G. (1976). *Aggression, anxiety and defense.* Lund, Sweden: Gleerup.

Yakovlev, P. (1948). Motility, behavior, and the brain. *Journal of Nervous and Mental Disease, 107,* 313–335.

# Part I Neuropsychological Interpretation and Clinical Applications

# 1
# Neofrontocerebellar Evolution in Regard to Computation and Prediction: Some Fractal Aspects of Microgenesis

PAUL D. MACLEAN

The traditional view has been that the cerebellum is involved in purely motor functions. In a provocative paper of 1974, Robert Dow cited a number of observations that were difficult to reconcile with this view. Some of the reasons for his questioning will be specified later. But his main question was this: If the cerebellum is altogether concerned with motor functions, how does one explain the substantial connections with cortical association areas of the frontal and temporal lobes? "Is the cerebellum," he asks, "in particular its hemispheral parts, a place where we store . . . motor patterns once they are learned?" (Dow, 1974, p. 111). Since then, he has collaborated with Leiner and Leiner in conducting research for testing the hypothesis that the frontal association cortex and neocerebellum participate in the "anticipatory use of cues" and "skillful manipulation of ideas" (Leiner, Leiner, & Dow, 1986; see also 1989).

Elsewhere in considering the functions of the frontal granular cortex, I have elaborated on the "Dow hypothesis" by suggesting that the advanced evolution of frontocerebellar systems in human beings may have provided neural circuitry for mathematical functions including those used in planning and prediction (MacLean, 1990). In the first part of the present chapter, I review anatomical, clinical, and other reasons for this suggestion. In the second part, I consider how an algorithmic functioning of neofrontocerebellar systems might apply to certain fractal aspects of cognitive microgenesis.

The language of words and the language of numbers both rank in the intellectual sphere as pinnacles of human achievement. If it is correct that the notches found on paleolithic tally sticks indicate that a capacity for tabulating numbers of things existed before an ability to devise verbal

---

Parts of this chapter are adapted from *The Triune Brain in Evolution: Role in Paleocerebral Functions* (pp. 545–552), by P.D. MacLean, 1990, New York: Plenum Press.

representations, then the knowledge of the underlying brain mechanisms seems to be developing in a reverse order. Compared with what has been learned about the cerebral substrate of verbal language, the neurological literature provides scant information about mathematical functions. Because of developments in computer-related sciences, it appears timely to renew efforts to obtain an understanding of cerebral mechanisms accounting for the field of mathematics that has had such a momentous influence on recent cultural evolution.

## Preliminary Considerations

The argument presented here is based first of all on evidence that the frontal "association" cortex plays a primary role in anticipation and planning. These functions are at the basis of certain other psychological manifestations identified with the frontal lobe, one of which may be regarded as indissociable from "planfulness": Planning would be a useless exercise if there were no recollection of what was planned. Moreover, two other memory processes usually enter into planning, regardless of whom or what the planning is for. These processes pertain to evaluations made according to (1) past experience and (2) ongoing experience. Hence, the planning process commonly depends on an integration of past experience, present experience, and actions to be taken in the future. According to the needs of the situation, the time involved may vary from moments to years. Although the focus of the present Chapter is on planning and the development of computation used in prediction, it is in no way intended to discount the role of the frontal lobe in generating affects associated with anticipation as it applies both to foreseen and unforeseeable events. In concluding these preliminary considerations, illustrative case material will be given in regard to (1) planning and (2) anticipation.

### *Illustrative Case Material*

#### Planfulness

From the voluminous literature on frontal lobe functions, I will use a single classic case to illustrate the kind of deficit in planning that may occur when a patient is bilaterally deprived of a large amount of the frontal granular cortex. The case is that of a 20-year-old man who was seen for evaluation by Dr. S.S. Ackerly because of a history of aberrant behavior and charges against him of stealing a car (Ackerly & Benton, 1948). Findings on a pneumoencephalogram led to a neurosurgical exploration that revealed "cystic degeneration of the left frontal lobe [and] absence of prefrontal lobe on the right" (p. 480), a condition that may have resulted from complications at birth. Hence, the case is particularly instructive because it indicates how bilateral frontal deficits affect human psychological development. The history revealed that since the age of 3, the patient failed in repeated instances to foresee the consequences of his actions and to learn from experience. This deficiency could not have been complicated by poor recollection, because he had an excellent memory for details of a book that he had read or a movie that he had seen. Although poor in arithmetic, his abilities as a student were such that he was regarded as having "scholastic promise," particularly in the languages. Clinical testing revealed no memory deficit, but his performance of the Porteus mazes indicated a defect in "planning ability and foresight," bearing out his reputation as having an inability to take the future into account (Ackerly & Benton, 1948).

In regard to the patient's criminality, his physicians argued that it was impossible for him to commit a premeditated crime because of his inability to plan and remember the steps to be taken in achieving the goal of the crime. This view was expressed despite the abundant evidence of the patient's ability to remember in considerable detail current and past happenings. It was as though premeditation required not only the ability to plan but also the step-by-step memory of what is planned, or as one might otherwise say, a "memory of the future" (MacLean, 1990, p. 560).[1]

### Anticipation

Because the human capacity to anticipate and to plan so greatly enlarges the realm of experience, it multiplies interminably the number of prospects that, at the affective level, can induce concern and anxiety or joyful expectation. During the medically bleak period when frontal lobotomy was performed extensively as a treatment of mental illness, a clinical consensus developed that relief of anxiety was the main benefit of the operation (see, e.g., McIntyre, Mayfield, & McIntyre, 1954). Anxiety strictly applies to the disagreeable affect variously denoted as "tension," "apprehension," "dread," and the like associated with anticipated happenings of a planned or unplanned nature. The incorporation of *anxiety* into the term *anxiolytic*, for drugs alleviating tension, has led to *anxiety* being used alternatively for *fear* because pharmacologists commonly test these agents on animals such as mice or rats in immediately fear-inducing situations. There is no evidence that such animals with poorly developed granular frontal cortex experience fear of happenings much beyond the immediate situation. Ideally, therefore, the use of the word *anxiety* should be reserved for fear of things outside of and beyond the current situation. The well-recognized capacity of unilateral or bilateral lobotomy to relieve chronic pain serves to illustrate this point. Because such patients actually have a reduced

---

[1] Since the present paper went to press, I have learned that Ingvar used this same expression in the title of a paper published in 1985 (see Ingvar, 1985).

threshold for painful stimuli (Chapman, Rose, & Solomon, 1948), physicians tend to attribute the benefit of lobotomy to a relief of anxiety generated by the prospect of continued suffering, rather than to an actual relief of pain.

# Anatomical Background

## *Frontal "Association" Cortex*

The so-called frontal association cortex is generally considered to be coextensive with the granular cortex, which is characterized by a thin, but definite, granular layer IV. It may be topographically defined as the cortex lying rostral to the agranular motor areas 4 and 6, as well as the transitional dysgranular cortex of area 8 identified with the "frontal eyefields" (see Akert, 1964). Figure 1.1 shows the outlines of cytoarchitectural areas that Brodmann (1907–1908) demarcated in the human brain. In a rostroventral direction, the granular cortex of the lateral surface (Fig. 1.1A) includes most of area 8, together with areas 9, 10, 46, 11, 47, 45, and 44. On the medial surface (Fig. 1.1B), it includes areas 8, 9, 10, 11, and the forward part of 12. The garnular cortex is frequently referred to as the *prefrontal cortex*, but because *prefrontal* means "at the tip," this designation should be reserved for the polar parts of areas 9 and 10.

## *Neocerebellar Structures*

The ventral pons is the cortical gateway to the hemispheral parts of the neocerebellum, which, in Dow's words, "reaches such enormous size" in the human brain (Dow, 1974, p. 110). As illustrated in Figure 1.2, a parasagittal section through the human brainstem reveals the great expansion of the ventral pons, which, at first glance, resembles a tumor squeezing off the overlying brainstem. In Figure 1.2, note also that the red nucleus reaches tumorous proportions. This nucleus forms a main link in the pontocerebellar system, receiving its major input via the roof nuclei of the cerebellum and from the motor and sensory neocortex. The red nucleus previously was believed to relay impulses to parts of the thalamus innervating the frontal motor cortex, but the anatomical findings of Hopkins and Lawrence (1975) in monkeys failed to provide evidence of such circuitry. Rather, the main projections of the red nucleus arise from the massive parvocellular division and descend to the inferior olive, while those originating in the small, magnocellular part constitute the rubrotegmentospinal tracts (see Carpenter, 1981).

Dow (1974) also emphasizes the development of a distinctive part of the dentate nucleus that is found in the great apes and humans but not in the less advanced primates (see also Larsell & Jansen, 1972). The upper arrow

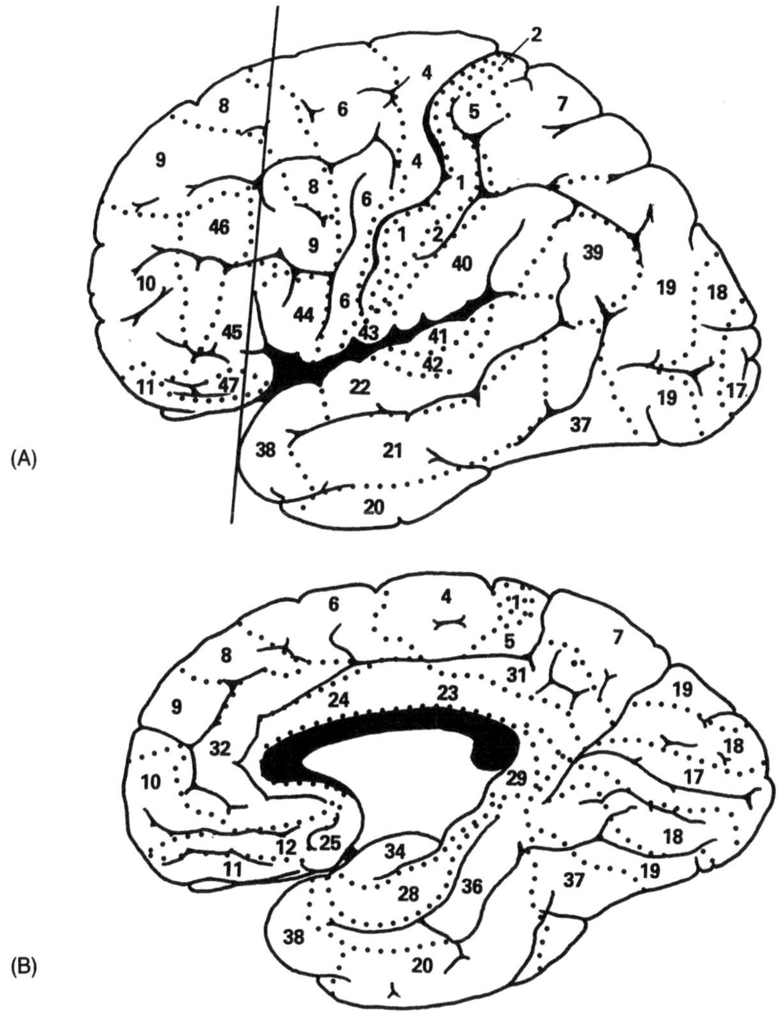


FIGURE 1.1. Simplified version of Brodmann's (1908) cortical cytoarchitectural scheme for the human brain. (A) Left lateral and (B) right medial views are shown. Dotted lines with enclosed arabic numerals show the limits of areas depicted in Brodmann's original drawings by ornate shading. Greater part of the frontal granular cortex is located rostral to the vertical line in upper drawing, showing approximate plane of section of the once-used standard frontal lobotomy. See text. From Denny-Brown, 1951, adapted in *The Triune Brain in Evolution: Role in Paleocerebral Functions* by P.D. MacLean, 1990, New York: Plenum Press.

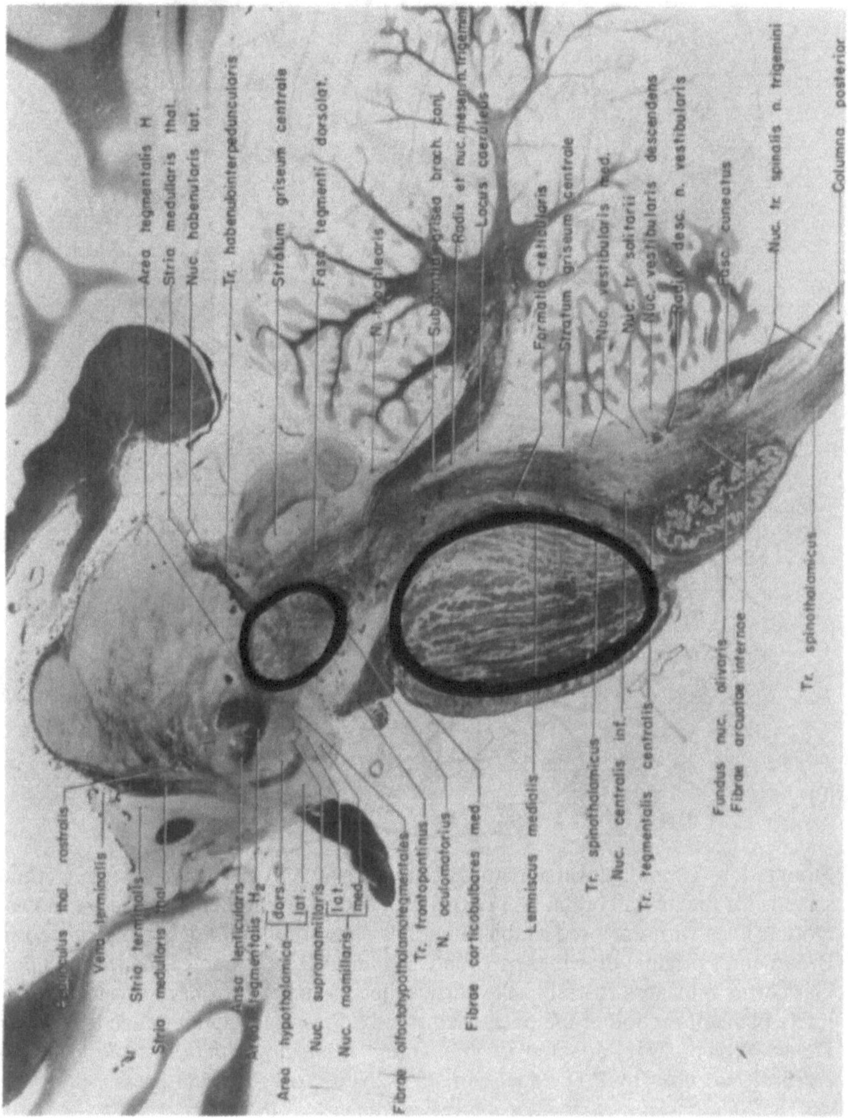
Vena terminalis
Stria terminalis
Stria medullaris thal.
Ansa lenticularis
Area tegmentalis H$_2$
Area hypothalamica
dors.
lat.
Nuc. supramamillaris
Nuc. mamillaris
lat.
med.
Fibrae olfactohypothalamotegmentales
Tr. frontopontinus
N. oculomotorius
Fibrae corticobulbares med.
Lemniscus medialis
Tr. spinothalamicus
Nuc. centralis inf.
Tr. tegmentalis centralis
Fundus nuc. olivaris
Fibrae arcuatae internae
Tr. spinothalamicus
Area tegmentalis H
Stria medullaris thal.
Nuc. habenularis lat.
Tr. habenulointerpeduncularis
Stratum griseum centrale
Fasc. tegmenti dorsolat.
N. trochlearis
Substantia grisea brach. conj.
Radix et nuc. mesenc. trigemini
Locus caeruleus
Formatio reticularis
Stratum griseum centrale
Nuc. vestibularis med.
Nuc. tr. solitarii
Nuc. vestibularis descendens
Radix desc. n. vestibularis
Fasc. cuneatus
Nuc. tr. spinalis n. trigemini
Columna posterior

in Figure 1.3 points to the new development of the dentate nucleus as it appears in a transverse section of the human brain. In contradistinction to the old dorsomedial part of the dentate nucleus with its microgyri and large cells, the new part forms a ventrolateral division with large gyri and smaller cells. As first shown histochemically by Gans in 1924, the new part is further distinguished from the old division by a greater content of iron. While inspecting Figure 1.3, note also the great development of the inferior olive (lower right-hand arrow) that serves inter alia to interconnect the ruber with the cerebellum.

## *Interconnections of Neofrontal Cortex with Thalamus and Cerebellum*

Cytochemical tracing techniques have augmented the knowledge of interconnections of the frontal neocortex with the thalamus and cerebellum. For present purposes, attention focuses on two sets of anatomical findings—namely, (1) those clarifying connections with the cerebellum and (2) those relevant to the "diffuse thalamic projection system" and its functional influence on the association areas of the frontal, temporal, parietal, and occipital lobes.

### Cerebellar Linkup

In the macaque monkey, the cerebellar cortex has been shown to project via the roof nuclei to the cell-sparse parts of a thalamic nucleus identified in 1909 as the "Noyau ventral intermediaire" by Cecile Vogt (1909; see also Asanuma, Thach, & Jones, 1983). This ventral intermediate nucleus of Vogt includes subdivisions of thalamic nuclei that Olszewski (1952) demarcated as the oral part of the ventral posterolateral nucleus (VPLo) and the caudal and "postrema" (VLps) parts of the ventral lateral nucleus (VLc), as well as a paralamellar part, which he called "area X." Cytochemical tracing techniques have shown that cerebellar influence on the motor cortex of area 4 derives from the main body of VPLo (Jones, Wise, & Coulter, 1979; Strick, 1976) while VLc and area X innervate the lateral surface distribution of area 6 and the eyefields of area 8.

With respect to the medial surface, a consensus had existed that the supplementary area (area 6 and part of area 8) received all of its connec-

FIGURE 1.2. Sagittal section of the human brain showing the greatly developed pons and red nucleus outlined in black. The pons gives the impression of compressing the overlying brain stem. From Singer and Yakovlev, 1954, adapted in *The Triune Brain in Evolution: Role in Paleocerebral Functions* by P.D. MacLean, 1990, New York: Plenum Press.

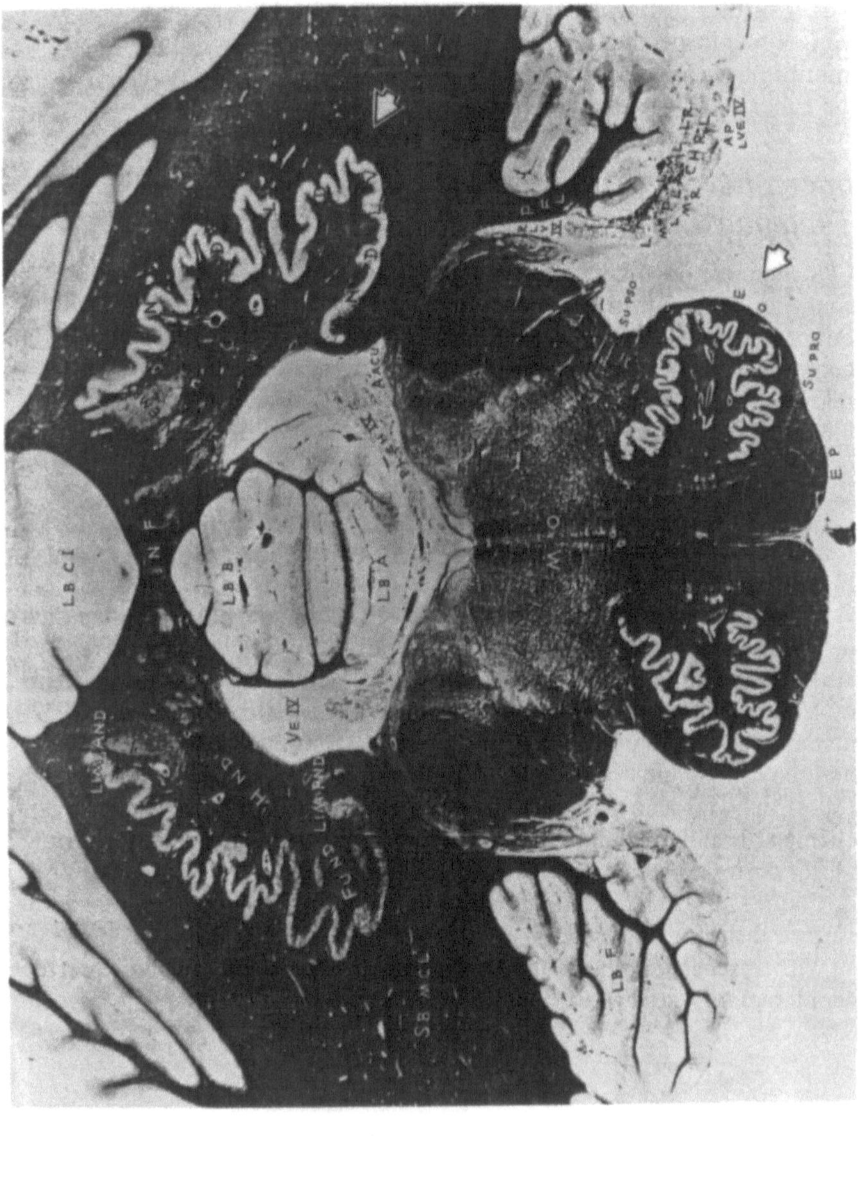
LB CI
LB B
LB A
Ve IX
LB E
Su PRO
EP

tions from the oral part of VL (VLo) innervated by pallidal projections, but recent evidence indicates that the rostral supplementary area also comes under cerebellar influence via VLc and the paralamellar part of area X (Wiesendanger & Wiesendanger, 1985).

In regard to cerebellar influences on the frontal granular cortex, Miyata and Sasaki (1983) have shown by retrograde labeling that the caudal part of area 9 receives connections from a paralamellar strip of area X. In anatomical studies following frontal lobotomies rostral to the vertical line in Figure 1.1A, A. Meyer, Beck, and McLardy (1947) and Yakovlev (1954) found degeneration of frontopontine pathways. This evidence of projections of granulofrontal cortex to the ventral pons has been confirmed experimentally in monkeys by both anterograde (Brodal, 1978) and retrograde (Glickstein, May, & Mercier, 1985) labeling.

### Linkup With Diffuse Thalamic Projection System

Based on studies of retrograde degeneration, it was believed until recently that the dorsolateral granular frontal cortex and a large area of the midline frontal cortex were athalamic, or at best received only collaterals (see Akert, 1964). Because the ventral anterior nucleus (VA) is regarded as central to the diffuse thalamic projection system, it is of special historical interest that, in 1970, Carmel reported that following small lesions placed in different parts of this nucleus, he could trace sparse, fine, degenerating fibers to widespread areas of the frontal cortex. Since then, with the use of cytochemical tracing techniques, several workers have demonstrated robust connections of VA, as well as midline thalamic nuclei, with both limbic and neocortical areas of the frontal lobe (see MacLean, 1987, p. 130, and 1990, p. 538, for summary). In my own studies employing cytochemical tracing techniques in Saimiri monkeys, the hilar limbic cortex appears to be innervated largely by cells of the magnocellular division of VA, and the labeling, extends more and more laterally into the parvocellular part with tracer applied toward the frontal pole and then caudally toward the supplementary motor area (SMA) (MacLean, 1988, 1990). The findings on SMA compare to what Jürgens (1984) had previously reported in Saimiri monkeys and what Goldman-Rakic and Porrino (1985) described in macaques.

---

FIGURE 1.3. Transverse section through the human cerebellum and pons, illustrating the greatly developed dentate nucleus. Upper right arrow points to recently evolved ventrolateral division of the nucleus; lower arrow identifies the greatly expanded inferior olive. See text regarding comparative and clinical implications. From Riley, 1960, adapted in *The Triune Brain in Evolution: Role in Paleocerebral Fuctions* by P.D. MacLean, 1990, New York: Plenum Press.

Goldman-Rakic and Porrino (1985) also studied the thalamic retrograde labeling after multiple injections of horse radish peroxidase (HRP) into the granular cortex of the outer convexity—namely, the granular cortex contained in the areas (1) above and (2) below the principal sulcus, and (3) the area of the lateral, inferior convexity. After such applications, the number of labeled cells was far less in VA than after injections in the dorsomedial part of the superior gyrus. The labeled cells were respectively located from above downward in the magnocellular part of VA.

## Questions Regarding Neocerebellar Functions

### *Traditional Views*

In the anthropoid apes, all the cerebellum-related structures illustrated in Figures 1.2 and 1.3 appear greatly enlarged when compared with the corresponding parts of the simian brain. But the enlargement is modest by comparison with the human brain. What might account for the extreme condition in the human brain? All of the traditional views relate to the demands of some special kind of motor performance. The ones most commonly considered are (1) the human adoption of an upright posture; (2) human dexterity involving very fine movements of the fingers; and (3) the unique requirements of speech.

Gordon Holmes, the well-known English neurologist, was unequivocal in stating that the "main function of the cerebellum is the control of muscular contractions" (1922a, p. 1177). He further elaborated by saying that the "chief function of the cerebellum as a whole is to concentrate and organize the different forms of afferent impulses outside consciousness for the service of other parts of the nervous system" (1907, p. 486). His sole emphasis on the role of the cerebellum in the control of muscular contractions must be considered in the light of certain negative experimental and clinical findings. Dow (1974), for example, points out that in monkeys with lesions carefully restricted to the neocerebellum, the classic signs of cerebellar ataxia seen with damage of other parts of the cerebellum failed to develop. Moreover, he observes that when stereotaxic surgery was used as a means of destroying cerebellar structures in patients with movement disorders, there were no signs of cerebellar deficits subsequent to "purely dentate lesions" (Dow, 1974).

#### Upright Posture and Manual Dexterity

In regard to the part played by upright posture in neocerebellar development, it has not been explained why the neocerebellum should undergo such extreme enlargement, rather than an expansion of the older midline structures involved in axial posture and movement. Nor is it clear why manual dexterity would require such massive neocerebellar development unless, as in the case of playing the piano without a musical score, memory were to involve the same mechanisms.

REQUISITES OF SPEECH

If, as just noted, memory is a required function of the same mechanisms, the mnemonic demands of an extensive vocabulary, together with the speech process itself, would provide an attractive explanation of the great enlargement of the neocerebellum and related structures. Lieberman (1985) has noted that the motor control patterns of speech "are probably the most complex maneuvers that the human being can master" (p. 659). He points out that speech affords the transmission of vocally phonetic segments "at an extremely rapid rate, up to 25 per second" (1989). In contrast to speech, it is not possible to identify other kinds of sounds at rates exceeding seven to nine items per second. Hence, he states, the high transmission rate of speech allows the communication of complex thoughts "within the constraints of short-term memory." Darley, Aronson, and Brown (1975) have calculated that speech production requires no less than 140,000 neuromuscular events per second.

These mechanical and mnemonic considerations would be more persuasive if the clinical evidence were less equivocal. As Fulton (1949) points out, disturbances of speech are usually associated with lesions of the paleocerebellum. "It would be more logical," he observes, "to believe that speech was integrated by the newer parts of the cerebellum since speech is one of the latest capacities to develop in evolutionary history" but "from clinical experience it is clear that speech is not seriously affected except with very large lesions of the cerebellum affecting the deeper nuclei" (p. 535). As Holmes (1907) had commented 40 years earlier, "[T]he delicately coordinated mechanism of speech is rarely affected by even extensive unilateral lesions of the cerebellum, but its disturbance may be a prominent symptom when the lesion involves both sides. . . . " (p. 487). In his experience, alterations in speech were most commonly associated with lesions of the vermis but might also occur with "disease strictly limited to one lateral lobe" (1922b, p. 63).

Holmes's (1907) observations on members of a family with apparent primary involvement of the cerebellar cortex are of basic interest in regard to cerebellar pathology in disorders of speech. Four of eight siblings developed locomotor signs of cerebellar disease, in their 30s. In addition, they developed alterations of speech variously characterized as "slow and drawling," "slow, jerky, and explosive." One patient (Case 2) said of himself that his speech was slow and thick because his tongue was awkward and got "twisted in his mouth." In the one case (No. 4) in which there was a postmortem examination, the cerebellar cortex was diffusely atrophied. The pons and inferior olive were also much reduced in size. Significantly, the roof nuclei, including the dentate, appeared about normal in size and "were well provided with cells." The description of the cerebral gyri is also of special interest regarding this Chapter: All appeared normal except those of the "medial and lateral prefrontal area," which suggested "a certain amount of general atrophy."

## Question of Neofrontocerebellar Role in Computation and Prediction

### *Preliminary Comment*

During World War II, problems arose concerning communication and control of anti-aircraft that brought together physicists, physiologists, and mathematicians. Norbert Wiener (1948) introduced the term *cybernetics* (derived from the Greek word for *steersman*) to denote the speciality dealing with "control and communication in animals and machines." In this respect, negative feedback became a popular expression, and in the discussion of animal behavior, the cerebellum was a focus of interest because of its recognized role in the smooth operation of the body and its extremities in goal-directed behavior. A favorite illustration was that of a frog with a meager cerebellum that would snap directly at a fly, as opposed to a cat with a well-developed cerebellum that would extrapolate the direction and speed of its prey and pounce accordingly. How much superior was the extrapolative ability of a baseball player in catching a high and long fly ball! It was as though the brain had a built-in calculus (MacLean, 1990, p. 550).

Some neurophysiologists use the expressions *long-term* and *short-term planning* to distinguish between the premovement role of the cortical association areas and the corrective control attributed to cerebellar nuclei once a movement has started (see, e.g., Allen & Tsukahara, 1974). In terms of function, however, there is in addition the obvious consideration that human beings foresee their actions not just in the immediate future, as when anticipating where to run when catching a fly ball, but also foresee their movements days, months, and years into the future. In conjunction with such anticipation, either intuitive or arithmetic calculation may be employed as a means of increasing the accuracy of prediction. Intuitive calculation is illustrated by a South Seas islander who walks to the shore, raises a wet finger to the wind, and then navigates a boat to a pinpoint island 50 miles away; whereas the formal logistics in preparing for D day provide an example of an opposite extreme. For most plannd events to be successful, the individual must have a memory of the successive events that are to transpire at a future time (MacLean, 1990, p. 551), or as one might say for short, a memory of the future.

### *Clinical Insights*

One cannot introduce the memory factor without recalling the frequent clinical impression that patients with prefrontal lesions suffer from a failure of memory. It was such impressions that led to the introduction of the delayed response test as a means of assessing memory in experimental work with nonhuman primates. As Luria (1969) has emphasized, however, careful examination shows that patients actually can remember, but in reporting what is remembered, they may relate it inappropriately to other happenings and thereby give the impression of memory failure. At any rate, the introduction of the expression "memory of the future" forces one to inquire how the underlying mechanisms might differ from those involved in the memory of past events and the memory of ongoing experiences.

### Clinical Evidence of Granulofrontal-Cerebellar Connections

Since the original observations of Bruns in 1892, it has been recognized that lesions of the frontal lobe may be accompanied by cerebellar symptoms, usually manifest as an ataxia of gait. Physicians have tended to attribute such symptoms to complicating increased intracranial pressure resulting in dysfunction of the pons and cerebellum. J.S. Meyer and Barron (1960), however, reported a study on seven patients in whom an increase of intracranial pressure was unlikely and in whom there was a disturbance of gait. Those authors suggest that the motor deficit is owing to a disturbance of abstraction. For example, a patient proves to be capable of kicking a ball, but finds it impossible to execute the same movements if asked to kick an imaginary ball. J.S. Meyer and Barron do not explain why they attribute the deficit to a disconnection of cortical association fibers rather than to interference with prefrontal pontine projections mentioned under Anatomical Background.

### Evidence of Role of Frontal Cortex in Calculation

When one considers the importance of numerical calculations in human activities (education, science, and commerce), it is surprising how rarely neurologic writings refer to this subject. Indeed, one may search the indexes of many textbooks and find no word alluding to calculation, arithmetic, or mathematics. The one term most reliably listed is *acalculia*, an expression introduced by Henschen (1920, 1922) for the inability to perform simple calculations. The condition may be mentioned only in passing or is dealt with as a subject that must be briefly described for the sake of completeness.

Without any other comment, Alpers (1958) states that in cases of frontal lobe tumor "disturbances in mathematical ability" may occur (p. 558). Significantly, Luria (1969) has written: "Perhaps the disturbances of intellectual activity in patients with a 'frontal lobe syndrome' are seen most clearly when they try to solve arithmetical problems" (p. 750). As an example, he cites a patient's response to a question about how many of 18 books would be on two shelves if there were twice as many on one shelf as the other. The patient immediately hears the word *twice* and gives the answer 36 + 18 = 54. Unlike the acalculias associated with occipital, temporal, and parietal lesions and owing, respectively, to visual, auditory, and spatial factors, the acalculia occurring with frontal lobe lesions appears to be secondary to inabilities in abstraction. But the deficits in simple calculation of the kind described would hardly seem to be exacting for the kind of mechanisms that will allow some individuals to perform in a matter of seconds (and with the accuracy of a calculator) computations involving large numbers (see Smith, 1983).

### Questioned Role of Cerebellum

In view of what has been said about the extrapolatory role of the cerebellum in goal-directed behavior, it would not be surprising if it eventually proves to be involved in numerical calculations ranging from the simplest type to the most complex of which the human is capable. Cases are described of patients with olivopontocerebellar atrophy in whom dementia or "intellectual deterioration" developed, but the extent that the disease of cerebellar circuits—as opposed to complicating lesions elsewhere—contributed to the mental disability remains ambiguous. Perhaps cases of agenesis of the cerebellum would provide the least complicated picture of human potential in the absence of the greater part of the cerebellum. Rubinstein and Freeman (1940) describe a remarkable case of cerebellar agenesis in a 72-year-old man who had shown no sign of motor disability before a vascular lesion in the left parietal region. The postmortem examination revealed that the cerebellum consisted of two small nubbins measuring no more than 8 × 7 × 5 mm. The patient had worked all his adult life either as a handyman, repairman, or gardener. As a boy, he had apparently participated in games without attracting attention because of disability. But most notably, he never went to school and was described by his brother as always being "mentally subnormal." His ability in arithmetic is not mentioned.

The question of brain mechanisms of computation leads naturally to the question of the cerebral status of so-called "idiot savants" who have such remarkable abilities in calculation. Because some such individuals have a diagnostic label of "autism," it is of relevant interest that in the 1980s there were both neuropathological and radiological reports of cerebellar changes in autism. Because none of the short case reports referred to numerical ability, only the nature of the cerebellar changes will be summarized here. In one study of four cases with mental retardation, the findings were generally negative, except in one in which a general reduction of Purkinje cells was mentioned (Williams, Hauser, Purpura, DeLong, & Swisher, 1980). Bauman and Kemper (1985) described one case in which there was "atrophy of the neocerebellar cortex with marked loss of Purkinje cells." These reports led Ritvo et al., (1986) to focus on cell counts in the cerebellum. In each of the four cases examined, there was a significant reduction of Purkinje cells as judged by counts in "comparison subjects." In 1984, a brief description appeared of three severely retarded patients with autism, for whom computerized tomography of the brain showed "hypoplastic" changes in the cerebellum (Jaeken & Van den Berghe, 1984). In a subsequent study employing magnetic resonance imaging (MRI) in 14 autistic patients ranging from 4 to 19 years, there was only a suggestion that the cerebella were smaller than those in the comparison group (Gaffney, Tsai, Kuperman, & Minchen, 1987). An MRI examination of a 21-year-old man with autism without mental retardation but with a marked alteration of speech indicated the presence of hypoplasia of the posterior vermis as well as of the medial part of each cerebellar hemisphere (Courchesne, Hesselink, Jernigan, Yeung-Courchesne, 1987). Finally, in another MRI study, focusing on the pons, there was no difference between 41 autistic cases and 36 "normal controls" (Hsu, Courchesne, & Press, 1989).

In regard to actual function under normal and abnormal conditions, improved tomographic scanning techniques promise to be enlightening. Significantly, Roland (1987) has said that in a task involving continuous subtraction of 3 (starting at 50), he and his colleagues observed increased blood flow, along with an increase in oxygen metabolism, in the lateral part of the cerebellum in conjunction with an increase in the prefrontal cortex.

It is also relevant to the topic of the present article that Roland, Larsen, Lassen, and Skinhoj (1980) observed variable increases in cerebral blood flow in the "inferior part of the frontal lobe" during silent counting as well as signs in the SMA indicative of a role in programming a motor finger sequence test. The SMA is interconnected with frontal granular cortex (see Pandya & Barnes, 1987).

## Microgenesis

Regardless of what remains to be discovered about the function of frontocerebellar systems, the proposed role in computation invites a consideration of the phylogeny of the forebrain and cerebellum in light of developing microgenetic theory as it promises to be further illuminated by the developing science of fractals. For this purpose, an explanation follows of the intended use of the terms *microgenesis* and *fractals*.

### *The Term* Microgenesis

What is microgenesis? The term itself has a twisted history. According to Liza Catán, it derives indirectly from the term *Aktualgenese*, which Sander (1930, cited by Catán), a Leipzig psychologist, used descriptively with respect to his own studies on the temporal evolution of percepts. He presumed that the realization of a percept developed according to a logical process that perhaps could be demonstrated experimentally by exposing a subject to suboptimal stimuli, as might be done by showing a picture tachistoscopically or in dim light. Suzanne Langer (American psychologist), in translating Sander's paper into English, interpreted the rarely used German word *Aktual* to mean *realize* (see Catán, 1986, p. 254), with the whole term implying the "origin of realization."

Werner, in connection with his interest in *The Comparative Psychology of Mental Development* (Werner, 1948), sought to derive laws that would be applicable to the unfolding of psychological experiences that occur not only in a matter of seconds but also over prolonged periods of time (see Catán, 1986, p. 254). Improvising on methods used by Sander and others of the Leipzig school, he devised for experimental purposes a "micromusical scale" as one of several means in the attempt to "actualize . . . the development of internal representations and the mechanisms whereby they were constructed" (Catán, 1986, p. 256). In 1956, Werner appears to have introduced the word *microgenesis* as an approximate translation of *Aktualgenese*, giving no explanation as to why *Aktual* became *micro* and proceeding as though both terms "were familiar items of [one's] conceptual equipment" (Catán, 1986, p. 253).

In his writings, Jason Brown has dealt extensively with microgenetic theory because he thinks that it provides a useful approach for clarifying the development of different kinds of aphasia, while at the same time suggesting needed changes in older interpretations (1988). He defines Werner's term *microgenesis* as descriptive of "the microtemporal unfolding of object representations, conceived as a more or less instantaneous recapitulation in cognition of patterns laid down in phylo-ontogeny" (1988, p. 3). He points out that in the formulation of Werner, phylo-ontogeny was thought "to leave a track that was retraced each moment in the process of object formation." Brown emphasizes that as opposed to this regressive view, he himself regards microgenesis as a unidirectional forward flow from "archaic" to "recent" structures in a matter of milliseconds. "Microgenesis," he comments, "is a type of instantaneous evolution" (p. 6). Because his clinical application of microgenetic theory is more germane than strictly psychological work to the present topic, and because it invites consideration of the fractal aspects, I will return to it after a short comment on fractals.

## *Fractals*

One might say that given any object, *fractals* applies to any dimensional scale right down to atomic limits. It is a word introduced by the French mathematician Benoit Mandelbrot in 1977 and relates to the word *fraction* derived from the Latin verb *frangere*, meaning to break. In the organic world, the fractal nature of things is most clearly illustrated by the branching of trees, whether elm tree, bronchial tree, or the tree-like shape of a nerve cell and its processes. Each branch has a similarity to the branch from which it stems—a condition that Mandelbrot (1977) referred to as *self-similarity*. In the bronchial tree, however, after a branching greater than 10 generations, self-similarity decreases because of the increasing number of irregularities (West & Goldberger, 1987). Hofstadter (1979) characterized the self-similarity in such complexity as "sameness-in-differentness."

The tree example also illustrates how the concept of fractal time enters the picture–as for instance, the slowing down of the nerve impulses as they propagate into the finer and finer branches of a nerve cell. It is evident how a lesion or disease of a nerve trunk or of its processes might lead to alterations in the timing and the flow of nerve impulses (see West & Goldberger, 1987).

It is the strength of fractals that it has made it possible to deal mathematically with both the relatively simple as well as the complex geometry that has been described. The applications of the subject in computer graphics has been useful not only in promoting that field but also in providing simulation of many physical conditions. Starting with a simple algorithm, one can build up a picture that rapidly increases in complexity. As Oppenheimer has illustrated (1985), such amplification can be obtained by using an algorithm involving recursions. In the case of decimals, for example, one might obtain either a 10-times increase or decrease with every recursion. It becomes evident how such principles might apply in regard to so-called self-reexciting loops of neurons as they might exist within cortical structures or in nuclear–cortical loops or in nuclear–nuclear loops.

In two articles on "neurological positivism" (1988, 1990), Vandervert presents evidence for suggesting that the brain has inherent algorithms that "might be regarded as self-organizing, optimizing fractal generators of experience." (1990, p. 6). Later, he speaks of "science's erroneous placement of the world outside the skull" (1990, p. 9). In saying this, he is not denying the existence of "a world out there." Rather, he contends that our experience is owing to what we realize by means of built-in algorithms of the brain. As an illustration, one might say that when a mathematician discovers an equation for solving a problem, it is not a "discovery" but an awareness of something that surfaces because the pre-existing mechanism for the algorithm afforded the solution. It seems that some mathematicians resemble talented musicians, being capable by introspection of "hearing the melody" of their equations. One might say that those conducting experiments involving microgenesis are looking for cerebral algorithms. In language of further relevance to microgenesis, Vandervert speaks of the *fractal hypothesis* in regard to the evolution of bifurcations. "In the brain," he states, "the time dimensions for the creation of bifurcations . . . would be *moment to moment*" (1990, p. 6; emphasis added).

## *Neofrontocerebellar Mechanisms in Terms of "Fractogenesis"*

As a contraction for the expression "fractal aspects of microgenesis," I shall use the term *fractogenesis*, because it will refer to both the somatic and temporal aspects of microgenesis. I will also use the term *algorithm* in the expanded sense of Vandervert, who, in his first article on neurological positivism, defines an algorithm as "any set of rules, including those which govern chaotic dynamical systems, that perform translational or transformational operations (mathematical, mechanical, linguistic, neurobiological, metaphorical) which link problems, input data, and solutions" (1988, p. 321).

Regardless of whether or not the cerebellum is implicated in high-order mathematical functions, its demonstrated role in goal-directed behavior involving varying degrees of extrapolation (prediction) means that its neural circuits are functioning according to some inherent algorithms. As has been mentioned, the feat of a baseball player's catching a high fly ball suggest that the brain has "a kind of built-in calculus." From the standpoint of the role played by nerve impulse conduction and axoplasmic flow in such goal-directed behavior, it is evident also that the bifurcations of both dendritic and axonal processes in neural networks must be critically significant regarding both the fractal somatic and fractal temporal aspects.

The same considerations apply to the frontal cortex regarding the cerebellum-related functions discussed earlier. As mentioned, patients with frontal lesions involving the granular cortex prove capable of kicking a ball but are unable to kick an imaginary ball. Moreover, as opposed to the cerebellum, there is definite clinical evidence that the granulofrontal cortex is involved in mathematical ability, as illustrated by what was said about deficits pertaining to abstraction and acalculia.

At this point, it is pertinent to comment about a distinction between the functions of the so-called cortical association areas and other areas. Except for the association areas, it seems that for adaptations to the external world, the algorithmic functioning of other cortical areas usually requires a continuous feedback from what is being perceived. On the contrary, the association areas seem to provide their own "screen" for the reflecting associational forms of cerebration. And it seems in particular that the frontal granular cortex evolved as a screen to reflect associations about unseen things to appear in the future.

## *Microgenesis in Terms of Phylogenesis*

In turning now to Brown's writings on microgenesis, it is necessary to comment briefly on cerebral evolution, because he gives far greater emphasis to phylogeny than ontogeny in his formulations. Figure 1.4 serves as a

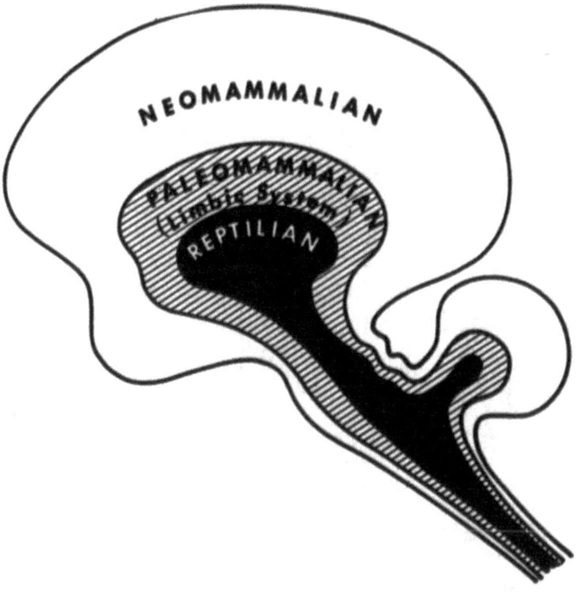


FIGURE 1.4. Symbolic representation of the triune phylogeny of the forebrain and cerebellum leading to advanced mammals. Labeling identifies three intermeshing evolutionary formations of the forebrain, which in structure and chemistry reflect a relationship to reptiles, early mammals, and late mammals. Corresponding developments of cerebellum could have been labeled archi-, paleo-, and neocerebellum. See text for implications in regard to microgenesis. From "The Brain in Relation to Empathy and Medical Education" by P.D. MacLean, 1967, *Journal of Nervous and Mental Disease*, *144*, p. 377.

symbolic representation of the evolutionary development of the forebrain and cerebellum in terrestrial vertebrates. The forebrain consists of the telencephalon and diencephalon, which together form the cerebral hemispheres lying rostral to the midbrain. The figure is intended to suggest that the forebrain of advanced mammals has expanded as a triune structure that anatomically and chemically reflects commonalities with reptiles, early mammals, and late mammals (MacLean, 1970, 1973, 1990). The three neural assemblies comprise (1) the striatal complex, including most of the basal ganglia, (2) the evolutionarily old cortex of the limbic lobe and its primary brainstem connections (limbic system); and (3) the neocortex and brainstem structures with which it is primarily connected. The reptilian core structures are basically implicated in species-typical forms of behavior used in the daily master routine and subroutines, as well as in the four main forms of prosematic (nonverbal) communication (MacLean, 1990). Experimental and clinical evidence suggest that the limbic system provides an intelligence that guides behavior on the basis of emotional feelings. The evolutionary transition from the mammal-like reptiles (therapsids) to mammals involves the development of a family-centered society entailing three cardinal forms of behavior identified as (1) nursing, conjoined with maternal care; (2) audiovocal communication for maintaining maternal–offspring contact; and (3) play (MacLean, 1990). The evolution of the neomammalian brain might, in computer language, be likened to the progressive enlargement of a central processor providing an expanding memory and intelligence for increasing the chances of survival.

As also schematized in the diagram, three corresponding evolutionary developments of the cerebellum develop in parallel with those of the forebrain. In Larsell's scheme (1937), the archi- and paleomammalian cerebellum would both be alluded to as paleocerebellum.

Regarding the phylogenetic substrate of microgenesis, Brown (1988) refers to four main levels involving, respectively, (1) the basal ganglia and midbrain; (2) the limbic system; (3) the "generalized" neocortex of both hemispheres; and (4) the "focal," contralateral neocortex. In his scheme, both in regard to the psychogenesis, on the one hand, and the expressive aspects on the other, microgenesis always entails an upward progression involving all four levels in a matter of seconds or fractions of a second.

Brown uses two quite synonymous terms—namely, *action* and *movement*—for very different connotations. His *action* is more akin to Sander's *Aktual*—realization. He defines an action "as a cognitive structure consisting of multiple representational planes, each of which is reconstituted moment to moment" and "read off into movements." An action, he states, "instantiates a movement in physical space." Viewed phylogenetically, an action "proceeds" bottom up "as a type of propagated wave from a core system in the upper brain stem and basal ganglia" (Brown, 1988, p. 303). The action becomes progressively patterned and "toned" with affects via the medial limbic cortex. In preparation for intended performance, the bilateral frontal "generalized" cortex further differentiates the action with respect to three-dimensional space. Finally, the contralateral precentral cortex carries the action forward by specifying the final, fine movements of the distal limb and vocal musculature.

As opposed to the classic Jacksonian (1958) view that derangements of function at higher levels give release to behavior mediated at lower levels, Brown (1988) contends that according to microgenetic theory, the symptoms and manifestations seen as a complication of brain lesions need not be regarded either as a release of lower levels of function or a regression to such levels. Rather, he suggests that the lesions may act "like an obstruction or partial blockage in a river" that results in a turbulence and divergence of flow. With respect to various aphasias, this analogy has special appeal. The mention of turbulence reminds the reader of a new science, "Chaos," concerned with nonlinear systems. Other of his figures of speech—"microgenetic trees," "phrase structure trees," and the like—

also remind one of fractal geometry and its later development, fractal biology.

## "Fractogenesis" in Regard to Neofrontocerebellar Systems

Returning now to the questioned role of neofrontocerebellar systems in both intuitive and notational computation, one thinks of at least three topics concerning which fractals are conceptually provocative: recursions, bifurcations, and phylogenesis.

### Recursions

As mentioned, computer graphics provide an example of how, starting with a simple algorithm, one may construct infinitely complicated patterns resembling trees, snowflakes, coastlines, and the like. This has led to the illustrative statement that one may enclose a *finite* area by a line of *infinite* length. Algorithms specifying recursions recall the interest generated in the 1930s in "self-re-exciting chains" of neurons existing at all levels of the nervous system. Such circular loops as Lorente de Nó (1934) schematized on the basis of his cytoarchitectural studies of the entorhinal cortex suggested to various workers how transient memories might be kept alive. Nowadays, such recursive neuronal networks might equally suggest a possible function in multiplication or division, whether in regard to dimensions, time, or numbers. That the human alpha-rhythm disappears during computation does not mean that its waxing and waning excitation is not occurring during the process; rather, it may be masked by the seemingly disorderly activity of neurons brought into play. The range of the alpha-rhythms between 8 and 12/s also raises questions as to how they might relate to preferred systems of counting, as say, the decimal system and its possible relation to the 10 fingers used in counting.

As an example of how recursions might apply to the microgenesis of thought processes, one could use a quotation that Hofstadter (1979, p. 560) employs in another context. It is from Stanislaw Ulam's autobiography, *Adventures of a Mathematician*:

> There must be a trick to the train of thought, *a recursive formula.* A group of neurons starts working automatically, sometimes without external impulse. *It is a kind of iterative process with a growing pattern.* It wanders about in the brain, and the way it happens must depend on the memory of similar patterns. [emphasis added]

### Bifurcations

One of the wonders of cerebration pertains to the ability of some individuals to carry out calculations with large numbers and to achieve speedily and repeatedly accurate answers without benefit of pencil and paper (see

Smith, 1983). The nature of the underlying mechanisms seems all the more baffling to anyone who has recorded unit nerve activity reflecting variations and irregularities in the number and timing of nerve impulses conducted in neuronal networks. However the repeated accuracy is achieved, it is evident that the fractal nature of neuronal branching must be a significant factor, both in regard to axoplasmic flow and the slowing down of nerve impulses as they propagate into the finer and finer bifurcations. Reference was made earlier to idiot savants, some of whom are labeled autistic. If such individuals, with their capacity to perform various difficult calculations, proved to have cerebellar damage like that reported in some autistic individuals (see preceding discussion), it will be against the argument that the cerebellum plays a pivotal role in numerical computation.

### Phylogenesis

The arborization of a tree is symbolic of factors that may be significant both at microscopic and macroscopic levels. In the case of trees or cladograms depicting phylogenetic development, how may distance from the main trunk affect the survival or extinction of species? A parallel question applies to neuronal trees at the microscopic level. For example, in Alzheimer's disease, the evolutionarily newest areas of the frontal and temporal cortex appear to be the most severely affected. The extensive involvement of the archicortex of the hippocampus might seem to be an exception, but there is considerable newness of development in the prosubiculum (MacLean, 1990, p. 306). How does distance from the main trunk(s) influence the disease process? Ramón y Cajal, in his research on degeneration and regeneration of nerve tissue, noted that abnormalities tended to occur at the "bifurcations" (1928/1959, p. 121), a word much used by those concerned with catastrophe theory when discussing evolution and related questions.

## Discussion

On the basis of Catán's review (1986), one might assume that the origins of microgenesis could be traced to the Leipzig school, presumably because the techniques used by Sander and by Werner were so much influenced by attitudes and methods identified with the "first psychological laboratory" of Wundt, the so-called "father of physiological psychology" (see Pillsbury, 1929). But Jason Brown (1988) and, Hanlon & Brown, 1989 seem to give greater emphasis to the introspectionists of the "Würzburg group" and their well-known work on processes of imageless thought for the concepts leading to the development of microgenetic theory. Brown himself has relied very much on his studies of aphasia in considering mechanisms of microgenesis. Regarding methodology, it is surprising that workers in this field do not seem to have given attention to the potential of observations in the neurosurgical operating room to provide clues about the "unfolding process" in microgenesis. An account given by Kubie (1953), a psychoanalyst, of observations he made during a visit to the Montreal Neurological Institute serves as an example. He went "under the drapes" to record the words of a young woman during diagnostic brain stimulation:

> Shortly after the exposure of the temporoparietal areas, a series of pictures were presented to the patient. These were simple line drawings of familiar objects, which she was asked to name. She did this quite readily until Dr. Penfield stimulated the area in the lobe which caused an arrest of speech. This occurred just as she had been shown the drawing of a human hand. At the moment of electrical stimulation all speech ceased as though frozen into immobility. . . . Then as the current was turned off, she began first to make mouthing movements and then slowly and hesitatingly said in sequence:"five, five . . . five horses . . . five horses . . . five pigs . . . five pigs . . . five fingers . . . hand." (1953, p. 45)

Kubie also notes that in both this and other cases, "stimulation deep in the temporal lobe produced interchangeably music, animal figures, human figures, smells, gastrointestinal sensations." (1953, p. 43).

## *Microgenetic Processes Regarding the Future*

The consideration of microgenesis calls attention to special problems regarding the psychological unfolding of anticipation and planning. Although cases of patients devoid of the frontal granular cortex do not have the requisite mechanisms for analysis of the processes, they are instructive with respect to the missing but necessary ingredients. The introductory case of the young man who was deprived of most of the granulofrontal cortex from a very early age serves as an example. As mentioned, his physicians argued that he was incapable of committing a premeditated crime because of his inability to plan and to recall the sequential acts involved. This view was expressed despite the clinical history and psychological testing that showed that he had a good memory for both ongoing experiences and past happenings. This case suggests that premeditation requires not only the ability to plan, but also the step-by-step memory of what is planned, or as one might otherwise say, "a memory of the future." A like kind of situation applies to any plan that is at all complicated.

When the expression "memory of the future" is used, one is inclined to ask, "How can there be a memory of something that has not yet happened? Isn't *planning*, rather than *memory* the appropriate term?" Planning, however, represents a developing, ongoing process. It is the blueprint in the *drawing stage*, not the blueprint itself. A game such as football provides an illustration. On introducing new plays to a team, the coach draws diagrams showing the position of each player and course of action in advancing the ball. For the quarterback to invent such plays while the game is in process would usually be ineffectual. What is important is to remember the "blueprint" that provides a foreknowledge of where each player is supposed to be. In terms of cerebellar mechanisms, the analogy is appealing because, for the runners in particular, what is required is a "mind-set" of the number and directions of turns and running distances.

The type of planning illustrated by the game metaphor can be characterized as intuitive, being performed according to the brain's built-in algorithms and requiring no calculator to deal with distances and the times involved. When, but a short time ago in cultural evolution, it proved desirable to use numerical calculation as a means of refining prediction, it is inconceivable that the frontal lobes would not have been implicated both with respect to the need and the development of methods. It is impossible to imagine, for example, that the development of probability statistics within the last 250 years would have occurred without a frontal lobe concern for the future.

Regarding mechanisms of planning and "memory of the future," the new anatomical findings that were mentioned with respect to the connections of the ventral anterior nuclear complex with the frontal granular cortex are of special interest because they help to clarify the electroencephalographic observations by Starzl and Magoun (1951) and of Hanbery and Jasper (1953) in the early 1950s. Recordings of the cat indicated that the rostral thalamic pole appeared to be the most effective site for activation of the diffuse "thalamic projection system" of Morison and Dempsey (1942; Dempsey & Morrison, 1943), with the recruited responses being most pronounced in the frontal association cortex but also occurring in the association areas of other lobes. Subsequently, Starzl and Whitlock (1952) reported that the responses in the frontal association areas were much greater in the monkey then in the cat. The integration of activity in the association areas would seem essential for global functions of the frontal lobe, including those depending on the integration of past memory and memory of ongoing experience as they relate to planning and a "memory of the future."

Of other questions that arise, one of foremost interest is whether or not there is something peculiar to the memory of the future that does not apply to other forms of memory. Based on information obtained during the period of frontal lobotomy, evidence accrued that even a unilateral lobotomy is effective in relieving an agonizing dread of death (see MacLean, 1990, p. 530). The recurring human awareness and concern with respect to one's own eventual death is an example of a strongly entrenched memory of the future. For human beings, one might conjecture that the loss of memory that one is going to die would be the last to occur with a general loss of memory.

Finally, answers as to whether or not the frontal lobes and cerebellum play a special role in computation and prediction will require an unusual degree of alertness on the part of neurologists for potentially revealing cases (MacLean, 1990, p. 552). In the past, incomplete case histories and only partial examination of the brain have restricted the amount of knowledge that can be obtained regarding correlates of psychological processes. Unlike other disciplines, medicine is in the unfortunate position that advances in knowledge depend on an analysis of conditions involving sickness and suffering. Hence those in the profession are all the more under the obligation to wrest from human and animal misery information that will help to relieve the suffering of all living things. Hopefully, neurologists of the future not only will be experts in neurology but will also be sophisticated in psychodynamics and human ethology and thereby will provide sufficient details in cases of unusual interest to make it worthwhile to study serial sections of the entire brain with the aid of computer-assisted analysis. In addition, it may be expected that improvements in various applications of computerized tomography will yield valuable information about the chemistry and function of both normal and disordered cerebral structures.

## *References*

Ackerly, S.S., & Benton, A.L. (1948). Report of case of bilateral frontal lobe defect. *Research Publications—Association for Research in Nervous and Mental Disease*, *27*, 479–504.

Akert, K. (1964). Comparative anatomy of frontal cortex and thalamofrontal connections. In J.M. Warren & K. Akert (Eds.), *The frontal granular cortex and behavior* (pp. 372–396). New York: McGraw-Hill.

Allen, G.I., & Tsukahara, N. (1974). Cerebrocerebellar communication system. *Physiological Reviews*, *54*, 957–1006.

Alpers, B.J. (1958). *Clinical neurology*. Philadelphia: F.A. Davis.

Asanuma, C., Thach, W.T., & Jones, E.G. (1983). Cytoarchitectonic delineation of the ventral lateral thalamic region in the monkey. *Brain Research Review*, *5*, 219–235.

Bauman, M., & Kemper, T.L. (1985). Histoanatomic observations of the brain in early infantile autism. *Neurology*, *35*, 866–874.

Brodal, P. (1978). The corticopontine projection in the rhesus monkey: Origin and principles of organization. *Brain*, *101*, 251–283.

Brodmann, K. (1907–1908). Beiträge zur histologischen Lokalisation der Großhirnrinde. VI. Mitteilung. Die Cortexgliederung des Menschen. *Journal für Psychologie und Neurologie (Leipzig)*, *10*, 231–246.

Brown, J.W. (1988). *The life of the mind*. London: Lawrence Erlbaum [See also the author's book review: *Journal of Nervous and Mental Disease*, *178*, 59–60, 1990].

Bruns, L. (1892). Über Störungen des Gleichgewichtes bei Stirnhirntumoren. *Deutsche medizinische Wochenschrift (Stuttgart)*, *18*, 138–140.

Carmel, P.W. (1970). Efferent projections of the ventral anterior nucleus of the thalamus in the monkey. *American Journal of Anatomy*, *128*, 159–183.

Carpenter, M.B. (1981). Anatomy of corpus striatum and brain stem integrating systems. In V. Brooks (Ed.), *American physiology handbook of "motor control"* (pp. 947–995). Baltimore, MD: Williams & Wilkins.

Catán, L. (1986). The dynamic display of process: Historical development and contemporary uses of the microgenetic method. *Human Development, 29*, 252–263.

Chapman, W.P., Rose, A.S., & Solomon, H.C. (1948). Measurements of heat stimulus producing motor withdrawal reaction in patients following frontal lobotomy. *Research Publications—Association for Research in Nervous and Mental Disease, 27*, 754–768.

Courchesne, E., Hesselink, J.R., Jernigan, T.L., & Yeung-Courchesne, R. (1987). Abnormal neuroanatomy in a nonretarded person with autism. Unusual findings with magnetic resonance imaging. *Archives of Neurology, 44*, 335–340.

Darley, F.L., Aronson, A.E., & Brown, J.R. (1975). *Motor speech disorders*. Philadelphia: W.B. Saunders.

Dempsey, E.W., & Morison, R.S. (1943). The electrical activity of a thalamo-cortical relay system. *American Journal of Physiology, 138*, 283–296.

Denny-Brown, D. (1951). The frontal lobes and their functions. In A. Feiling (Ed.), *Modern trends in neurology* (pp. 13–89). New York: Harper & Row.

Dow, R.S. (1974). Some novel concepts of cerebellar physiology. *The Mount Sinai Journal of Medicine, 41*, 103–119.

Fulton, J.F. (1949). *Physiology of the nervous system*. New York: Oxford University Press.

Gaffney, G.R., Tsai, L.Y., Kuperman, S., & Minchin, S. (1987). Cerebellar structure in autism. *American Journal of Diseases of Children (Chicago), 141*, 1330–1332.

Gans, A. (1924). Beitrag zur Kenntnis des Aufbas des nucleus dentatus auf zwei Teilen, namentlich auf Grund von Untersuchungen mit der Eisenreaktion. *Zeitschrift für die Gesamte Neurologie und Psychiatrie, 93*, 750–755.

Glickstein, M., May, J.G., & Mercier, B.E. (1985). Corticopontine projection in the macaque: The distribution of labelled cortical cells after large injections of horseradish peroxidase in the pontine nuclei. *Journal of Comparative Neurology, 235*, 343–359.

Goldman-Rakic, P.S., & Porrino, L.J. (1985). The primate mediodorsal (MD) nucleus and its projection to the frontal lobe. *Journal of Comparative Neurology, 242*, 535–560.

Hanbery, J., & Jasper, H. (1953). Independence of diffuse thalamocortical projection system shown by specific nuclear destructions. *Journal of Neurophysiology, 16*, 252–271.

Hanlon, R.E., & Brown, J.W. (1989). Microgenesis: Historical review and current studies. In A. Ardila & P. Ostrosky-Solis (Eds.), *Brain organization of language and cognitive processes* (pp. 3–15). New York: Plenum.

Henschen, S.E. (1920). *Klinische und Anatomische Beiträge zur Pathologie des Gehirns* (Vols. 5–6). Upsala, Sweden: Almquist & Wicksell.

Henschen, S.E. (1922). *Klinische und Anatomische Beiträge zur Pathologie des Gehirns* (Vol. 7). Stockholm: Nordiske Bokhandeln.

Hofstadter, D.R. (1979). *Gödel, Escher, Bach: An eternal golden braid*. New York: Random House.

Holmes, G. (1907). A form of familial degeneration of the cerebellum. *Brain*, *30*, 466–489.
Holmes, G. (1922a). The Croonian Lectures on the clinical symptoms of cerebellar disease and their interpretation. Lecture I. *Lancet*, *1*, 1177–1182.
Holmes, G. (1922b). The Croonian Lectures on the clinical symptoms of cerebellar disease and their interpretation. Lecture III. *Lancet*, *2*, 59–65.
Hopkins, D.A., & Lawrence, D.G. (1975). On the absence of a rubrothalamic projection in the monkey with observations on some ascending mesencephalic projections. *Journal of Comparative Neurology*, *161*, 269–294.
Hsu, M., Courchesne, E., & Press, G. (1989). Absence of brainstem abnormality in study of autistic patients using magnetic resonance imaging. *Society for Neuroscience Abstracts*, *15*, 1334.
Ingvar, D.H. (1985). "Memory of the future": An essay on the temporal organization of conscious awareness. *Human Neurobiology 4*: 127–136.
Jackson, J.H. (1958). On some implications of dissolution of the nervous system, in: *Selected Writings of John Hughlings Jackson*, Vol. 2 (J. Taylor, ed.), Basic Books, New York, pp. 29–44. (Original work published 1882)
Jaeken, J, & Van den Berghe, G. (1984). An infantile autistic syndrome characterised by the presence of succinylpurines in body fluids. *Lancet*, *2*, 1058–1061.
Jones, E.G., Wise, S.P., & Coulter, J.D. (1979). Differential thalamic relationships of sensory-motor and parietal cortical fields in monkeys. *Journal of Comparative Neurology*, *183*, 833–882.
Jürgens, U. (1984). The efferent and afferent connections of the supplementary motor area. *Brain Research*, *300*, 63–81.
Kubie, L.S. (1953). Some implications for psychoanalysis of modern concepts of the organization of the brain. *Psychoanalytic Quarterly*, *22*, 21–68.
Larsell, O. (1937). The cerebellum: A review and interpretation. *Archives of Neurology and Psychiatry (Chicago)*, *38*, 580–607.
Larsell, O., & Jansen, J. (1972). *The comparative anatomy and histology of the cerebellum: The human cerebellum, cerebellar connections, and cerebellar cortex* (Vol. 3). Minneapolis, MN: The University of Minnesota Press.
Leiner, H.C., Leiner, A.L., & Dow, R.S. (1986). Does the cerebellum contribute to mental skills? *Behavioral Neuroscience*, *100*, 443–454.
Leiner, H.C., Leiner, A.L., & Dow, R.S. (1989). Reappraising the cerebellum: What does the hindbrain contribute to the forebrain? *Behavioral Neuroscience*, *103*, 998–1008.
Lieberman, P. (1985). On the evolution of human syntactic ability. Its pre-adaptive bases—motor control and speech. *Journal of Human Evolution*, *14*, 657–668.
Lieberman, P. (1989). Origins of some aspects of human language and cognition. In P. Mellars & C.B. Stringer (Eds.), *The human revolution: Behavioral and biological perspectives on the origins of modern humans* (pp. 391–414). Edinburgh: University Press.
Lorente de Nó, R. (1934). Studies on the structure of the cerebral cortex: I. The area entorhinalis. *Journal für Psychologie und Neurologie*, *45*, 381–438.
Luria, A.R. (1969). Frontal lobe syndromes. In P.V. Vinken & G.W. Bruyn (Eds.), *Handbook of clinical neurology* (Vol. 2, pp. 725–757). Amsterdam: North-Holland Publishing.

MacLean, P.D. (1967). The brain in relation to empathy and medical education. *Journal of Nervous and Mental Disease, 144*, 374–382.
MacLean, P.D. (1970). The triune brain, emotion, and scientific bias. In F.O. Schmitt (Ed.), *The neurosciences. Second study program* (pp. 336–349). New York: Rockefeller University Press.
MacLean, P.D. (1973). A triune concept of the brain and behavior, Lecture I. Man's reptilian and limbic inheritance, Lecture II. Man's limbic brain and the psychoses, Lecture III. New trends in man's evolution. In T. Boag and D. Campbell (Eds.), *The Hincks Memorial Lectures* (pp. 6–66). Toronto: University of Toronto Press.
MacLean, P.D. (1987). The midline frontolimbic cortex and the evolution of crying and laughter. In E. Perecman (Ed.), *The frontal lobes revisited* (pp. 121–140). New York: IRBN Press.
MacLean, P.D. (1988). Cytochemical tracing of cerebral connections of midline frontal cortex in Saimiri monkeys. *Society for Neuroscience Abstracts, 14*, 692.
MacLean, P.D. (1990). *The triune brain in evolution: Role in paleocerebral functions.* New York: Plenum.
McIntyre, H.D., Mayfield, F.H., & McIntyre, A.P. (1954). Ventromedial quadrant coagulation in the treatment of the psychoses and neuroses. *American Journal of Psychiatry, 3*, 112–119.
Mandelbrot, B.B. (1977). *Fractals: Form, chance, and dimension.* San Francisco: W.H. Freeman.
Meyer, A., Beck, E., & McLardy, T. (1947). Prefrontal leucotomy: A neuroanatomical report. *Brain, 70*, 18–49.
Meyer, J.S., & Barron, D.W. (1960). Apraxia of gait: A clinico-pathological study. *Brain, 83*, 261–284.
Miyata, M., & Sasaki, K. (1983). HRP studies on thalamocortical neurons related to the cerebellocerebral projection in the monkey. *Brain Research, 274*, 213–224.
Morison, R.S., & Dempsey, E.W. (1942). A study of thalamo-cortical relations. *American Journal of Physiology, 135*, 281–300.
Olszewski, J. (1952). *The thalamus of the macaca mulatta: An atlas for use with the stereotaxic instrument.* New York: Karger.
Oppenheimer, P. (1985). The genesis algorithm. *The Sciences, 25*, 45–47.
Pandya, D.N., & Barnes, C.L. (1987). Architecture and connections of the frontal lobe. In E. Perecman (Ed.), *The frontal lobes revisited* (pp. 41–72). New York: IRBN Press.
Pillsbury, W.B. (1929). *The history of psychology.* New York: W.W. Norton.
Ramón y Cajal, S. (1959). *Degeneration and regeneration of the nervous system* (Vol. 2) R.M. May (Trans. & Ed.). New York: Hafner. (Original work published 1928)
Riley, H.A. (1960). *An atlas of the basal ganglia, brain stem, and spinal cord.* New York: Hafner.
Ritvo, E.R., Freeman, B.J., Scheibel, A.B., Duong, T., Robinson, H., Guthrie, D., & Ritvo, A. (1986). Lower Purkinje cell counts in the cerebella of four autistic subjects: Initial findings of the UCLA-NSAC autopsy research report. *American Journal of Psychiatry, 143*, 862–866.
Roland, P.E. (1987). Changes in brain blood flow and oxidative metabolism during mental activity. *News in Physiological Sciences, 2*, 120–124.

Roland, P.E., Larsen, B., Lassen, N.A., & Skinhoj, E. (1980). Supplementary motor area and other cortical areas in organization of voluntary movements in man. *Journal of Neurophysiology*, *43*, 118–136.
Rubinstein, H.S., & Freeman, W. (1940). Cerebellar agenesis. *Journal of Nervous and Mental Disease*, *92*, 489–502.
Sander, F. (1930). *Structure, totality of experience and "Gestalt" in: Murchison. The psychology of the thirties.* Worcester: Clark University Press.
Singer, M., & Yakovlev, P.I. (1954). *The human brain in sagittal section.* Springfield, IL: Charles C Thomas.
Smith, S.B. (1983). The great mental calculators. New York: Columbia University Press.
Starzl, T.E., & Magoun, H.W. (1951). Organization of the diffuse thalamic projection system. *Journal of Neurophysiology*, *14*, 133–146.
Starzl, T.E., & Whitlock, D.G. (1952). Diffuse thalamic projection system in monkey. *Journal of Neurophysiology*, *15*, 449–468.
Strick, P.L. (1976). Anatomical analysis of ventrolateral thalamic input to primate motor cortex. *Journal of Neurophysiology*, *39*, 1020–1031.
Vandervert, L.R. (1988). Systems thinking and a proposal for a neurological positivism. *Systems Research*, *5*, 313–321.
Vandervert, L.R. (1990). Systems thinking and neurological positivism: Further elucidations and implications. *Systems Research*, *7*, 1–17.
Vogt, C. (1909). La myeloarchitecture du thalamus du cercopitheque. *Journal für Psychologie und Neurologie*, *12*, 285–324.
Werner, H. (1940). *Comparative psychology of mental development.* New York: Harper & Row.
Werner, H. (1956). Microgenesis and aphasia. *Journal of Abnormal Social Psychology*, *52*, 347–353.
West, B.J., & Goldberger, A.L. (1987). Physiology in fractal dimensions. *American Scientist*, *75*, 354–365.
Wiener, N. (1948). *Cybernetics, or control and communication in the animal and the machine.* New York: John Wiley & Sons.
Wiesendanger, R., & Wiesendanger, M. (1985). The thalamic connections with medial area 6 (supplementary motor cortex) in the monkey *(Macaca fascicularis)*. *Experimental Brain Research*, *59*, 91–104.
Williams, R.S., Hauser, S.L., Purpura, D.P., DeLong, G.R., & Swisher, C.N. (1980). Autism and mental retardation: Neuropathologic studies performed in four retarded persons with autistic behavior. *Archives of Neurology*, *37*, 749–753.
Yakovlev, P.I. (1954). Anatomical studies in frontal leucotomies: II. Cortical origin of the fronto-pontine tract and organization of the thalamo-frontal projections. *Transactions of the American Neurological Association*, 53–56.

# 2
# Microgenetic Theory and the Dual Premotor Systems Hypothesis: Implications for Rehabilitation of the Brain-Damaged Subject

GARY GOLDBERG

## Rehabilitation as an Empirical Practice in Search of Workable Theory

It should be recognized from the outset that rehabilitation has historically been an empirical practice seeking practical results. The orientation has been clinical and patient based because modern rehabilitation has arisen out of the need to address with immediacy the disabling consequences of chronic disease. Practical solutions to the practical, everyday problems that the disabled person encounters is the focus of clinical rehabilitation. Thus, the clinical need has driven the development of the field, both in the modern era as well as historically. Rehabilitation has been an historical human empathic response to the ravages of disease and injury. No apology for this is needed. The quality of life of countless individuals has been addressed through this orientation and emphasis. The trial-and-error approach has tended to be the driving method and has been successful to some degree in identifying important innovations. Because of the immediacy of the need, however, rehabilitation science with a viable theoretical framework has been slow in developing, and rehabilitation as an academic, knowledge-based discipline remains in its infancy, ripe for development. There has been relatively little opportunity and, for some, perceived need, to step back from the clinical interface and theorize constructively.

The formulation of a theoretically driven rehabilitation science, however, is problematic. Rehabilitation is a dynamic process of experientially driven change analogous to education. Theorizing about rehabilitation and theorizing about education are necessarily related endeavors. The goal of rehabilitation, in a general sense, is the optimization of human functionality, a broad goal, indeed, and one that is not easy to conceptualize succinctly. The need to develop testable scientific theory for rehabilitation is clearly a major project that would help to drive the field forward through a balanced interaction of theory and experiment. What will be required for a workable theory for rehabilitation? This will depend critically on how one views and conceptualizes "human functionality." For the purposes of this discussion, I will assume that an important component of the functionality of living systems is the ability to act successfully (Reed, 1982).

## Conceptualizing Action as an Emergent Interaction Between Intentionality and Environmental Affordance

In a very general sense, theoretical development for rehabilitation science will depend on an adequate modeling of the functioning human body as a dynamic system, a problem traditionally dealt with in the science of physiology. I will begin to narrow the focus by asserting that human functionality is closely tied to human performance and that performance, understood as "adaptive behavior," can be viewed as a "product" of cognition. Adaptive behavior as a product of cognition will be further viewed as a generalization of the concept of biological action, and the view put forward here will be an action-oriented conceptualization of human performance. Action is conceptualized here as a basic *goal-directed dynamic process defined in space and time: a time-dependent change in the physical configuration of the body in relationship to the environment.* This process can be viewed as involving the whole body functioning in concert to alter its interactive relationship with the environment. Action can also be considered as the process of solving a specific motor problem of functional relevance to the organism through the simultaneous satisfaction of emergent constraints that arise from a variety of sources, both intrinsic and extrinsic to the organism, on a variety of different time scales, ranging from phylogenetic to microgenetic (Yakovlev, 1948; this statement will be clarified to some extent in the following discussion). These lawful constraints serve to select the act through a "self-organizing" (Prigogine 1980; Yates 1986) process in which the potentially available degrees of freedom for an act are progressively peeled away so that the performance itself is low dimensional. Thus, the system remains stable, controllable, and ordered in its behavior in spite of its complexity and many potential degrees of freedom. Self-organization refers to this spontaneous emergence of order in complex systems operating far from thermodynamic equilibrium. Through the application of constraints to the system in a nonequilibrium state, cooperativity between autonomous elements emerges in a complex system. This cooperativity may itself be driven through inherent variability or fluctuations that become selectively amplified (Kugler & Turvey, 1987; Mpitsos et al., 1988; Prigogine, 1980). Furthermore, this fluctuation or "noisy" variability critical to the process of self-organization may be produced through nonlinear dynamic behavior within the system, thus having a deterministic or lawful basis rather than being totally random (Crutchfield, Farmer, Packard, & Shaw, 1986).

Action thus is defined here through an emergent process that satisfies a specific goal of biological relevance to the organism through *an interaction between the intentionality of the organism* (i.e., a directedness toward the achievement of a state of goal satisfaction at some future point in time: an increase in the probability of a particular outcome—Searle, 1984), which applies intrinsically originating constraint, and the affordances offered by the environment (which provide the organism with the potentialities for structuring a strategy for goal satisfaction), which apply extrinsically originating constraint. It should be noted that extrinsic constraints relate to both natural, physical constraints as well as cultural conventions that govern acceptable social behavior within a particular cultural context (Norman, 1988). As a bottom line, this process must, at all levels and at all points in time, be constrained by physical law (e.g., conservation of energy, laws of dynamics, etc.). This condition necessarily applies not only to microgenesis but also to ontogenesis and phylogenesis, the time scales of development and evolution into which the microgenetic time scale is embedded. It is the recognition of this fact that may open the way to a unification of the physical and biological sciences, at least as they apply to biological action (Brooks & Wiley, 1988; Kugler & Turvey 1987; Yates 1987). The laws of biological evolution apply further historical constraints that relate to the basic asymmetry between extant and extinct organisms, existence and nonexistence; behavioral capacities of extant organisms have been selected for their successful adaptation to environmental conditions at the ecological interface.

Furthermore, a theoretical approach to action will be viewed as closely related to the active "information-processing" capacity of the nervous system. This idea of information-processing ability, however, is rarely dealt with in a formal theoretical sense in the context of neuropsychology, even though information theory is a well-accepted formalism in the physical sciences closely linked to the process of "communication." Here, "information" is formally defined mathematically in the context of dynamical systems theory as a change in the *predictability of system behavior*: information gain is formally defined as a specific distance measure between the a priori ("expected") and subsequently known a posteriori ("actual") probability distributions for a system variable. Thus, the gain in information provides a means of quantifying predictability in a stochastic system: A peaked probability distribution has a high information content relative to a flat distribution. Furthermore, information theory can be applied to time-evolution of dynamic systems by postulating that the system dynamics serve to communicate information stored in the current state of the system into the future (Shaw, 1981). One of the tasks that will be attempted here will be to link the formal "information theory" of the physical sciences to the problem of conceptualizing brain dynamics and cognition, with, hopefully in the process, some light shed on microgenetic theory. To do this, we will call on the emerging sciences of complex systems, dynamic systems theory, and nonequilibrium physics (Nicolis & Prigogine, 1989; Prigogine,

1980)—theoretical approaches that have arisen out of applied mathematics and the modeling of the evolutional dynamics of physical systems functioning far from thermodynamic equilibrium using time-dependent differential equations. This will be part of an attempt to outline a theory for the development of a rehabilitation neuroscience consistent with a physical biology that draws on a variety of sources, especially the "ecological psychology" of J.J. Gibson (1979) and the "physiology of activity" of N.A. Bernstein (1966), in addition to the concepts of dynamic systems theory, which specify physical law in the form of systems of differential equations that permit a formal approach to the modeling of complex system dynamics operating under nonequilibrium conditions (Nicolis & Prigogine, 1989; Prigogine, 1980; see also Kugler & Turvey, 1987).

The major underlying context from the biological sciences is the theory of biological evolution, through which the dynamics of biological function have been defined by the historical interaction of necessity and chance. Biological evolution itself may be viewed in the context of nonequilibrium physics as a self-organizing process. Similar processes involving selection applied to diversified variants may apply as well to the ontogenetic and microgenetic time scales (Edelman, 1987). It is proposed that the development of a theoretically oriented rehabilitation neuroscience that draws on a synthesis of the relevant physical and the biological sciences (long headed in opposite directions—see Yates, 1987) directed toward a theoretical conceptualization of human performance may be helpful in guiding practice and experiment as applied specifically to the rehabilitation of the brain-injured subject.

## The Application of Dynamic Systems Theory to Microgenetics

The microgenetic theory of cognitive processes can be viewed as an approach to the organization of neural dynamics underlying cognition. Microgenetic theory proposes that these dynamics are intrinsically constrained by the phylogenetic and ontogenetic processes in which the microgenetic process is embedded (Brown, 1988; see also Katz, 1983). These processes are linked to each other continuously in the time domain. Emphasis is placed on dynamic process rather than content, and the symptoms associated with brain injury are viewed as revelations of normal process not adequately constrained so as to reduce the likelihood of error. Thus, the symptom itself is an "error" that reveals normal process prematurely erupting to the surface (see also Canguilhem, 1989, for a general discussion of the concept of error in the context of medical pathology). Microgenesis is thus the process through which constraints emerge that specify the behavior and thus limit the likelihood of alternative behavior or "error." Microgenesis is fundamentally associated with *information gain*: a "battle" between deterministic forces, actively structuring and specifying the behavior-to-be through constraint application directed toward increasing the predictability or likelihood of a specific outcome (i.e., goal) at a future point in time, and the second law of thermodynamics, which resists this process of specification by making all possible outcomes equally likely and dissolving any differentiating constraints (thus maximizing the "entropy" or "unpredictability" of the system). From this basic thermodynamic consideration, microgenesis is an energy-consuming irreversible process that must involve specific patterns of brain "work" or "activation" involved in the structuring of specific system instabilities. The appearance of the overt act itself may actually represent a "relaxation" of the potential state generated through the microgenetic process, with associated dissipation of energy (Kwan, 1988; Kwan, Yeap, Jiang, & Borrett, 1990). The microgenetic process of "setting up" the performance, however, would require the active selection of boundary conditions and the structuring of the singular set in the state space of the dynamics being prepared. This suggests a certain complementarity in terms of energy flows between microgenetic preparation and the overt performance of the act. Performance is inherently probabilistic, and biological organisms are fundamentally stochastic (i.e., "noisy") in nature. Thus, to err is a fundamental property of a living system, and the possibility of error is itself intrinsic to life processes (Foucault, 1989). Surviving systems have a built-in capacity selected through the evolutionary process to statistically assure survival through adequate control of error. They are structured so as to survive and reproduce in spite of the possibility of error.

The symptom of the brain-damaged subject can be viewed as an "error" revealing impairment in the specification process: a result of the ever-present dialectic between predictability (information gain) and unpredictability (entropy gain), which more frequently leads to error in the presence of brain damage. Furthermore, the nature and frequency of the errors and the degree to which they are systematic in their structure may provide important clues to understanding the normal process whereby error-controlling constraints are elaborated and how such constraints may be faulty in the presence of brain damage. A careful analysis of the nature and structure of "errors of action" can provide important insight into the impairment of the constraint-generating mechanism in the damaged brain (Mayer, Reed, Schwartz, Montgomery, & Palmer, 1990; Norman, 1981; Norman, 1988; Reason, 1979; Schwartz, Reed, Montgomery, Palmer, & Mayer, 1990; Shallice, 1982). This information may also be used to innovatively restructure environmental affordances so as to reduce the likelihood of error. In addition, this view of symptomatology places the symptom in a functional holistic context and suggests that the process of rehabilitation may be viewed as reducing the frequency of errors produced as a manifestation of the brain damage (Mayer et al., 1990). This can be approached through the careful study of the errors made and an analysis of how constraint-generating mechanism has failed to avoid these errors. Learning can be viewed as the experientially related emergence of intrinsically elaborated constraint that reduces the probability of error. The recovery process following brain damage may be similarly conceptualized as the restoration of a faulty constraining mechanism in the error-controlling processes.

How can dynamical systems theory assist in the understanding of microgenetic process? How can we apply principles derived from nonequilibrium thermodynamics (Prigogine, 1980) and the study of self-organizing physical systems (Yates, 1987) to understand human cognition? The concept of self-organization in dissipative structures (i.e., entities that consume energy obtained from their surround) is an extremely important one that provides a fundamental underpinning for a new holism in the study of the behavior of complex systems. In complex dissipative structures (such as life forms) that include nonlinear interactions in their dynamics, coherent ordered behavior emerges that is highly dependent on the global features of the system. This is very different from system behavior at equilibrium, where behavior depends exclusively on the linear summation of short-range interactions between system components. This latter view—compatible with the simple Euclidean concept of space-time as homogeneous and isotropic—has been a driving force throughout Western science, but one that is becoming more and more difficult to defend, particularly when considering the study of complex biological phenomena that involve emergent highly ordered cooperative behaviors with coordination of the system as a whole entity (Prigogine, 1980). As Prigogine (1980, p. xiv) notes, "(biological) space is functional, not geometrical." The modern theory of dynamical systems, however, is beginning to provide a new geometry of bifurcation and attractor structures that can be applied to the organized world of biological function (Nicolis & Prigogine, 1989).

Some of the general principles of dynamic systems theory may provide valuable insights. One general concept is that of the representation of dynamics through the topological structure of a phase–space representation. In this manner, the dynamics is viewed as a time-dependent trajectory traversing the state space of the system. *This mathematical conceptualization allows system dynamics to be interchangeably transformed to geometric structure*. In dissipative systems in which available energy is consumed in an irreversible process, trajectories representing system dynamics are "attracted" to specific regions of the phase space referred to as "attractors" or singular solutions to the system dynamics, as phase–space volume contracts and the system "relaxes." These "objects" in phase space represent stable, asymptotic solutions of the defining system of differential equations and may be characterized using geometric formulation. This illustrates the interchangeability of system dynamics and geometric structure in phase space. This equivalence opens up means for the visualization of complex dynamic processes and their geometric characterization. Furthermore, it suggests a new interpretation of structure–function interaction within adaptive living systems, where there is always the tendency to separate form from function and to distinguish anatomy from physiology. It suggests a much more plastic or fluid interactive relationship between form and function within biology over the various time scales (phylogenetic, ontogenetic, and microgenetic) than is generally recognized and an ongoing tension between stability and adaptability reflected in this interaction between form and function. In this conceptualization, form and function are the same thing distributed across a spectrum of temporal rate of change. Stability and change are both relative in evolutionary time. This suggestion also has important implications for understanding the response to brain damage and, in particular, the important influence of the behavioral context in which the brain-damaged subject performs.

## Information Theory and Brain Dynamics

In conceptualizing voluntary action in the preceding terms, one can view the central nervous system as an information source that specifies the patterns of activation of the neuromuscular apparatus in the course of producing an act. This type of information is specificational as opposed to indicational–instructional. Specificational information is derived from dynamic considerations (i.e., it is time or rate dependent), while indicational–instructional information exists as a physical array or symbol string (i.e., it is static or rate-independent) communicating a state of affairs often through linguistic representational encoding (Collier, 1986; Kugler & Turvey, 1987; Pattee, 1977; Reed, 1981; Shaw, 1981). If we then refer to this dynamic form of information as "carried in the evolving *geometry* of structured energy distributions" (Kugler & Turvey, 1987, p. 9, emphasis added), then specific action patterns may be associated with specific informational content captured in the geometric representation of the associated dynamics. One can then begin to talk about the informational content of an action pattern and relate this to the demands placed on brain dynamics necessary to produce the act. Effortful action may thus be related to the level of information content (related to the dimensionality of the resulting dynamics) being elaborated in the production of the act. The information content specifying the action will be related to both the spatial extent and accuracy of the movement as well as the temporal rate of change of muscle activation and the complexity of the spatial pattern of muscle activation.

The nervous system can equivalently be viewed as applying specific *boundary conditions* to the system of differential equations capturing the dynamics of the ecological system that involves the organism interacting with its immediate surround (Kugler & Turvey, 1987, p. 424). These boundary conditions define the set of attractors or singularities in the phase space of the ecological dynamical system that specify the instabilities of the system, and this "singular set provides a low-dimensional control space description that can be mapped into a high-dimension machine space description *to form an efficient, controllable system*—that is, a low-dimension information description constrains a high-dimension neuro-muscle-joint description" (Kugler & Turvey, 1987, p. 425, emphasis added). The transformation of system dynamics produced by brain damage can be viewed as an alteration in the capacity of the nervous system to specify boundary conditions, which results in a change in the structure of the singular set imposed by these conditions in the dynamics of the ecological system. An inability to adequately specify singular "solution" states in the dynamics results in an impairment in the acquisition of goal states. In the context of goal-directed behavior, if the nervous system is unable to specify constraints so that a state of goal satisfaction is reliably and consistently achieved, then the result is an increased probability of error, or equivalently, an increase in the unpredictability of system performance and, therefore, an increase in system entropy. This change can be framed in terms of *a degradation of the ability of the nervous system to maintain the predictability of the dynamics of the ecological system in a goal-oriented context* and, equivalently, an impairment of the ability of nervous system dynamics to generate sufficient information *at an adequate rate* to constrain behavior so as to reduce and control error.

## The Dual Premotor Systems Hypothesis

How might the process of action specification through the elaboration of constraints proceed with reference to brain structures? The major functions of the organism are attained ultimately through the control of energy flows at the ecological interface between the organism and its surround. These flows are of two fundamentally different forms. The first type is a low-energy *perceptual coupling* in which external information sources are coupled into the organism through "receptors" that transduce energy flow fields conveying information generated by external sources. This external source of informational constraint may then be applied to neural structures so as to constrain their activity in the microgenetic process through which the sensory percept emerges and information is extracted about external conditions. The second type is a coupling in which informational constraints generated centrally in the nervous system are transformed into high-energy mechanical couplings with the surround in the microgenetic process through which voluntary action emerges and internal sources of potential energy are specifically deployed (Kugler & Turvey, 1987). These couplings are potentially highly interactive within the nervous system. Furthermore, it is proposed that there are two major sources of informational constraint used to control this second type of coupling: an intrinsic source related to the intentionality of the organism and an extrinsic source related to the existing external conditions. The first source enables the organism to function in an *anticipatory* adaptive mode using information that is derived from intrinsic models structured from past experience, while the second source enables motor responses that are *reactive* to environmental conditions (see Rosen, 1985). Thus, both sources are concerned with linking conditions for action to the executive mechanism, but they do so in different modes. Similarly conditional responses can be separated into those that are anticipatory or expectant ("forward-directed") versus those that are reactive or "backward-directed" (Perruchet, 1984). The dual premotor systems hypothesis states that there are separable premotor systems in the brain associated with these different behavioral modes. (Goldberg, 1985a, 1985b, 1987a). It does not, however, argue for a strict functional dichotomy but rather a relative subspecialization of different brain subsystems.

The hypothesis will not be fully repeated here. The main issues have been published in the form of a review with commentary (Goldberg, 1985a) and have been further elaborated more recently (Goldberg, 1987a). Expressions of similar concepts have been made by Kornhuber (1980, 1984), Passingham (1987), and others in various contexts (e.g., Brown & Marsden 1988; Frith 1987; Taylor, Saint-Cyr, & Lang, 1986). Related hypotheses regarding the function of the supplementary motor area (SMA), the frontal region, corresponding to the putative medial premotor system (see following), have been put forward: the proposal that the initiation of all voluntary movement occurs in this region (Eccles 1982a, 1982b) through an as-yet poorly understood mechanism involving interaction between "mental" and "physical" entities (Eccles, 1986; Popper & Eccles, 1977); the idea that the SMA is specifically involved in the selection of the timing of voluntary acts (Kornhuber & Deecke, 1985); and the idea that anticipatory postural adjustments preceding voluntary movement are organized through SMA activity (Wiesendanger, 1986; Wiesendanger & Wiesendanger, 1984).

A conceptual framework with regard to how premotor systems participate in determining the conditions for action is proposed. The hypothesis basically synthesizes a broad array of data gathered from a variety of perspectives regarding the relationship of behavior and brain function to support the notion that conditions for action can be categorized as being externally oriented or internally oriented and that there are separable neural substrates, termed *premotor systems*, through which these different conditions are integrated and brought to bear in the course of the microgenetic production process.

It is contended that this process involves the coupling of informational constraints arising from two major sources:

1. Endogenous factors arising from within the organism that relate to internal state, memory, and the *self-generated* aspects of action detected

through the monitoring of efferent outflow by way of recurrent transmission to sensory regions (corollary discharge)
2. Exogenous factors that relate to environmental conditions

It is proposed that willed, self-initiated voluntary movement involves an *anticipatory* activation of the medial premotor system that enables *prospective* control of behavior (i.e., following a "plan") and permits the perceptual differentiation of "active" self-generated activity from "passive" response to external forces through the generation of a "corollary discharge" (Sperry, 1950). This central message from efferent to afferent brain regions informs the perceptual centers in advance regarding forthcoming self-generated activity and anticipated consequences, so that the perceptual products of the activity (e.g., "re-afferent" proprioceptive discharge) can be appropriately determined to be originating either from within or outside the organism (Amassian, Cracco, & Maccabee, 1989; Phillips & Porter, 1977; Teuber, 1972). This may be one of the major functions of the preparatory set of the organism.

It is further proposed that these internal and external constraints on movement are coupled to the process of organizing movement through different brain systems that can be considered "premotor" to the extent that they influence the structure of efferent flows that impinge on the motor unit. These premotor systems are proposed to be in a state of mutually inhibitory balance that may shift with context. It is thus postulated that the nervous system differentiates in a fundamental way between actions made in relationship to external conditions and actions performed in a prospective, "willed" manner through the elaboration of internal goals.

Considerations from evolutionary cortical architectonics (Pandya & Barnes, 1987; Sanides, 1964, 1970) suggest the fundamental hypothesis that the six-layered isocortex has evolved from two primary sources of undifferentiated cortex: the archicortex of the hippocampus and the paleocortex of the olfactory cortex (Sanides, 1970; see also Pandya & Barnes, 1987 for review). The lateral premotor system, derived from its phylogenetic origins in primitive olfactory paleocortex, gives rise to the sensory cortices of the lateral aspect of the hemisphere and conditionally relates sensory conditions to motor cortex in the monkey brain by way of the arcuate premotor area (APA). An equivalent region in the human brain may be the lateral inferofrontal "negative motor area" anterior to the face region of the motor strip identified in human epileptic subjects using cortical stimulation methods (Lüders et al., 1988). In the isolated operation of this system, a specific stimulus is linked to the action that operates in a "responsive" mode. This mode of action is opportunistic and "data-driven" rather than planned: The behavior results from and takes advantage of current conditions (Norman, 1988). This system facilitates orientation toward external information and is important when the conditions for action depend critically on external signals. When this system is "released" or disinhibited in the presence of frontal lobe damage, compulsive automatisms that are directed toward object use or that may be imitative, are released (Lhermitte, 1983; Lhermitte, Pillon, & Serdaru, 1986). With bihemispheric release of this system with extensive bilateral prefrontal damage, a condition in which the patient loses the ability to unhinge behavior from prepotent social environmental context develops. The patient loses personal autonomy and responds in an *obligatory* manner to external cues. This condition has been described by Lhermitte (1986) as the "environmental dependency syndrome." With release of this system, there is a loss of an active self in the maintenance of balance between the occurrence of actions that are either correlated or uncorrelated with externally originating performance constraints. This can be equivalently viewed as a disorder of intentionality or "will." With limited lesions of the medial frontal lobe, involving the anterior cingulate cortex and the SMA, the patient may retain a good deal of insight and show a striking dissociation between actual and intended action (Goldberg & Bloom, 1990; Goldberg, Mayer, & Toglia, 1981).

The medial system, whose phylogenetic origins can be traced to primitive hippocampal cortex, is used to control action when temporal structure is present and memory (i.e., some form of internal model) can be used in conjunction with selective perception to allow anticipatory prospective control of behavior. To act prospectively, there must be anticipation based on prior experience or "recalled" information: a memory-driven mode as opposed to a data-driven mode of performance (Norman & Bobrow, 1975). The appearance of the act is preceded by specific intentional content, and because intentionality implies the capacity to act in accordance with a plan, it is primarily through the operation of the medial system that a sense of volitional control over action emerges and the capacity to act autonomously—with selective rather than obligatory dependence on external information—develops. The major premotor structure in the medial system is the SMA on the medial surface of the frontal lobe. Damage to this system may result in a reduction in spontaneous initiated acts or hypokinesis in the performance of self-initiated movement. Release of this system with damage to the lateral parietal regions of the lateral system results in an excessive dependence on intrapsychic data and a lack of awareness or even an active avoidance of the external world. External information is not able to access the motor mechanism as readily and the patient does not actively orient to this information. This is typically what is observed in the attentional disorder of sensory neglect.

The dual premotor systems hypothesis can be related to the idea of cortical "tropisms" elaborated by Denny-Brown (1966). Denny-Brown proposed a sensorimotor theory of cortical control over action in which the lateral parietal cortex is viewed as a center for facilitating approach behavior to respond to and access external information, while the medial frontal cortex is viewed as a center that facilitates withdrawal from and avoidance of external stimuli. These two centers operate in a state of mutual inhibition that serves to maintain an "approach–avoidance equilibrium" with respect to current environmental conditions. In normal behavior, these two systems are constantly interacting as shifting back and forth between the active capturing and release of external stimuli occurs. In terms of sensorimotor linkages, actively capturing sensory information requires a positive feedback between the afferent and efferent flows so that increasing afference produces increasing efference in response to the afference so as to enhance the initial afference, thus drawing the sensory information into focus and "locking on" to it. Active release of stimuli requires an inhibition of this coupling or even a reversal of this coupling mechanism so that the efferent flow can effect an "escape" or withdrawal from the current stimulation at hand. This "unlocking" is a necessary first step in moving the sensory focus or "searchlight" from one site to another. These concepts were used to explain the release of various "reflexive" responses that occur in the presence of specific brain damage (e.g., grasping) as well as different forms of apraxia (Denny-Brown 1958).

The separation of these modes of behavior was also suggested by Bernstein (1984) who proposed two different modes of perceptual modeling necessary for the guidance of behavior: "[t]he model of the past-present, or what has happened and is happening, and the model of the future . . . these are necessarily distinct from each other, chiefly because the first type of model is single-valued and categorical, while the latter can only operate by means of future extrapolation to some or other degree of confidence or probability" (p. 455). Thus, responsive action requires a categorical model of factually existing reality of the extrapersonal spatial world as its stands in the present, while projectional action requires a temporal probabilistic model of the future in order to support anticipatory control (see Rosen, 1985, for a detailed discussion of reactive versus anticipatory adaptive control).

Recently, a number of lines of investigation have produced additional evidence supporting the dual premotor systems hypothesis. Recording cortical unit activity from the SMA, the APA, and the primary motor cortex (MI) in monkeys, Okano and Tanji (1987) found a unique population of units in the SMA, which fired selectively with a premovement latency of several hundred milliseconds before self-paced upper limb movements. Units that fired with a usually shorter premovement latency in advance of movements made in response to a visual signal were found in the SMA, APA, as well as MI. These authors indicated that their data identified a unique role for the SMA in self-paced movement but that a complete double dissociation between SMA and APA neuronal activity could not be supported. They also found the SMA to participate in visually triggered movement together with the APA. This finding suggests that the dual premotor systems do not function in a truly dichotomous fashion but rather that the medial system participates in all voluntary action, including that triggered by external information, with additional participation from the lateral system, depending on the extent to which external conditions must be integrated into the preparatory process. The medial system tends to organize self-initiated endogenously based actions more selectively. Passingham (1987) has pursued the investigation of function of premotor areas using the technique of identifying the effects of selective cortical lesions on performance in trained monkeys. Bilateral lesions of the arcuate premotor area were found to disrupt learned behaviors that depend on the learning of a conditional rule dependent on differentiation of external stimuli (Halsband & Passingham, 1985; Petrides, 1986), whereas bilateral lesions of the SMA were found to disrupt learned behaviors that were dependent on endogenous proprioceptive information about limb position (Thaler & Passingham, 1988). These findings suggest that another way of viewing the proposed differentiation of medial and lateral premotor systems may be in terms of reference informational systems for action. The medial system may be especially important for the organization of actions in an *egocentric*, or body-based, informational reference system, whereas the lateral system participates when an *exocentric*, or environmentally based, informational space-time reference, system is additionally required for successful completion of an act. This approach appears to be supported by recent information accumulating with respect to the cortical participation in saccadic eye movement control. Schlag and Schlag-Rey (1987) have reported the discovery of an eye movement area anterior to the SMA representation in the monkey frontal cortex, which they have labeled the supplementary eye field (SEF). Microstimulation of this region of cortex produced saccades. Stimulation mapping of this region suggests that it may encode for eye position in a head-based reference system so that gaze is biased toward a particular part of space, independent of initial gaze direction. The saccades thus produced by stimulation at some points in the SEF converge to a region of space, whereas saccades produced by stimulating at a point in the frontal eye field (FEF) on the lateral surface of the frontal lobe generally produce movements in a fixed direction. Unit behavior in the SEF is similar to that found for the SMA by Okano and Tanji (1987), in that a population of units can be found that fire with long premovement latencies and a gradual buildup of activity before exploratory eye movements performed during visual search in the dark—that is, in the absence of visual targets. This form of activity is quite different from that found in the FEF. In the FEF, activation of units appears to relate to the presence of an external visual target to which the saccade is directed (Bruce, Goldberg, Buschnell, & Stanton, 1985). Moster and Goldberg (1990) have reported electrophysiological evidence of this differentiation of medial and lateral cortical presaccadic activity in a study of normal human subjects using topographic mapping of presaccadic brain electrical activity. It thus appears that the differentiation of a medial and lateral cortical system for limb movement may be extended to the volitional control and context-dependence of voluntary saccadic eye movements.

## Implications for Rehabilitation

The ideas reviewed here begin to provide a basis for a theoretical approach to the study of human performance and to the amelioration of performance deficits through a training process. Performance is viewed as an emergent phenomenon appearing through an interaction between intentionality and environmental affordance carried out in a social context (Gibson, 1979, 1982). The specific behavior is selected through a self-organizing process involving the satisfaction of multiple constraints. Normal physiological capacity confers a large number of potential degrees of freedom available for the solution of motor problems. Self-organization leads to the emergence of low-dimensional ordered dynamics, whereby, through cooperativity, the number of effective degrees of freedom in the emerging act is reduced. Brain damage can be viewed as reducing the dimensionality of the initial space out of which the performance dynamics are selected. Furthermore, as noted previously, brain damage can be viewed as leading to impaired goal-directed behavior through a failure to apply centrally originating intentional constraints to the performance. This leads to decreased predictability of the successful achievement of the goal state and thus an increased probability of error. Identification and understanding of the impact of brain damage in everyday life can be pursued through a careful study of the nature and frequency of errors occurring during the performance of routine activities of daily living (Mayer et al., 1990; Norman, 1988).

Furthermore, the dual premotor systems hypothesis suggests that the central nervous system is organized so as to couple externally versus internally originating informational sources through separable brain systems. This may lead to different forms of performance errors, depending on whether the damage incurred selectively involves one system as opposed to the other. These systems operate in a complementary fashion and may be able to provide a degree of compensation for each other in the course of performance. Furthermore, environmental structuring and cuing can be used to enhance performance by enriching possibilities for affordance (e.g., provision of a wheelchair in an accessible building), enhancing the salience of important environmental factors, or reducing the potential for error by creating the environmental conditions naturally compatible with and supportive of the action (Norman, 1988). Thus, the greatest demands on intentionality are placed when the patient must traverse what Norman (1988) calls the "gulf of execution," whose breadth depends inversely on the degree to which an intention of the actor is supported by compatible unambiguous environmental conditions. Similarly, Norman (1988) defines the "gulf of evaluation" as depending inversely on the ease with which the state of the environmental conditions can be perceived and interpreted in reference to the intentions and expectations of the actor. Thus, it is possible to deliberately organize and design the environment so as to specifically support a particular behavior. Similarly, ambiguities in the environmental affordances in relationship to the intentions of the actor can lead to error. The degree to which successful performance of a task relies on informational constraints from the surround as opposed to informational constraints "in the head" can vary significantly, and this variability can be used to enhance performance in the presence of brain damage (Norman, 1988).

Rehabilitation can be viewed as an educational process whereby the ability of the person to perform tasks of importance to them is improved. Rehabilitation is directed toward the amelioration of disability. Disability refers to the reduced capacity of the affected individual to successfully perform essential routines of daily living that are expected, in accordance with social norms. In this context, it thus is helpful to define the behavioral impairment associated with brain damage in the context of the performance of routine daily activities such as dressing, washing, feeding, and grooming rather than using formal means of testing for apraxia (Mayer et al., 1990). The errors that occur in attempts to perform these activities may be observed and systematically encoded as a way to begin to identify and characterize the nature of the impairment and its specific impact on daily activities (Mayer et al., 1990; Schwartz et al., 1990). Furthermore, it may be possible to interpret the generation of these errors in the context of the conceptual framework presented here. Memory-driven as opposed to data-driven modes of performance may be differentially affected by different pathophysiologic processes and by differential impairment of the premotor elements. For example, the general effect of aging appears to be a selective impairment of the memory-driven, projectional mode of action (Rabbitt, 1981; Rabbitt & Vyas, 1980), and a similar view also may be applied to the performance deficits seen in Parkinsonism (Brown & Marsden, 1988; Taylor et al., 1986). In traumatic brain injury, in which selective damage to frontal lobes and medial brain structures is frequently observed, affected individuals have difficulty acquiring anticipatory, memory-dependent behaviors even though they maintain the ability to respond to motivating stimuli in avoidance tasks (Freedman, Bleiberg, & Freedland, 1987). This may in turn relate to the finding of a reduced amplitude of the contingent negative variation in patients with closed head injury, suggesting reduced anticipatory activation of the cerebral cortex in the context of learned expectancy (Rugg et al., 1989). A detailed behavioral analysis of routine daily activity in a patient with medial frontal damage indicated that his deficit could be characterized as a problem in the formulation, maintained activation, and realization of intentions (Schwartz et al., 1990). In such situations, where impairment may selectively involve the medial premotor system, the possibility of compensatory strategies relying more heavily on data-driven processing modes than memory-driven modes can be considered, provided that sensory channels are functionally intact and operative and that the environment can be structured so as to be more effective in guiding performance. Furthermore, successful performance may be facilitated through teaching sensory imaging as a compensatory strategy for direct performance. On the other hand, patients with damage selectively involving the lateral premotor system classically are able to generate intentions but may appear to act without awareness of important external conditions. In such cases, training should focus on using the intact intentional control mechanism to train the patient to compensate for a lack of awareness of external factors by intentionally scanning (usually into a particular hemispatial region) to search for this information. It should be noted, however, that damage to the medial system, with its important role in the formulation and control of planned action (i.e., "intentionality"), can lead to a fragmentation of action and errors related to the interference generated by low-level environmental affordances that inappropriately capture the control process and disrupt the activity (see Norman, 1988; Schwartz et al., 1990). These problems can produce behavior that appears "confused" and error-prone and can significantly interfere with the ability to successfully perform routine daily activities.

An additional issue that is central to the rehabilitation of the brain-damaged person and has not been considered yet will be only briefly mentioned here. This relates to the inherent capacity of nervous systerms to restructure in an adaptive manner in response to experience. This may be referred to as *adaptive neurodynamics*, or "*neuroplasticity*" (e.g., Bach-y-Rita & Bach-y-Rita, 1990; Boyeson & Bach-y-Rita, 1989; Goldberg, 1987b), an idea that has been somewhat foreign to the mainstream of neuroscience for most of the last 130 years, because of the dominance of strictly static localization concepts. Consideration is given here to the inherent capacity of the nervous system to adapt in response to experience in the processes of development, learning, and in the recovery of function following brain damage. This adaptive capability can be viewed as an inherent possibility for the nervous system to effectively modify its own structure so as to reduce the likelihood of performance error, that is, its ability to support "learning". The nervous system is a dynamic organ that is constantly undergoing change in its own organization in response to changes in experience, not only during the course of development but also throughout adult life (Jenkins, Merzenich, Ochs, Allard, & Guíc-Robles, 1990). It will be crucial to the development of a rational rehabilitation neuroscience to better understand how these adaptive changes occur, what are the physiological controls in the nervous system that maintain the critical balance between stability and adaptive change, and how these controls may be manipulated through an interaction of training experience and receptivity to change within the nervous system to effect a functional reorganization of neural mechanism supporting recovery of function.

## Summary

Microgenetic theory involves study and interpretation of the neural dynamics involved in the elaboration and organization of behavioral structures. Human functionality depends on the success of adaptive goal-oriented behavioral structures operating in the context of everyday life. Such success does not come easily, depending on an adaptive dynamics produced through a circular interaction of intention and affordance, which emerges through a process that is, to a great extent, subconscious. Furthermore, this conative process involves an active structuring of the future that guides the system toward the goal state in predictable fashion. Failure of this process results in error and may occur in a variety of ways in normal as well as in brain-damaged subjects. The rehabilitation of the brain-damaged patient must begin with a careful characterization and understanding of the manner in which error occurs in the performance of daily activities using action-coding systems (Mayer et al., 1990; Schwartz et al., 1990). The dual premotor systems hypothesis may be helpful in providing a heuristic framework in which to interpret and classify such errors and relate them to specific distributions of brain damage. It may also serve as a heuristic framework in which to develop specific rehabilitative treatment programs directed toward the restructuring of behavioral dynamics so as to reduce the likelihood of error in the performance of daily activities.

*Acknowledgments.* The development of this paper has benefited through opportunities to interact in discussion of these issues with H.C. Kwan, M.F. Schwartz, E.S. Reed, and N.H. Mayer. The author was supported in part through a grant from the Whitaker Foundation, the Staff Research Fund of Moss Rehabilitation Hospital, and Moss Rehabilitation Medicine, Inc.

## *References*

Amassian, V.E., Cracco, R.Q., & Maccabee, P.J. (1989). A sense of movement elicited in paralyzed distal arm by focal magnetic stimulation of human motor cortex. *Brain Research, 479*, 355–360.

Bach-y-Rita, P., & Bach-y-Rita, E. (1990). Biological and psychosocial factors in recovery from brain damage in humans. *Canadian Journal of Psychology, 44*, 148–165.

Bernstein, N.A. (1966). *The coordination and regulation of movements.* New York: Pergamon Press.

Bernstein, N.A. (1984). Trends and problems in the study of investigation of physiology of activity. Republished in Whiting HTA (Ed.): *Homan motor actions, Bernstein reassessed* (pp. 441–466). Amsterdam: North-Holland.

Boyeson, M.G., & Bach-y-Rita, P. (1989). Determinants of brain plasticity. *Journal of Neurological Rehabilitation, 3*, 35–57.

Brooks, D.R., & Wiley, E.O. (1988). *Evolution as entropy. Toward a unified theory of biology* (2nd Ed.). Chicago: University of Chicago Press.

Brown, J.W. (1988). Introduction: Microgenetic theory. In *The life of the mind* (pp. 1–26). Hillsdale, NJ: Lawrence Erlbaum.

Brown, R.G., & Marsden, C.D. (1988). Internal vs external cues and the control of attention in Parkinson's disease. *Brain, 111*, 323–345.

Bruce, C.J., Goldberg, M.E., Buschnell, M.C., & Stanton, G.B. (1985). Primate frontal eye fields: 2. Physiological and anatomical correlates of electrically evoked eye movements. *Journal of Neurophysiology, 54*, 714–734.

Canguilhem, G. (1989). *The normal and the pathological.* (C.R. Fawcett & R.S. Cohen, Trans.). New York: Zone Books.

Collier, J. (1986). Entropy in evolution. *Biology and Philosophy, 1*, 5–24.

Crutchfield, J.P., Farmer, J.D., Packard, N.H., & Shaw, R.S. (1986, December). Chaos. *Scientific American*, 46–47.

Denny-Brown, D. (1958). The nature of apraxia. *Journal of Nervous and Mental Diseases, 126*, 9–32.

Denny-Brown, D. (1966). *The cerebral control of movement.* Liverpool: Liverpool University Press.

Eccles, J.C. (1982a). The initiation of voluntary movements by the supplementary motor area. *Archiv fur Psychiatrie und Nervenkrankheiten, 231*, 423–441.

Eccles, J.C. (1982b). How the self acts on the brain. *Psychoneuroendocrinology, 7*, 271–283.

Eccles, J.C. (1986). Do mental events cause neural events analogously to the probability fields of quantum mechanics? *Proceedings of the Royal Society of London. Series B: Biological Sciences, 227*, 411–428.

Edelman, G.M. (1987). *Neural darwinism. The theory of neuronal group selection.* New York: Basic Books.

Foucault, M. (1989). Introduction. In *The normal and the pathological.* New York: Zone Books.

Freedman, P.E., Bleiberg, J., & Freedland, K. (1987). Anticipatory behaviour deficits in closed head injury. *Journd of Neurology, Neurosurgery and Psychiatry, 50*, 398–401.

Frith, C.D. (1987). The positive and negative symptoms of schizophrenia reflect impairments in the perception and initiation of action. *Psychological Medicine, 17*, 631–648.

Gibson, J.J. (1982). Notes on affordances. In E. Reed & R. Jones (Eds.), *Reasons for realism. Selected essays of James J. Gibson* (pp. 401–418). Hillsdale, NJ: Lawrence Erlbaum.

Gibson, J.J. (1979). *The ecological approach to visual perception.* Boston: Houghton Mifflin.

Goldberg, G. (1985a). Response and projection. A reinterpretation of the premotor concept. In E.A. Roy (Ed.), *Neuropsychological studies of apraxia and related disorders* (pp. 251–266). Amsterdam: North-Holland.

Goldberg, G. (1985b). Supplementary motor area structure and function: Review and hypotheses. (*Behavioral and Brain Sciences, 8*, 567–616.

Goldberg, G. (1987a). From intent to action. Evolution and function of the premotor systems of the frontal lobe. In E. Perecman (Ed.), *The frontal lobes revisited* (pp. 273–306). New York: IRBN Press.

Goldberg, G. (1987b). Principles of rehabilitation of the elderly strok patient. In R.E. Dunkle, J.W. Schmidley (Eds.), *Stroke in the elderly. New issues in diagnosis, treatment and rehabilitation* (pp. 103–143). New York, Springer-Verlag.

Goldberg, G., & Bloom K.K. (1990). The alien hand sign. Localization, lateralization and recovery. *American Journal of Physical Medicine and Rehabilitation, 69*, 228–238.

Goldberg, G., Mayer, N.H., & Toglia, J.U. (1981). Medial frontal cortex infarction and the alien hand sign. *Archives of Neurology, 38*, 683–686.

Halsband, U., & Passingham, R.E. (1985). Premotor cortex and the conditions for movement in monkeys *(Macaca fascicularis). Behavioural Brain Research, 18*, 269–277.

Jenkins, W.M., Merzenich, M.M., Ochs, M.T., Allard, T., Guíc-Robles, E. (1990). Functional reorganization of primary somatosensory cortex in adult owl monkeys after behaviorally controlled tactile stimulation. *Journal of Neurophysiology, 63*, 82–104.

Katz, M.J. (1983). Ontophyletics: Studying evolution beyond the genome. *Perspectives in Biology and Medicine, 26*, 323–333.

Kornhuber, H.H. (1980). Introduction. In H.H., Kornhuber & L. Deecke (Eds.), *Motivation, motor and sensory processes of the brain: Electrical potentials, behaviour and clinical use. Progress in brain research* (Vol. 54, pp. ix–x). Amsterdam: Elsevier.

Kornhuber, H.H. (1984). Mechanisms of voluntary movement. In W. Prinz & A.F. Sanders (Eds.), *Cognition and motor processes* (pp. 163–173). Berlin: Springer-Verlag.

Kornhuber, H.H., & Deeclce, L. (1985). The starting function of the SMA. *Behavioral and Brain Sciences, 8*, 591–592.

Kugler, P.N., & Turvey, M.T. (1987). *Information, natural law, and the self-assembly of rhythmic movement.* Hillsdale, NJ: Lawrence Erlbaum.

Kwan, H.C. (1988). Network relaxation as behavioral action. Some conjectures on the control of movement by the nervous system (Technical Report RBCV-TR-88-26). Toronto: Department of Computer Science, University of Toronto.

Kwan, H.C., Yeap, T.H., Jiang, B.C., & Borrett, D. (1990). Neural network control of simple limb movements. *Canadian Journal of Physiology and Pharmacology, 68*, 126–130.

Lhermitte, F. (1983). Utilization behavior and its relation to lesions of the frontal lobes. *Brain, 106*, 237–255.

Lhermitte, F. (1986). Human autonomy and the frontal lobes: 2. Patient behavior in complex and social situations: The "environmental dependency syndrome." *Annals of Neurology, 19*, 320–325.

Lhermitte, F., Pillon, B., & Serdaru, M. (1986). Human autonomy and the frontal lobes. Part I. Imitation and utilization behavior: A neuropsychological study of 75 patients. *Annals of Neurology, 19*, 335–343.

Lüders, H., Lesser, R.P., Dinner, D.S., Morris, H.H., Wyllie, E., & Godoy, J. (1988). Localization of cortical function: New information from extraoperative monitoring of patients with epilepsy. *Epilepsia, 29* (Suppl. 2), S56–S65.

Mayer, N.H., Reed, E., Schwartz, M.F., Montgomery, M., & Palmer, C. (1990). Buttering a hot cup of coffee. An approach to the study of errors of action in patients with brain damage. In D.E. Tupper & K.D. Cicerone (Eds.), *The neuropsychology of everyday life: Assessment and basic competencies* (pp. 259–284). Boston: Kluwer Academic Publishing.

Moster, M.L., & Goldberg, G. (1990). Topography of scalp potentials preceding self-initiated saccades. *Neurology*, 644–648.

Mpitsos, G.J., Creech, H.C., Cohan, C.S., & Mendelson, M. (1988). Variability and chaos. Neurointegrative principles in self-organization of motor patterns. In J.A.S. Kelso, A.J. Mandell, & M.F. Shlesinger (Eds.), *Dynamic patterns in complex systems* (pp. 162–190). Singapore: World Scientific.

Nicolis, G., & Prigogine, I. (1989). *Exploring complexity. An introduction*. New York: W.H. Freeman.

Norman, D.A. (1981). Categorization of action slips. *Psychological Reviews, 88*, 1–15.

Norman, D.A. (1988). *The psychology of everyday things*. New York: Basic Books.

Norman, D.A., & Bobrow, D.G. (1975). On data limited and resource limited processes. *Cognitive Psychology, 7*, 44–64.

Okano, K., & Tanji, J. (1987). Neuronal activities in the primate motor fields of the agranular frontal cortex preceding visually triggered and self-paced movement. *Experimental Brain Research, 66*, 155–166.

Pandya, D.N., & Barnes, C.L. (1987). Architecture and connections of the frontal lobe. In E. Perecman (Ed.), *The frontal lobes revisited* (pp. 41–72). New York: IRBN Press.

Passingham, R.E. (1987). Two cortical systems for directing movement. *CIBA Foundation Symposium, 132*, 151–164.

Pattee, H.H. (1977). Dynamic and linguistic modes of complex systems. *International Journal of General Systems, 3*, 259–266.

Perruchet, P. (1984). Dual nature of anticipatory classically conditioned reactions. In S. Kornblum & J. Requin (Eds.), *Preparatory states and processes* (pp. 179–198). Hillsdale, NJ: Lawrence Erlbaum.

Petrides, M. (1986). The effect of periarcuate lesions in the monkey on the performance of symmetrically and asymmetrically reinforced visual and auditory go, no-go tasks. *Journal of Neuroscience, 6*, 2054–2063.

Phillips, C.G., & Porter, R. (1977). *Corticospinal nevrones. Their role in movement*. London: Academic Press.

Popper, K.R., & Eccles, J.C. (1977). *The Self and Its Brash*. New York: Springer International.

Prigogine, I. (1980). *From being to becoming. Time and complexity in the physical sciences*. New York: W.H. Freeman.

Rabbitt, P.M.A. (1981). Cognitive psychology needs models for changes in performance with old age. In J. Long & A. Baddeley (Eds.), *Attention and performance* (Vol. 9, pp. 555–573). Hillsdale, NJ: Lawrence Erlbaum.

Rabbitt, P.M.A., & Vyas, S.M. (1980). Selective anticipation for events in old age. *Journal of Gerontology, 35*, 913–919.

Reason, J.T. (1979). Actions not as planned. The price of automatization. In G. Underwood & R. Stevens (Eds.), *Aspects of consciousness* (Vol. 1, pp. 67–89). London: Academic Press.

Reed, E.S. (1981). *Indirect action*. Unpublished manuscript, Center for the Study of Human Learning, University of Minnesota.

Reed, E.S. (1982). An outline for a theory of action systems. *Journal of Motor Behavior, 14*, 98–134.

Rosen, R. (1985). *Anticipatory systems. Philosophical, mathematical and methodological foundations*. New York: Pergamon Press.

Rugg, M.D., Cowan, C.P., Nagy, M.E., Milner, A.D., Jacobson, I., & Brooks, D.N. (1989). CNV abnormalities following closed head injury. *Brain*, *112*, 489–506.

Sanides, F. (1964). The cyto-myeloarchitecture of the human frontal lobe and its relation to phylogenetic differentiation of the cerebral cortex. *Journal für Hirnforschung*, *6*, 269–282.

Sanides, F. (1970). Functional architecture of motor and sensory cortices in primate in the light of a new concept of neocortical evolution. In C.R. Noback & W. Montagna (Eds.), *Advances in primatology*, (Vol. 2, pp. 137–208). New York: Appleton-Century-Crofts.

Schlag, J., & Schlag-Rey, M. (1987). Evidence for a supplementary eye field. *Journal of Neurophysiology*, *57*, 179–200.

Schöner, G., & Kelso, J.A.S. (1988). Dynamic pattern generation in behavioral and neural systems. *Science*, *239*, 1513–1520.

Schwartz, M.F., Reed, E.S., Montgomery, M., Palmer, C., & Mayer, N.H. (in press). The quantitative description of action disorganization after brain damage: A case study. *Cognitive Neuropsychology*.

Searle, J. (1984). *Minds, brains and science*. Cambridge, MA: Harvard University Press.

Shallice, T. (1982). Specific impairments of planning. *Philosophical Transactions of the Royal Society of London*, *B298*, 199–209.

Shaw, R.S. (1981). *The dripping faucet as a model chaotic system*. Santa Cruz, CA: Aerial Press.

Sperry, R.W. (1950). Neural basis of the spontaneous optokinetic response produced by visual inversion. *Journal of Comparative and Physiological Psychology*, *43*, 482–489.

Taylor, A.E., Saint-Cyr, J.A., & Lang, A.E. (1986). Frontal lobe dysfunction in Parkinson's disease: The cortical focus of neostriatal outflow. *Brain*, *109*, 845–883.

Teuber, H.-L. (1972). Unity and diversity of frontal lobe functions. *Acta Neurobiologiae Experimentalis*, *32*, 615–656.

Thaler, D.E., & Passingham, R.E. (1988). The supplementary motor area and internally directed movement. In A.R. Crossman (Ed.), *Neural mechanisms in disorders of movement*. London: Libbey.

Wiesendanger, M. (1986). Recent developments in studies of the supplementary motor area of primates. *Reviews of Physiology, Biochemistry, and Pharmacology*, *103*, 1–59.

Wiesendanger, M., & Wiesendanger, R. (1984). The supplementary motor area in the light of recent investigations. *Experimental Brain Research*, (Suppl. 9), 382–392.

Yakovlev, P. (1948). Motility, behavior and the brain. *Journal of Nervous and Mental Diseases*, *107*, 313–335.

Yates, F.E. (Ed.) (1986). *Self-organizing systems. The emergence of order*. New York: Plenum.

Yates, E.E. (1987). Forward. Physics and biology. In P.N. Kugler M.T. Turvey *Information, natural law, and the self-assembly of rhythmic movement*. (pp. xiii–xix). Hillsdale, NJ: Lawrence Erlbaum.

# 3
# Mental States and Perceptual Experience

Jason W. Brown

*In the human spirit, as in the universe, nothing is higher or lower; everything has equal rights to a common center which manifests its hidden existence precisely through this harmonic relationship between every part and itself.*

—Goethe

Are mental events independent of brain activity? One way of approaching this question is to ask whether mind can be altered without a change in brain. There was a time when mental illness seemed pertinent to this issue, but now we view such disorders as an effect of altered brain chemistry or physiology. Are there purely mental causes of mental change, such as telepathy? (see Koestler, 1972) This seems to be the crucial test of mind–brain interaction because telepathy and other psychic phenomena involve an effect of mind "at a distance," an effect of mind on objects or other minds in a way that cannot be mediated by brain states. Telepathy gets around the problem of whether a brain determines, or can be affected by, a change in mind when that change is not driven by a corresponding brain state, as required in a two-way (brain → mind, mind → brain) causality.

Clinical studies indicate that mind is not a product of the entire brain, at least not in equal proportions. Sherrington spoke of a mental brain and a nonmental brain. Every region of the brain is not equally linked to mind. Parts of the brain can be removed or destroyed without a demonstrable change in mind. Even large portions can be lost, and awareness and intentionality seem to remain intact. Because mind survives the loss of some brain elements, it is not the brain as a whole or even its elements that form the brain half of the mind—brain equation. Of course, the absence of change with the loss of an area does not speak to the activity of the area itself. The sound of a violin alone cannot be predicted from the sound of an orchestra, whereas if a single violin is removed from an orchestra, the

This also appears in *Self and Process* by Jason W. Brown, 1991, New York: Springer-Verlag. 

difference can scarcely be noticed.[1] If one does not know the function of an area to begin with, determining its function when it is removed is like experiencing an object from its absence. It is like a blind man describing a color.

Is the brain state a composite of myriad groups (columns, modules) of nerve cells? A slab of cells in the cortex continues to be active when it is isolated from other regions. Could this population generate a partial or rudimentary mental state? What is the difference between the activity of this population and another process in the brain that does not participate in the elaboration of mental states? Presumably, such a (nonmental) process has the status of other processes in the body, such as the electrical function of cells in the heart. Do such processes differ from those that participate in mental states? Brain states underlying mentation must differ from nonmental brain states in more ways than just complexity. The mental state depends on *organized* patterns of brain activity. If such patterns unfold over stages, isolated cell groups, even if quite large, could not elaborate (even part of) a mental state. The activity of separate brain elements would have to be embedded in, or configured by, the activity of the brain as a whole.

Thus, small areas of the brain probably cannot mediate partial mind states, large areas can be sacrificed without discernible effects, while damage to small but strategic regions can result in a disturbance of vital components. The specificity of the brain or the importance of focal brain areas does not imply that mind is a composite of brain elements. Even in cases where damage to focal areas has a devastating impact, for example, a disruption of language or object perception, the damage leads to a qualitative change, not a piecemeal dissection.

It would not seem possible to map a mental state to an underlying brain state because the existence of the brain state is *inferred* by a self within its mental state. Similarly, a component in mind would not predict the activity in a corresponding piece of the brain. Nor can mental phenomena be predicated on specific brain states. In epileptic patients, for example, the stimulation of limbic areas can produce psychic experiences, but the effect is inconsistent and the nature of the required brain activity is unclear. Presumably, *configural* aspects of the process elaborating the brain state correspond with configural properties in the structure of the mental state.

The problem is that brain states are conceived in relation to the process through which they develop; there is no "content" in the brain state. Mental states, however, are described in terms of content only, such as the content of a representation, not in relation to the process leading to that content. The resultant asymmetry—brain process versus mental content—is taken to reflect a discrepancy between the mental and physical series. It follows that an account of brain state correlates of the content of, for

[1] This analogy was first suggested by Penfield.

example, a perception (or a proposition) requires an artificial immobilization of activity in brain so as to pinpoint the "state" and an artificial stasis in the flow of cognition to pin down the "content."

From this perspective, a process model of the mind–brain is a theory on the origin of a class of mental contents, not an explanation of the neural basis for a given content. The mind—brain mapping is configurational. There is no part-to-part or whole-to-whole correspondence, no algorithm for the translation between the activity of a given brain state and the content of the corresponding mental state.

The concept of a mental state implies a minimal or irreducible cognitive moment. Because brain and mental activity have the nature of a continuum, there is no state in the sense of a static slice that can be designated, but rather there is a process distributed in space and time. What is important in this process is the flow from one mind—brain state to another. This is the problem of continuity in relation to the snapshot-like encapsulation of mental frames or segments, that is, the temporal context of the state. There is also the matter of the distribution of components within a state—the compositional or spatial context of the state. Finally, there is the relation across moments in the mind—brain series: the volitional, purposeful, and automatic series in action or the contrast between images and objects in perception.

These issues are often sidestepped in philosophical writings in pursuit of the more general relation between mind and brain. An understanding of the *structure* of the state itself, however, is important for a theory of mind. Wittgenstein (1953) said that to "talk of processes and states and leave their nature undecided [is] . . . the decisive movement in the conjuring trick." Perhaps mental states are vastly different from the assumptions of folk psychology, perhaps mental events as such, as *events*, do not even occur. It seems prudent to explore the nature of mind and brain states before speculating too much on their identity, correlation, or the interaction between them.

## The Content of Mind

The mental life has a depth beneath awareness and a surface punctuated by conscious events. The subconscious is not a form of mentation *complementary* to consciousness but a preliminary stage in the derivation of consciousness. That the contents of awareness rest on and develop out of subsurface mentation is evident from dream analytic work, psychopathological case study, and the effects of brain injury (Brown, 1988).

In contrast to subconscious cognition, the conscious "surface" of mind is usually held to consist in the content of introspection. On the microgenetic view, however, introspection—unique to man, the "highest" stage of mentation—is not an addition to a cognitive end point but is an accentuation at a more preliminary phase, (Brown, 1988, pp. 30–33, 149–151). The surface of mind, the terminus of the mental state, is filled with developing objects, not just the images of private space anticipating those objects but the rich abundance of forms that make up the perceptible world. This world, the surface of mind as the skin is the surface of the body,[2] changes instantly according to what is perceived. I glance at the field before me, and that is my mind. I turn and take in the road and farmhouse, and that is my mind. What mind perceives is the substance of what mind is for the moment of that perception. A perception is not a space punctuated by objects; there is no empty space out there, only one enormous object, the world.

At the same time there are inner events, awareness, feelings, a reminiscence of the past that objects call up, thoughts, commentaries, and other private states, all of which as "mind" seem set against the field of perception. But acts and objects and the memories and mental images that precede them are not part of an outer and an inner world but points on a continuum of transformation; they are not projected into the world but build up and articulate the world as part of the representational space of mind.

From pathological cases, it is known that a loss of objects entails a disruption of image content in the damaged modality (Brown, 1988, pp. 249–251). The patient with cortical blindness and a "loss" of the object world has a disturbance of visual imagery; cases with neglect for objects on one side of perceptual space show a similar disruption of imagery. Awareness is inconceivable if the world should suddenly disappear or if mind could no longer generate that world (Brown, 1988, pp. 198–205, 264–269). The disorientation that occurs in snow blindness or sensory deprivation is due to the loss of sensory modeling (see following discussion) and the loss of external objects. Introspection, even if focused on imagery, requires an object world, otherwise there is a dream cognition. The surface of mind is a continuation of the process through which inner states are elaborated. The gap from private to public is a psychological deception, not a basic epistemic division.

Mind, therefore, extends over the inner and outer contents of awareness as well as stages leading to awareness on which those contents depend. Both surface and depth have an equal share in mind. The concept of a stratified cognition is central to the notion of a mental state, for it estab-

---

[2]There is, in fact, a deep analogy between the world as the surface of mind and the skin as the surface of the body. Skin and brain are stratified and stem from common germinal ectoderm. The lifeless outer layer of skin is formed of cells rising out of subcutaneous fields. Object representations also develop out of fields submerged beneath waking awareness; objects individuate as they emerge to the surface, where they too die, making way for newly developing contents. The object world is the lifeless crust or rind of mind, a skin for mental structure.

lishes the *formative direction* of the state. This entails an unfolding from depth to surface, not from one surface to the next, a direction crucial to agency and the causal or decisional properties of consciousness.

In sum, mind includes perceptual objects, acts, emotions, ideas, and other subjective images, everything in the center of awareness and on the periphery, as well as the complete series of formative levels or incipient minds out of which these contents emerge. The formative direction and thus the dynamic structure of a mental state is from subsurface mentation through private events to the perceptual surround.

## Mental States

A mental state is the minimal state of a mind, an absolute unit from the standpoint of its spatial and temporal structure. It is the briefest duration over which a mind can be elaborated and includes elements that need to be incorporated in the duration for the events to have mental characteristics. This entails a medium within which representations can develop and some form of awareness. The state also has to include the prehistory of the organism. The state is my state, in *my* mind, an instance of *my* mind in action, not just a segment of mental activity. The concept of a mental state implies a fundamental unit that has Gestalt-like properties, in that specific contents—words, thoughts, percepts—appear in the context of mind as a whole. The concept is not inconsistent with the idea of mental components, but the unitary nature of the state across components and relations between components within the state need to be explained. A mental state is not a piece of a mind or a slice that can be demarcated but a structure that is active over time. It is assumed from clinical studies that this structure unfolds from a core to a distributed surface over hierarchic (evolutionary) layers, each stage forming a background out of which the next individuates (Fig. 3.1).

Cognitive levels are not superimposed but have emergent properties (Brown, 1988, pp. 357–359). The content of a stage that is transformed is not lost in the progression to a later stage but is embedded in the final representation. Antecedents of the field of awareness, subconscious layers beneath the surface content, are as much a part of the mental state as the objects and ideas to which they lead. The content at the surface is not waiting *in status nascendi* to be activated but is derived from stages that prefigure and shape the final representation.

The transformation over levels and the distributed nature of content at each level reflect the spatiotemporal character of the mental state. The *temporal* aspect is the transition from depth to surface over a fraction of a second. Though preliminary phases are ineffective by the time the transformation reaches the surface, such phases are still active in cognition after

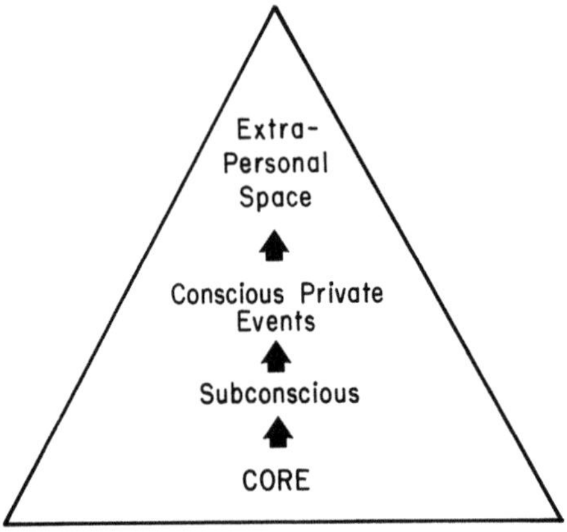


FIGURE 3.1. The structure of the mental state.

they have been traversed.[3] The mental state requires a certain duration of the immediate past (within that state). The duration of the unfolding is the time required for a single transition through the microgenetic structure of the state. The state is not an open-ended chain but an obligatory sequence that is reiterated, the minimal duration of which is the time elapsed for one complete traversal.

The mental state also has a *spatial* or cross-sectional character. Each phase generates incipient content in several domains, in action, in language, and in the different perceptual modalities. Each phase in each component is part of a distributed system linked to stages in evolutionary growth. The entire multitiered system arborizes like a tree, with levels in each component linked to corresponding levels in other components. For example, an early (e.g., limbic) stage in language (e.g., word meaning) is linked to an early stage in action (e.g., drive, proximal motility) and perception (e.g., hallucination, personal memory) so that a given level across components is a stage in the evolutionary structure of mind, not just a phase in the microgeny of that component.

In sum, a description of the spatial and temporal features of a *single* unfolding series amounts to a description of the minimal unit of mind, the *absolute* mental state.

On this view, consciousness and its objects are the expanding rim of an outward-flowing mind. Like a river pouring into its tributaries, mind is constantly resurrected, the nature of the state each moment reflecting the degree to which the revival is successful. An incomplete transformation

[3] This is also true for preceding states. The suspension of the physical past in the duration of the mental present—the transcendence of the now over the passage of physical time—is a (the) crucial problem in mind–brain theory.

fails to realize the world of waking objects, and mind is centered in the subjective. Objects, inner states, awareness—all withdraw as one to a private world of dream.

Each of the potential minds submerged within the surface has a share in the self. The complete series of traversed and realized configurations constitutes a dynamic vertical envelope within which life is played out. Successive waves flowing from the core guarantee that each state falls in the same self. The continuity of mind, the perpetuation of the self over time and over gaps in awareness, owes to the generation of surface content out of the core. The transition from one mental state to another is a replacement of each state by the next rising from below, a succession of vertical unfoldings reiterated each moment throughout life (see following discussion).

## Brain States

It is argued that a mental state has a structure that may be mapped to the structure of the brain with a correspondence between psychological levels and levels in physiological structure. Specifically, the series of planes in the derivation of acts and objects is taken to correspond to a matched series of physiological transformations. The theory obligates that stages (distributed levels) are entrained in a succession, retracing phyletic growth. The base of the brain state is organized around ancient neural formations, the phyletic endowment and early experience; its surface is organized around structures recent in phylogeny that elaborate ongoing perceptions. In every object, the progression from past to present reenacts the history of the earliest life experiences. There are minds within minds and brains within brains, with a precise configurational mapping between the two.[4]

The brain state begins with a configuration in the brain stem that is derived through limbic formations and basal ganglia to generalized neocortex and belt areas surrounding the "primary sensory and motor" regions. Reciprocal connections across parallel levels (e.g., between stages in action or object formation) and from one level to the next within the same

[4] If one slices through the "tree" of the mind–brain state at a given level intersecting the main branches, the theory predicts that neural events at each phase will be simultaneous *across* each cognitive domain; i.e., across the different branches. For example, events at an early limbic stage in the brain state will be simultaneous for each domain sampled (action, perception, etc.). Studies of the visual system in monkey (Merzenich & Kaas, 1980) show simultaneity across different cortical visual areas. A study in man by Fried et al. (1981) indicates simultaneity across anterior and posterior language areas. Of course, documentation of the model can only come from physiological evidence of serial entrainment of these putative levels in a given behavior.

component (e.g., between levels in object formation) maintain levels (processing stages) in the different components in phase, provide "feedback" or upstream modulation, and presumably constrain downstream flow.

## Sensory Determinants of Perceptions

The model entails that a brain state is an *intrinsic* series that elaborates a mental state. There is no gradualist appearance of events underlying brain states. An activity does not become more like or part of a brain state. Input and output systems are discontinuous from those generating the brain state. An important part of the theory is that the mind–brain state is distinct from its sensory determinants and its behavioral effects.

The difference between a sensory and a perceptual process is inherent in this distinction. A perception is the outcome of a composite of brain states. A sensation is a physical series that shapes but is extrinsic to the brain state. We are not aware of sensations, only their presumed effects on perceptions. A sensation is an inference about the origins of a perception.

It is usually assumed that percepts are constructed out of sensations, with the difference between sensation and perception a matter of degree. The idea of a series of stages in visual cortex mediating shape specification is grounded in this approach. This way of thinking about the boundary of sensory and perceptual events poses many theoretical and clinical problems.

Though it is necessary to distinguish physical (sensory) events linked to real objects from physical (brain state) events linked to mental representations of those objects, there is no clear way of conceptualizing a transition from one order of events to the other. At what point in a sensory chain do unconscious events in the physical construction of the object become mental objects in consciousness? How do we know what objects to look at if the object we see is the first stage in perceptual awareness? Clinical study shows that objects do not break into constituent (sensory) elements but degrade to preliminary representations (Brown, 1988, pp. 173–205). Image phenomena, illusion, and hallucination can only be understood in relation to a concept of representational levels (Brown, pp. 206–251).

In perception, a series of stages in image formation leads to object representations if sensory information is driving the perceptual process. The difference between the image and the object is the greater autonomy of the former and the bond with sense information in the latter. This approach opens the way for a concept of sensation as a set of *constraints* on percept formation. The constraints determine the degree to which an object is approximated. Sensations impinging on each stage in the object formation sculpt the process to model a physical object (Brown, 1988, pp. 258–259).

Imagine breathing into a balloon constricted at various points. The shape of the balloon is not determined by the internal force but the external constrictions that restrict its freedom of form. The constrictions also limit other possibilities of development. In the same way, constraints on the elaboration of the mind–brain state determine the form taken by the state but are not part of the internal form-building process.

## Motor Outcomes of Actions

Movement and action are analogous to sensation and perception. Movements are physical events read off levels in action. The part of the brain state through which an action is represented is the physical referent of the action, not the external events associated with the actual movements. These are the implied outcomes of action representations (Brown, 1988, pp. 313–315). The action in awareness is a perceptual model laid down in the action discharge. That is, the awareness of a movement is a secondary perceptual awareness, not a direct apprehension of the physical movement. The irony is that an action in awareness is neither an action nor a movement but a perception generated by the initial action representation and its motor outcome.

More precisely, levels in the brain state constitute the action structure. As it unfolds, this structure generates the conviction that a self-initiated act has occurred. This structure—the action representation—does not elaborate content in consciousness. Levels in the action representation are transformed through motor keyboards into movements. The keyboards drive the muscles through which the action is instantiated. This phase, the discharge of the keyboards and the actual movements, is outside awareness in physical space-time. As with the sensory–perceptual interface, the transition to movement occurs across an abrupt boundary. In some manner (Brown, 1988, pp. 303–304), perhaps through a translation of cognitive rhythms in the action to kinetic patterns in the movement, levels in the emerging act discharge into motor (physical) events (Fig. 3.2).

A secondary representation of the action develops perceptually through central and peripheral recurrent pathways. The perception of an action is the action that is experienced. This perception is simultaneous with the movement or follows after a brief delay. It arises like an object through sensory effects on object formation. The content of the action, the behavior that is happening, bodily changes one is aware of, plans and goals, even the decision to act, are ideas or objects in perception constructed out of the residues of the action microgeny.

In sum, a brain state consists in a brief overlapping series of act and object formations. This series unfolds from base to surface over strata in brain evolution and corresponds with psychological planes embedded in the mental state. Distributed around the system are successive tiers of

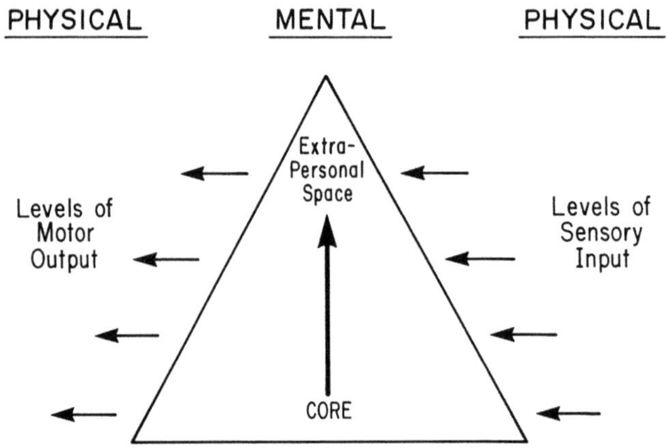


FIGURE 3.2. Sensory input at successive moments in the unfolding of the brain state constrains a configuration to model the external object. Similarly, motor keyboards discharge at sequential moments in the action representation, the discharge folding into the movement structure. This pattern of an emerging mental state interfacing with, but insulated from, a physical sensorimotor surround is reiterated at successive stages.

sensorimotor processors. These mediate transforms between physical systems elaborating movements and sensations outside the mind–brain state and physical systems elaborating cognition within the mind–brain state.

## Mind–Brain as a Living System

A structural description of mind–brain states as a hierarchy of levels or stages does not explain the bond between the mental and neural series. However, a change in function at a stage in the brain state is accompanied by a change in cognition at the same level in the mental state. In clinical studies, the change in mentation cannot always be anticipated because of the many variables involved (e.g., age, skill, degree of lateral asymmetry), (Brown, 1988, pp. 137–144) but taking these into account, the change is theoretically predictable. It is not a matter of faith but observation that the state of the brain corresponds with, elaborates, or constitutes a mind, that mind flows from brain even if the relation between mind and brain cannot be explained.

Two individuals cannot have identical mental states nor can an identical state recur in the same individual. The idea that two people could share the same mental state misses the point of what a mental state is. It is based on an account of the representation as identical to its propositional content. For example, if John and Mary believe that Reagan was President, they share that proposition and have that mental state in common. There is a similar problem with the argument that the same mental state can be realized through different physical systems (a brain, a computer). The nature of the mind–brain state, its emergence through levels in memory and personality, the persistence of these levels in the final representation, its evolutionary underpinnings and relation to phyletic and maturational growth trends, are all features of an organic living system linked to the life process and fundamentally different from the operations of (presently known) machines.

## The Continuity of Experience

How does the concept of a series of vertical mind–brain states explain the unity of conscious experience over the transitional series, as well as the unity across gaps in consciousness such as sleep or hypnotic trance? Attempts to deal with the problem of integration across perceptual moments usually take a movie-strip approach in which the rate of transition determines the smoothness of the flow. Studies of perceptual fusion and minimal perceptual duration suggest that the flow is laid down by rapid seriation. This approach is reinforced by the impression that the continuity from one mental state to the next is governed by logical or causal relations across conscious representations. That is, the continuity is maintained by the fusion that occurs when transitions are too rapid to be discriminated, and this continuity is bound up with the causal thread that ties together the content of waking experience. On this view, the "stream of consciousness" is sustained over longer durations by the persistence for many seconds of the content of the immediate past, by the gradual transformation of this short-term memory content to a long-term store, and by an accretion of the short-term content to that of the present moment.

The impression of a surface continuity, however, is a deception elaborated by the continuous replacement of unfoldings rising out of the same core (Fig. 3.3). The unity of experience is guaranteed by the commonality

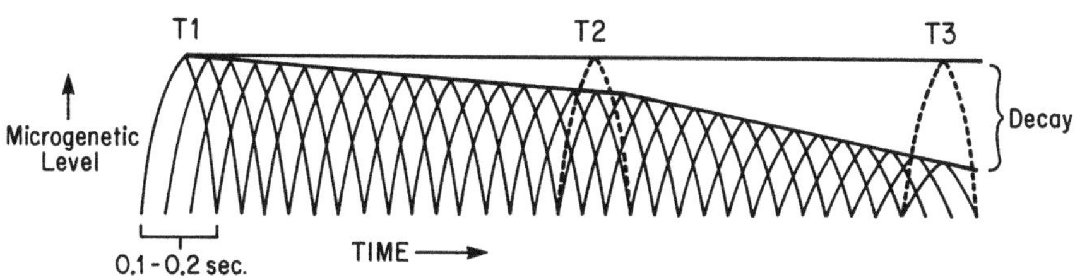


FIGURE 3.3. Each mind–brain state is replaced by the next in the series. The replacement is overlapping. The decay of the state (T1) within subsequent states (T2, T3) accounts for memory and time experience.

of the core across different surface contents. The crucial transition is from depth to surface, the bottom-up sequence, not across conscious representations. Conscious content is a product that serially exhausts a single deep concept embracing multiple surface representations.

The focus, therefore, is not on a rapid exchange across objects in consciousness but on the slow drift from one subsurface frame to another. Because the transition from one core to the next persists through sleep (in sleep, the microgenetic sequence is truncated), the integrity of the mental life is maintained in the absence of conscious experience.

This entails that unfoldings are not concatenated but overlapping. As a new wave rolls to the shore before the first has ended, so the content of an ensuing moment—the immediate future—begins its development as the present moment unfolds. Conversely, the present moment, the now of this instant, is past history even as it appears, for the moment that follows is already underway. The continuity of mind does not depend on a linkage of nows but a succession of present moments articulated out of the core.

Put differently, surface events are figures that realize over time a simultaneous or spatial ground too replete for expression all at once. The core of the microgeny, only partly expressed in the manifold of conscious moments, establishes a thematic that provides unity and coherence. Deep levels undergo slow transformation—gradual movement from one conceptual frame to another—a change obscured by the evanescent shifts at the surface. Attention is like a moving stream, the unseen depths of which run slowly. Waking objects are brief snapshots that dance over the glacial drifts of the core.

The picture is that of a dynamic, rëiterated, tree-like system, the base of which arborizes outward as the next series develops. Each wave issues from a core mediated by midline brain mechanisms and distributes into the world of perception. The progression from archaic strata in subconscious and primary process cognition through the private space of waking mentation to the external space of objects retraces a path from subjectivity to external objects, from the intrapsychic to the extrapersonal, renewing each moment the self, its prehistory, consciousness, and the world.

## Consciousness and the Self

Consciousness is central to the problem of mental states; indeed, it is difficult to imagine a nonconscious mental state or one that does not include some element of awareness. Consciousness is part of the definition of a mental state. If consciousness cannot be inferred, for example in the mental states of animals, we cannot be certain that behavior is accompanied by mentation. The consciousness that is inferred, of course, is modeled after our own experience. This experience is not just the awareness of objects, the introspective and intentional awareness of the waking state, but includes the consciousness of dream, even if this differs in many ways from that of wakefulness. Dream cognition is as pure a mental state as one can point to. The objects of a dream are clearly mental objects. If an animal was shown to have a dream awareness like our own, we would impute to that animal mental states.

A mental state is defined in relation to its conscious quality, but this is not the same as to define what it means to be conscious. The definition of consciousness is elusive, partly because there is more than one form. Consciousness is often restricted to the consciousness *of* an object or an idea. If we define consciousness in this way, however, we exclude the formative stages out of which it develops. Because the formative stages comprise the substructure of the state, there is no hope of understanding the nature of human or any form of consciousness if these stages are ignored. This is not only because we neglect the deep structure of consciousness and the context in which it appears but because the inclusion of a formative or microgenetic segment entails that self-consciousness is a product of subsurface mentation, the terminus of a momentary process, not the locus of a decision-making self.

Planes of conscious experience parallel stages in the realization of the mental state. The degree to which the state unfolds determines the content of the state as well as the mode of awareness within which the content is embedded. Vigilance or arousal, dream awareness, the unreflective awareness of objects and activity, introspection, are forms of consciousness that refer to stages in the unfolding. These stages are not aggregates of separate operations but a series retracing the path of object formation. Conscious experience is deposited in this process. The object formation lays down the different modes of consciousness, resultants, not faculties gazing out at incoming objects.

## *Self-Consciousness*

Self-awareness or introspection is not awareness of the self but the self aware of objects, the condition of being conscious that one is perceiving an object. This is not a self one is conscious of but a relation between a self and its objects, both image and object representations. Consciousness of self requires a self that is conscious and a self that is the object of that conscious state. The misapprehension that consciousness is distinct from the self—that the self can be an object for consciousness—introduces a regress of conscious states; one is conscious of being conscious and so on. The self is the subject of consciousness, and images and objects are what the self is conscious of. When one is conscious of being conscious, the object of consciousness is not the self but an idea or description of the self in a state of consciousness.

The self is conscious in the context of a perception. A relation is established between the self and other objects. Consciousness arises in the context of this relation. The relation determines the mode of consciousness that occurs, so ultimately, it is the relation between constituents that is the core of the conscious experience rather than the constituents on which the relation depends.

Consciousness takes as its object an external percept or an internal image. Introspection (awareness of images) and exteroception (awareness of objects) are different aspects of the same process. The same self can scan an object or an image so the content scanned is not crucial to a description of the state (see also Churchland, 1984), the content reflecting the degree to which the representation objectifies.

Consciousness of self is the end result of a historical process of consciousness development, but the prominence of the self as an inner event, and the fact that inner events are stages on the way to exteriorized objects, implies that self-consciousness is not a "higher" phase in human mentation but a retreat from external objects to preparatory (internal) phases in the object formation.[5] Self-consciousness requires a fully unfolded mental state, a state leading outward to independent objects, positioned not at the surface of the perception but at a penultimate (private) phase in the object formation.

Part of being conscious in this way—having a self that is conscious of something—is the idea of a self that endures, a persisting self that observes and changes slowly over time, even though the ideas and objects it surveys come and go. The self is an image that is remembered, an image of a memory, not a thing or item that is retrieved but the unrecollected background that embraces everything that is recalled, the context within which a specific memory appears. In a very real sense, the self is a repository of past memories and future expectations, a representation that expresses or stands for a personal history and an identity.

A second element is a feeling of distance or detachment between the self and other representations. The self is a representation out of memory that accompanies other acts and percepts. The self representation differs, however, from a concurrent idea or image—a difference that pervades the sense of what it means to have an independent self. Surely, part of this detachment is related to language and the ability to describe inner and outer events. But a commentary on events is not an essential feature of consciousness (total aphasics still appear to be conscious in a human way), but language does enable a more fine-grained conscious experience.

---

[5] This is consistent with the evolutionary principle that new formations occur as outgrowths of earlier layers, not as terminal additions.

## *States of Consciousness*

A theory of consciousness is wedded to a theory of perception. The microgenetic account of perception entails a series of moments in the developing object representation leading from upper brain stem to limbic and neocortical structures toward exteriorization and featural modeling at the level of visual cortex. Sensory or physical input at each stage constrains the developing configuration to model the external object. The perceptual series is autonomous; layers in the final object are intrinsic mental constructs sharply demarcated from the sensory inputs through which they are defined.

These layers—separate modes of existence—are successive planes in the same *mental* space. The percept begins and ends in mind. Similarly, the different types of consciousness and the varied expressions of the self linked to the different conscious states are embedded in a mental space laid down by the developing object. At least four planes of consciousness can be distinguished, corresponding to the described perceptual series (Brown, pp. 259–266).

### Pure Wakefulness

Arousal or vigilance is wakefulness unfocused on specific objects. Vigilance as a persistent state of consciousness occurs with damage to the upper brain stem. Such damage gives rise to coma or a condition in which the eyes are open but the patient is unresponsive. This is also coma, but because the eyes are open it is a state of *pure wakefulness*. This state is inferred to be a stage in object formation before the appearance of an object, before even a mental image, the earliest stage in the elaboration of consciousness, preliminary even to dream mentation. There is no self; there is no mental content for a self to contemplate. There is only a global, undifferentiated preobject preparatory for later conscious stages, implicit in these stages and an obligatory phase in their development.

What is the difference between coma and dreamless sleep? Discounting neurological impairments in comatose patients and looking only at the coma state, coma represents a sleep that is dreamless and interminable. Put differently, dreamless sleep occurs when the initial segment in object formation actualizes at the upper brain stem. In coma, this stage precipitates as a more or less permanent lid on the unfolding process. Damage to the brain stem results in coma through an attenuated object formation giving a vegetative or preparatory stage in the elaboration of consciousness. This phase, the state of dreamless sleep, reflects the initial configuration appearing normally with a suspension of sensation. In the brain-damaged patient, it is expressed in coma if the eyes are closed and in arousal if the eyes are open. The stage represents the earliest appearance of a preobject coextensive with the body and the immediate body surround in an unextended somatic space field.

## Dream Consciousness

Normally, a preliminary representation constrained by sensation at the upper brain stem is transformed to limbic and temporal lobe. The limbic traversal is marked by a relaxation of sensory input, allowing the forming object to undergo selection through a system of personal memory and dreamwork mentation. In this way, the object emerges through the life history. Dream and hallucination are the objects of this level, and the dreamy state is the mode of consciousness that dream objects elaborate. The dream image participates in the dreamer's mental space. Like the space of hallucination, it is plastic and changing and lacking in depth. The self of the dream has a passive quality.

The self of dream differs from wakefulness in other ways. It is charged with affect and shares affect with objects around it. Changes in the perceptual qualities or affective tonalities of dream images are accompanied by changes in the self. This is a sign of incomplete detachment in the affective life of the self and its objects. It shows that the image of the self and the image of objects in the world-to-be are part of a single world image at the point of divergence into the constituent objects and affects that build up the inner life of mind and the outer world of perception.

Dream appears on the continuum from intrapersonal to extrapersonal space. Images appear in an external moiety that is not in opposition to a private sphere of mentation. Inner and outer are indistinctly divided; a single medium is part of the hallucinatory content. Space is volumetric, egocentric, and dependent on the viewer. Space is also a kind of object. It has a tangible, perceptible quality and undergoes distortion. The boundaries between image and space are unclear, so images are also distorted. In addition to spatial distortions, there are conceptual derailments. The similarity of shape or overall configuration as a nexus between the real object and the dream image (e.g., knife—penis) owes to prior sensory information at the upper brain stem constraining the developing object. Though relations of shape predominate, dream images tend to represent the meaning of the object rather than its form. The content of the image is determined by conceptual, symbolic, or experiential relations between the object-to-be, only some physical parameters of which have influenced the object formation at this point, and the preparatory image of that object passing through the dreamwork. The dreamer "sees" the model that has so far evolved, a model that in waking perception is derived to an exteriorized object in which the meaning is buried in the representation of object form.

The view of images as preliminary implies that the shift to imagery or the withdrawal to the dream do not involve a secondary reworking of a perception but a destructuration or decay within the microgeny of the original object. In other words, the nightly regression to dream is an uncovering or a coming to the fore of a *transitional phase* in object formation. Put differently, every object in the world, in order to be there, survives a traversal and selection through a system of dreamwork mentation.

### Object Awareness

The image passing through dream or primary process cognition develops out of distant memory in the context of the life experience. The object takes on meaning in relation to the perceiver's life history and early knowledge of the world. As it develops, the image becomes more like an object; space becomes more like object space. The development leads from context to reference as the object clarifies, enlarging to a three-dimensional space of objects and object relations. This phase is mediated by parietal neocortex.

At this stage, space is extended and filled with external objects. We know from pathology that these objects are linked to the actions of the perceiver and are not yet truly independent (Brown, 1988, pp. 188–196). This is a space of limb action on objects in the immediate environment. There is consciousness of objects and actions on them, directed outward to extrapersonal space. This phase in perception and consciousness was described by Piaget in young children. Perhaps it is the consciousness of subhuman animals. There is a self-concept. Children and chimpanzees show self-recognition in a mirror (see Brown, pp. 218–220, and following discussion). The self is given up as images resolve into objects. The self is a product of the phase of imagery, left behind as a plane in mental representation as cognition moves outward in the laying down of object space.

### Analytic Perception and the Separation of Self and World

The gestalt-like percept along with an external space of relations between objects and viewer gives way to a fully independent space of "public" objects and featural detail, a space of infinite extent with objects that have a life of their own. The transition from a proximate space of object relations in the perimeter of the arm's reach to a solid world of real objects unaffected by an exploring eye or limb is accomplished through the influence of sensory input relaying information on the fine aspects of object form, input received in visual cortex and applied to an emerging object representation.

Unlike the preceding stage, which lays down a space linked to actions of the limb, this stage establishes a world indifferent to the perceiver's behavior. Mind does not affect this world. Actions are relations between objects that are real and do not depend on the perceiver's mind. The self needs objects that are independent; only through the representation of an external world can mind elaborate a feeling of agency that is not embedded in the world. The world has to be sought after and extracted from mind. The self is a kind of deposition bypassed in the object formation, marveling at a world of its creation.

## *The Self in Relation to Objects*

The achievement of an ostensibly real world distinct from mind accompanies the possibility of a self looking on and distinct from the world. One domain entails the other. The world exists in confrontation with mind; mind exists when there is a world the self is conscious of. The world and self appear as separate physical and mental modes of existence, but their boundary is a gradual transition. The self arises in this transition as the object develops from mental space to a location in externality. The self arises at a phase in the forming object before the resolution of clear mental images, because the self is more than any one image type. In the expansion of the mind outward, the self looks on as emerging configurations transform through a fringe of dependent objects to those that are fully exteriorized (Fig. 3.4).

With cognition fully unfolded and directed to objects, the self and the sphere of the imagination are unexpressed or transparent within the microgenetic stream. When a self-conscious stance is assumed, when the perceiver takes an introspective frame of mind, the focus of the object development withdraws from the external world and settles at an earlier stage of mental imagery. The object development is not arrested at this stage, but imagery or internal mentation now constitute the dominant mode of cognition. The withdrawal is incomplete, not as pervasive as in dream. The outer world remains but not in the foreground of attention.

The self is accentuated in moments of reflection. The level of the self is recaptured, is more emphatic, in the brief partial regression that takes place. The same occurs in dream, where the regression enhances an archaic mode of thought normally buried in waking mentation. In dream, however, there is a loss of the external world. The self of dream and the world of dream are all the dreamer has. In reflection, the observer moves back one step from the world of perception; the shift in attention accesses the self by approximating an earlier, bypassed level. The external world persists, unattended, implicit, a necessary soundboard against which the self can resonate.

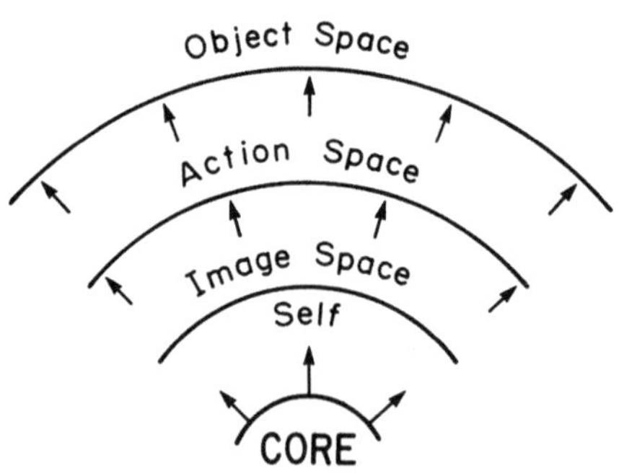


FIGURE 3.4. The mental state unfolds from core to world through the self and successive stages in space representation (see text).

William James (1890) wrote of the unity of the self and its intentional or purposive nature. These were core features of the self and established the mental status of a performance. The feeling of unity or centrality arises because the self actualizes all of what memory can deliver to the present. The self is the now of that moment, an image extending over all of the objects and modalities in the conscious field, an image of memory in action, one that anticipates those objects and out of which they devolve. The self has unity because there is nothing else in mentation at the moment the self appears except the potential objects the self will generate. The unity of the self is part of the definition of what it means to have a self, and this unity owes to the anticipatory, stem-like position that the self occupies in the microgenetic series.

Another feature James (1890) emphasized is an active, purposeful attitude. The sense of purposefulness, or volition, is enhanced by the fact that the self is a precursor of the object representations on which it acts. The self is laid down in the wake of forming objects, satisfying the need for a causal priority of the self in relation to other representations.

The object formation is important in goal-directed behavior not only because it contributes objects for volition to engage, but because it contributes the self as an agent leading outward to those objects. It also generates a feeling of passivity in relation to developing objects that complements the action development, ensuring that objects will be apprehended as external and independent.

The feeling of passivity can be examined over the continuum of the object development. Objects draw away from the self as actions go out to meet them. The deception of an object as a goal is elaborated in parallel with the deception that actions make a difference. Hallucinations and dream images arise spontaneously. Waking memory or imagination images are looked up voluntarily. External objects have been there all along. There is a different relation of the self to the image or object at each of these points. An active or passive self is as much a result of the type of image that develops as the image is a topic for the self.

At each level, the image undergoes increasing clarification. There is progressive loss of affect and narrowing or specification of object meaning. The relation between self and object goes through many changes. Dream images that arise unbidden in the subconscious overpower the self, which is more like an object for the images that surround it. The self of dream is passive to its own images. Gradually, the image unfolds to a stage of illusory control. Reverie marks the transition out of the dream state, where the effortless flow of images gives way to a feeling that one can direct the image stream. This leads to introspection or reflection, when we search through "memory banks" to evoke an image at will. We seem to hunt up the image when it is the image itself that is searching out its own expression. The self is no longer the victim of its images but has an active role in image construction. The play of conscious imagery that populates the self leads finally to a world of independent objects. Now the object is passive to the perceiver, "detached" and no longer part of the mental life.

The process of exteriorization does not involve the projection of an object from mind to world but the elaboration of a level in mental space that appears to be external. The self is left behind in the outward migration of objects. This is a gradual process with qualitative differences at each point in the transitional series. These differences, especially as revealed in the pathological material, help us to understand the microstructure of the series. The belief in the existence of real objects is a byproduct of this process. We are deceived into thinking that the objects we perceive are there for our enjoyment, deceived into thinking the self is a type of mental object, an Ego with meaning and substance that effects actions on real objects in a world that matters.

## Pathology of the Self

Whether the self or its objects are affected by pathology depends on the stage where the pathological change happens to fall. The deeper the impact, the more likely the self is disturbed; the more superficial, the more likely the disruption affects objects in a single modality. The self cannot survive unaltered the various forms of object breakdown. Disorders of object perception encroach on the self, and it undergoes change. In dementia, a progressive change in the self-concept accompanies the object disorder. In severe cases, the individual may not recognize himself in a mirror though other reflections are identified (Brown, 1988, p. 218). There is also a breakdown in mirror space. In dementia, the problem begins with a perceptual disorder and erodes into the self. In schizophrenia, the problem begins with a change in the self that erodes into perception.

"Pure" disorders of the self, as in psychotic cases, are not confined to changes in the self-concept but spill into perceptual functions. Schizophrenic patients experience derealization, loss of the reality of objects, as well as illusory and hallucinatory phenomena. The dissolution of the self is inseparable from these perceptual symptoms.

Regression in schizophrenia is not a return to a primitive state but an accentuation of an early stage in the microstructure of cognition. Behavior comes to be dominated by this early stage, that of the self and neighboring dream or limbic cognition. Initially, the withdrawal from objects may be expressed in an introspective tendency. The fixation on bodily space and hypochondriasis are the other side of the withdrawal. Derealization is a presentiment of the cognitive origins of objects, an incomplete gaining of reality in the object development. Déjà vu phenomena reflect the momentary apprehension that objects do not come to us from outside but are "remembered" into perception. The feeling of familiarity arises because the object is experienced as a reminiscence.

Hallucinations are truncated object developments; delusions, the play of word–meaning relations unencumbered by the drive toward reference and denotation. Paranoia has several roots. The fact that objects are attenuated, and the prominence in the object of limbic cognition, revive feelings of vulnerability to images as in dream. The helplessness we feel to our own hallucinatory objects invades the waking object experience. This is part of the passivity of the subject at this phase in the object formation. As in dream, the perceiver feels he is an object for his own mental images. The passive quality of the self, the loss of the world and with it the active nature of the self, invite the delusion that the schizophrenic is an object for his own images to persecute.

## The Nature of the Self

The self has the nature of a global image or early representation within which objects-to-be are embedded. As with other objects, there is a dynamic stratification, a different self at each level, each self corresponding with different configurations of images and a specific mode of consciousness. There is no bounded self. The self is the accumulation of all the momentary cognitions developing in a brain configured by heredity and experience in a particular way. When we speak of an "inner" and an "outer" self, an anxious, indecisive or troubled self, a search for one of the many different "selves" imminent within the unexpressed potential of a personality, we allude to the lamination of the self, the futility of the quest within the flow from one stratum to the next, and the presence in this lamination of a depth and an inchoateness that accounts for the wealth and ineffability of self-knowledge, shadowing and abiding within the fragment of the self that happens to surface.

The self, a preliminary object embracing all of the objects and images into which it develops, struggles toward understanding. The drive we all share to articulate the self or to "know one's self" reflects this precedence of meaning. The self is meaning without content, shape without internal topography. The self arises in cognitive renewal, where meanings latent in fully developed objects predominate. In perception, the self is a prefigural gestalt, in language, the background semantic content preceding phonological realization.

The deposition of a holistic representation filled with unanalyzed meaning laying down the self as it fractionates into partial contents—acts, images, and the separate perceptual modalities—creates the deception of a self that stands behind and propogates events. The feeling of the self as an agent is reinforced by the forward thrust of the process and the deeper locus of the self in relation to surface objects. The self appears to be an instigator of acts and images, when in fact it is given up in their formation. The self does not cause or initiate, it only anticipates.

Objects grow into the world, pieces of personal memory building up and populating an external image of reality; like the groping tips of tentacles, the mental organism reaches out to form and replenish an ever-changing surface. The self is the medium through which this process occurs, a segment in the object formation preparatory to the isolation of discrete contents. The self emerges as a momentary disclosure of the meaning of a life experience, an unclear form brimming with possibility, poised between the indistinctness of memories that have not yet risen to the surface and their final destination as objects in the construction of external space.

Beneath the introspecting self lies a world of the subconscious, beyond, a world shared with others. Subconscious content is given up in the formation of the self while the self is drawn out and lost in the world of perception. The subconscious is a mystery to its possessor, the world of perception a public world independent of the perceiver. These worlds—subconscious, self, and objects in perception—largely sealed off from one another, are planes in the construction of mental space, successive moments in the forming object and all part of a larger concept of the self.

The origins of the self can be traced to an early segment of the microgeny where the intrinsic configuration arising in the upper brain stem is transformed by incoming sensations to limbic structures. At this point, relatively free of sensory modulation, the configuration traverses a system of personal (long-term) memory and is selected to represent whatever is to emerge out of memory at that moment. The selection of the representation through layered fields or nets of experiential and conceptual object- and word-meaning relations guarantees that standing behind the surviving content is the entire network of relations that was traversed. This network constitutes the experiential sum of the individual.

In the course of the traversal, the content that is selected activates many potential configurations. Latent or unevoked configurations, or those transiently activated that have fallen by the way, persist as a surround of context and tacit knowledge within which the final representation actualizes. This context is the life record brought to bear on every cognition. When we think about an idea or reminisce on a percept, we revive this record, early stages implicit in the original representation. Because every object, every thought, utterance, or behavior develops out of personal memory, whatever passes through this system belongs to it, is part of it, and is part of the mind it elaborates and through which it unfolds.

This deep, still unconscious system of tacit knowledge and experience comprises the self. We distinguish the self from memory and the memory "store," but while the self is not what is actually retrieved or thought about, it is the implicit segment in knowing and remembering. Once a content is revived into consciousness, this phase has been traversed. The self is not composed of the contents we invoke to describe it, but of memories long forgotten and knowledge that fails to materialize.

At this (limbic) phase, the network of active and potential configurations constituting the self is insufficiently distinct from that of the contents against which the self is to be demarcated. That segment of the microgeny preceding the dreamwork contributes a unity and a directionality to the rudimentary self that is realized in dream cognition.

In the neocortical phase, there is increasing resolution and specificity. A phase of meaning relations gives way to one of object relations. This coincides with a resurgence of sensory constraint on the object formation. The self is deposited in the wake of the forming object, reasserted, and abandoned by the very objects to which it gives birth. As a child leaves a parent to make his way in the world, objects are borne, grow, and struggle out of mind, no longer to acknowledge the ancestry of which they are but a moments distillation.

## Consciousness as Relational

The inner bond between self, object, and mode of consciousness is so lawful that it can only mean they are not separate functions but manifestations of a common process. Self and object (or image) are points in the unfolding of a single representation, consciousness the relation between them. The relation between self and object is comparable to that between two objects in the visual field. When I see a chair and a table, the chair, the table, the entire scene are one enormous object articulated into elements. We can focus on one element or another or on the relation between elements, but the element is an artifact of the focus, not a constituent. The chair and the table are part of my perception at that moment, *horizontal* nodes in the same object.

Self and object can be approached in the same way but as *vertical* nodes in the same mental state. The relation between elements in an object depends on the elements. If the elements change, the relations change. In perception, the relations between elements are mental phenomena, as are the elements, but the elements and the world of which they are a part are perceived as physical events outside the mind. This is not the case for consciousness, which concerns the vertical relation between self and object or between a mental and a "physical" segment in the same object representation. Instead of a relation between two external objects, the relation involves two stages in the same object. This relation is construed as a linkage, not between two objects in external space but between mind and externality. This is because one element in the forming object, the self, has a foot in the mind; the other element, the external object, has a foot in the world, and consciousness straddles the two.

Most of the time attention is rivetted on objects. Objects are end points in the derivation of the self, the self is the source of the objects it perceives, objects are the self made explicit. With this phase in relief and the object derivation in abeyance, the self rises into prominence. At other times, the transition from self to object seizes the foreground. Consciousness is the intuition of a relation between levels in object formation, an intuition of the organic thread binding mind to world. Whether the focus is on the self, on objects or on the relation between them, it is only a matter of emphasis on a different aspect of the same mental representation.

## What Is the Purpose of Consciousness?

Karl Popper (1977) asked why consciousness evolved if it has no biological significance. If consciousness has survival value, it must have a purpose; if it has a purpose it is causal, not epiphenomenal. Microgenetic theory obligates that consciousness does not intercede in behavior but arises in the convergence of various aspects of the object development. From this point of view, Popper's question pertains not to consciousness but to its constituent features, consciousness being a collection of those features. Thus, the question is not the evolutionary status of consciousness but the elements of which it is composed: private events, the concept of the self, and the feeling of agency.

In a process model, elements of conscious experience, like other mental contents, can be described in relational terms; it is impossible to pin down a single element as the target of evolutionary advance. In componential models, this is done all the time. Take the case of scanning. This is another way of describing the self as an agent in relation to ideas and objects. Scanning is extracted from this context and assigned a role in evolution. The ability to scan images and ideas or survey objects in the world is reified as an encapsulated function with adaptive value. This notion appeals to everyday experience. Ideas in consciousness seem to propogate. There is awareness of motives and ends. Planned behavior and actions carried out are reviewed and reflected on. The preparation for action and the opportunity to edit actions that are forthcoming seem to assure the best possible outcome. But the scanning of private events is the same as that of external objects, one step removed. Scanning captures the diversity of potential or revived objects or ideas because consciousness incorporates that diversity before the resolution of the individual items.

Another way of thinking about consciousness in behavior is to ask, if conscious experience develops as a by-product of act and object formation, especially the elaboration of these components into language, is the evolution of language at issue, not consciousness, which is a byproduct? The experience of the self and the feeling of agency, however, are so real, vivid, and emphatic, it is hard to accept these attitudes as functionless auras of underlying adaptations. Consciousness and private experience must be there for a reason. One might ask whether a robot that is able to duplicate human performance but lacks internal representations is disadvantaged in relation to its human counterpart. Could a robot duplicate human performance? It is difficult to believe that consciousness does not count for something.

In humans, conscious behavior differs, even if subtly, from automatic behavior. This does not mean that consciousness contributes to the performance but, rather, that the performance contributes to consciousness. If there are qualitative differences between conscious and automatic behavior, a robot mind would have to be an *exact* duplicate of the human, instead of a purely formal resemblance, to attain an identical outcome. The behavior of the robot would have to develop through the same covert series for a verisimilitude in the overt phase. In other words, for humanlike performance, the behavior would have to lay down the contents and conditions that make consciousness possible. It may not be essential that consciousness drive a performance for that performance to be successful, but the achievment of that performance may not be possible without traversing the stage where consciousness is deposited.

These considerations imply that consciousness evolved for a reason even if its constituents do not have causal properties. I believe this reason is to be found not in the enhancement of certain behaviors that consciousness entails but in the different worlds elaborated in the unfolding of consciousness and the self. A self of some sort is a necessary condition for objects to develop. Animals, lacking reflection, still have an archaic or rudimentary self and a concept of autonomy. The animal fights to survive. The feeling of agency and the belief in the autonomy of a self set against objects—the elements of conscious experience—are necessary for survival in a perilous environment. The idea of a self that is real and substantial, a self that can be wounded or destroyed, a self that lives and dies, is an illusion needed for survival. Without this illusion, the self is embedded in a world of mental objects; the individual no longer exists, actions are purposeless, and autonomy dissolves.

The trend in the separation of self and world begins in lower forms of life, accentuates over the mammalian series, and extends still further into human consciousness. Language enhances this trend and helps to build up and protect the self-concept. The deception that objects exist independent of thoughts, that the self acts on objects, even that the self is independent of its own mental content, is essential if the individual is to struggle and survive. Objects have to matter; life depends on this. The self also has to matter. If the self lacks the conviction that it can will an action to pass, if actions are apprehended as enacted through rather than by the self, if existence is a dream, there is no drive to overcome, and life cannot be sustained.

The deception of the conscious self is lost in psychosis. The psychotic intuits the real situation of life. There is a loss of will because he understands that will does not play a part in action. He is traversed by the action, manipulated by invisible strings. Catatonics lose faith in the efficacy of action. The self is a conduit for actions passing through it. For psychotics, the world is replete with meaning. Objects are ridden with thought content and acknowledged as waking dreams. The self withdraws to a proximity with concepts guiding the action. These concepts surface and take on dream-like properties. The self apprehends the sources of action and the springs of its own nature in concepts lying deep beneath the appearance of autonomy and will.

## *References*

Brown, J.W. (1988). *The life of the mind: Selected papers.* Hillsdale, NJ: Lawrence Erlbaum.

Churchland, P. (1984). *Matter and consciousness*, Cambridge: MA, Bradford.

Fried I., Ojemann, G. & Fetz, E. (1981). Language related potentials specific to human language cortex, *Science, 212*, 353–356.

James, W. (1980). *Principles of Psychology*. Holt.

Kestler, A. (1972). *The Roots of Coincidence*. London: Hutchinson.

Merzenich, M., & Kaas, J. (1980). Principles of organization of sensory-perceptual systems in mammals, *Progress in Psychobiology and Physiological Psychology, 9*, 1–42.

Popper, K. (1977), Part I. In K. Popper & J. Eccles (Authors), *The self and its brain* (pp. 3–223). Berlin: Springer-Verlag.

Wittgenstein, L. (1953). *Philosophical investigations*. Macmillan.

# 4
# Meaning and Consciousness: Microgenetic Perspectives on Levels of Processing and Hemispheric Asymmetry

GEORGE KURIAN

The concept of levels in information processing or levels of awareness is one of the central themes in cognitive psychology. Literature in experimental psychology sufficiently documents the importance of levels of processing (see Broadbent, 1958; Hunt & Lansman, 1975; Sperling, 1967), though without making any explicit reference to the brain mechanisms involved. It is also acknowledged that, somewhere along the information processing sequence, meaning is captured first and conscious awareness is a much later outcome (Neisser, 1967). Although tacitly assumed, these intuitions were not sufficiently integrated in the models of cognition, and the neuropsychological models of hemispheric specialization also failed to pay sufficient attention to integrate the phenomena of primacy of meaning and levels of awareness within their framework.

Current literature in this field documents evidence that the meaning of a stimulus (a picture or word) is developed much earlier in the course of information processing than the conscious identification of it. Earlier research in subliminal perception (Dixon, 1971), its later reformulation as preconscious processing (Dixon, 1981), and the more recently argued semantic activation without conscious identification (Holender, 1986) all point to the possibility that meaning may be processed much earlier than the structural (syntactic or phonemic) processing of the stimulus. The microgenetic theory (Brown, 1977, 1983a, 1983b, 1985a, 1985b) offers a methodology and a viable conceptual framework within which phenomena such as preconscious semantic processing, levels of awareness, and hemispheric asymmetry may be captured.

Investigators have made several attempts to develop models of hemispheric specialization (Allen, 1983; Bradshaw & Nettleton, 1983; Corballis, 1983; Hellige, Cox, & Litvac, 1979; Jones, 1982; Kosslyn, 1987; Moscovitch & Klein, 1980; Sergent, 1982a, 1982b). In these attempts, however, the phenomena of preconscious semantic processing, hemispheric asymmetry, and levels of awareness are not explicitly captured within a unitary scheme. Such an attempt—as seen in microgenetic theory—is worthy of serious consideration in view of recent attempts to map the levels at which hemispheric asymmetries emerge (Hellige, Cox, & Litrac, 1979; Marzi, Stefano, Tassinari, & Crea, 1979; Moscovitch, 1983; Sergent, 1982b, 1983); recent theoretical positions advocating the multiple sources of asymmetry, which also imply that the hemispheres probably differ quantitatively rather than qualitatively (Bever, 1983); and more significantly, the issues raised on the nature and origin of consciousness (Bever, 1983; Brown, 1977; Corballis, 1983; Eccles, 1979; Harnad, 1982; Libet, 1987).

In this chapter, an attempt will be made to show how the microgenetic theory accounts not only for the observed phenomena of primacy of meaning in cognitive unfolding but also for the terminal and emergent nature of consciousness. This theory may yield powerful predictions concerning the varying degrees of asymmetry during the microgenesis of cognition as a function of the level or stage that is being tapped in a given experimental (clinical) setting.

## Levels of Processing and Hemispheric Asymmetry

Research on hemispheric specialization has shown that the two hemispheres may not differ at the sensory level (Moscovitch, 1983; Moscovitch & Klein, 1980; Sergent, 1983). Marzi et al. (1979), in their attempt to map the perceptual stage at which hemispheric asymmetries may emerge, found that asymmetries are not manifested at the level of iconic storage. They concluded that the "time decay of iconic storage of either alphabetical or pattern material is essentially similar in the two hemispheres" (p. 38). Hellige et al. (1979) proposed that the processing stage at which attentional shifts develop, resulting in laterality effects, occur beyond the early stages of processing and that attentional shifts take place at the postperceptual stage. There are suggestions that the attentional filter is located, not at the early part of information processing, but somewhere intermediate between the early and end stages of processing (Cowan, 1988), though there is no agreement among researchers on the function of the filter—to filter out information or to attenuate information (Treisman, 1964). Schwartz and Kirsner (1982) tested laterality effects in visual information processing and arrived at the conclusion that hemispheric asymmetries may be obtained at the postperceptual stages of visual information processing. They also noted that individual differeces effects may also be a function of processes at the postperceptual stages. Electrophysiological studies provide further support to the argument that hemispheric asymmetry may not be observed in the early stages of processing. Harter, Aline, and Schroeder (1982) found that the earlier portion of the visual-evoked potential (VEP) was distributed symmetrically over the center scalp region. Konstandov and Arzumannov (1986), studying event-related potentials (ERP) associated with emotional versus neutral stimulus processing, observed that when emotional processing was involved (which is a more primitive function in comparison to feature-analytic processing) the P-300 component of the ERP was found to increase diffusely over both the hemispheres. On the other hand, asymmetries were observed for the late components (Ruggs & Beaumont, 1978). McCarthy and Donchin (1978) found that the late components of the ERP were more pronounced centrally and asymmetric in distribution over the two hemispheres during the performance on tasks involving structural and functional visual matching. At least two components have been delineated corresponding to detection and recognition performances. Parasuraman and Beatty (1980) found that the process of detecting a stimulus begins long before identifying it. Those processes associated with recognition may give rise to hemispheric asymmetry.

Moscovitch and Klein (1980) have proposed a model that posits the levels at which hemispheric asymmetries may emerge. "The model . . . shows that the early stages of processing involved with the extraction of physical or sensory features from the stimulus are similar in both the hemispheres" (Moscovitch & Klein, 1980, p. 590). Simion, Bagnara, Bisiacchi, Roncato, and Umilta (1980) also make a similar suggestion. According to these investigators, the absence of asymmetry in the early stages of information processing indicate that these levels engage the processing mechanisms in both the hemispheres. It is also possible, however, that the absence of asymmetries in the early stages of processing may not be because the two hemispheres perform sensory analysis in a similar fashion or because the early levels engage the processing mechanisms in both the hemispheres but probably because the higher cortical structures are not involved in processing at this stage. It is worth noting that featural processing or structural processing is a higher order or second-order processing, as suggested by Brown (1983a, 1983b, 1985a) and Moscovitch (1983).

Evidence also shows that hemispheric asymmetries are not observed under very brief exposure, very short stimulus-onset asynchrony (SOA), and with reduced luminance, while asymmetries are manifested as higher order cognitive processing comes into play with enhanced exposure duration, heightened visual acuity (foveal vision), increased luminance, and increased interval between the stimulus and the mask (Moscovitch, 1983; Sergent, 1983). It has also been observed that increments in such state-limiting parameters as luminance, acuity, exposure duration, and SOA may lead to left hemispheric superiority, suggesting that the right hemisphere has an upper limit for these parameters and that additional increments may not enhance its processing capabilities.

According to Sergent (1982a), the right hemisphere superiority obtained under inferior stimulus presentation conditions is a spurious one "by default and may also reflect a left hemisphere disadvantage due to a low level of visual resolution, rather than a right hemisphere superiority per se" (p. 12). Sergent (1982a) argues that the right hemisphere processes early-available, low-spatial frequency components while a high degree of visual resolution is required for left-hemisphere processing. A similar argument can be found in Brown (1983a, 1983b, 1985a). He suggests that the early levels in cognitive processing yield a spurious right hemisphere superiority because the early levels in cognition "[represent] a ceiling on cognitive unfolding in the right hemisphere. However, the same cognitive level which is preliminary in the right hemisphere undergoes further analysis in the left hemisphere. That is why tasks that involve later or end stage processing yield a left hemisphere effect" (Brown, 1983a, p. 43). This is also in agreement with the suggestion that the left hemisphere mediates relational processing (Bever, 1983). Relational processing, involves accessing more than one unit in a cognitive domain, whereas a fast access of a single unit would be referred to as unitary processing, because no relational specifications are involved. The often-observed right-hemispheric superiority for unitary processing (otherwise referred to as *holistic processing*) is due to the left hemispheres' propensity to process stimuli by bringing into relationship several units of a cognitive domain as seen in syntactic and phonological processing. Kosslyn (1987) has recently shown that in the case of imagery processes such a phenomena also is observed. Bever (1983) thus attempts to solve the often-observed shifts in hemispheric superiority for the same or identical task as a function of the cognitive processing involved and the stage of processing accessed in a given experiment. Both Bever (1983) and Brown (1983a) argue that the left hemisphere is computationally more advanced than the right hemisphere and also that the left hemisphere is involved in the feature-analytic modeling of the object (cognition), leading to the conscious awareness of the percept. Corballis (1989) ascribes the function of "generativity" to the left hemisphere, though he is less definite about the relationship between generativity (or relational processing) and consciousness.

The primacy of global processing (or holistic/unitary processing) over local featural processing is also well documented in the literature. Hoffman (1980) found evidence for the global precedence hypothesis in which the low-spatial frequencies from a visual display were extracted first and the extraction of high-spatial frequency spectral components took place later. In the perception of apparent motion, the visual system has been found to process global features like texture, and low-spatial frequency components like brightness first, compared to edges and outlines (Ramachandran & Anstis, 1986). Treisman (1986) similarly suggests that the extraction of meaningful wholes precedes the analysis of parts and their properties in object perception. This progression from global to feature-analytic processing is explicit in the microgenetic account of cognitive unfolding (Brown, 1977, 1983a, 1983b, 1985a, 1985b). According to the microgenetic theory, cognition unfolds over a series of structural levels, and over a period of time when the earlier levels form a unitary system that may be involved in the extraction of meaning, while structural processing and conscious identification of the stimulus may occur at the end stages of cognitive microgenesis.

## The Primacy of Meaning

The early levels in cognitive processing may be mediated by the subcortical structures, and these structures probably are involved in the mediation of meaning, too. Brown (1985a) says, "a lexical representation—is derived, one could say retrieved, through a stage of word meaning toward a stage of phonological representation. The phonological representation elaborates the *conscious* perception of the word after its meaning is already understood" (p. 86). This is in agreement with Bever's (1983) rationale for relating relational processes to consciousness: both according to him, are mediated by the left hemisphere of the brain.

Although the issue of preconscious semantic processing is open to some amount of criticism on methodological grounds (e.g., Holender, 1986; Inhoff, 1982), sufficient experimental evidence supports the contention that affect and meaning are processed much earlier than the conscious experience of the stimulus. Such a process is strongly predicted by the microgenetic theory. According to Brown (1985a), "a word or an object is in some sense understood before it is perceived, and the subcognition responsible for these stages in perceptual microgenesis occurs prior to the final featural modelling at a cortical level" (pp. 85–86).

Seamon, Marsh, and Brody (1984) found that affect and meaning may be processed about 8 to 10 ms after the stimilus onset. They found that at very low exposure durations, both affect and recognition judgments were at chance level. At slightly more exposure durations, recognition judgments again remained at chance level, while affect judgments attained better than chance levels. This may be because, as noted earlier, the latter may depend on more primitive processes than those required for recognition judgments. Similarly, Kunst Wilson and Zajonc (1980) found that "individuals can apparently develop preferences for objects in the absence of conscious recognition and with access to information so scanty that they cannot ascertain whether anything at all was shown" (p. 558). Fowler, Worford, Slader, and Tassinary (1981) and Marcel (1983) also showed that meaning can be processed without accompanying consciousness of the stimulus. Whereas featural processing and conscious identification of the stimulus occur at a subsequent level, a pre-attentive global processing sufficient for the extraction of meaning. Humphreys (1981) suggests that even when conscious identification of the stimulus has been blocked by a mask, higher order category information was available to the subjects. Employing the dichotic listening technique, Lewis (1970) found that unattended messages were processed at the semantic level. Using pictorial material, McCauley, Parmelee, Sperber, and Carr (1980) showed that meaning from pictures was extracted long before sufficient information for the conscious identification of them was accumulated. To further attest to the methodological finesse of the study, these investigators found no interaction between threshold levels and relatedness of the prime to the target. They note that "the relatedness effect at zero threshold was identical to that at full threshold, despite the greatly different probabilities of prime identification at those exposure durations in the threshold setting session" (McCauley et al., 1980, p. 269). Semantic processing without identification of the stimulus has been demonstrated by Groeger (1984) using a forced error task also.

Studies on word-superiority effect also provide support to the notion of semantic primacy. For example, Krueger (1970) found that a target letter could be recognized faster when it was embedded in a word rather than in a random letter string. Visual search experiments also show that search performance was enhanced when the target word to be detected differed from the ground in which it was embedded in terms of semantic category (Lawrence, 1971). The implication is that visual features (in tachistoscopic presentation) have quicker access to lexical storage than to featural aspects. This is accomplished by a pre-attentive process that will be "able to pick out portions of the input that are worth synthesizing and to arrive at preliminary identification of these portions" (Neisser, 1967, p. 195).

Extraction of meaning without accompanying consciousness has a reflex-like, or automatic quality, as seen in lexical decision experiments and the now well-known "Stroop effect" (Stroop, 1935). For example, Carr, Posner, Pollatsek, and Snyder (1979) found that word–nonword judgments were performed much faster than phonetic judgments. Just like the syntactic module (Chomsky, 1980), access to meaning also appears to function like a tightly wired in process. This kind of a pre-attentive semantic access might have provided sufficient evolutionary advantage to those members of the species who possessed such a faculty, because apprehending the meaning of a stimulus—such as, for example, a prey versus a predator—would have been a decision about survival itself. Such inferences are more often based on very scarce and degenerate information. The literature in cognitive and experimental psychology discussed previously attests to such a possibility.

Altman (1978) has developed a model of brain and cognition that is in many ways similar to the microgenetic model. While characterizing the triarchic levels of brain organization in cognition, Altman (1978) places affect and meaning at the level of "pathic mentation" where the organism has as outputs only binary choices like flight versus fight, affiliation versus dissociation, and so on, leading to equally polarized action patterns that typify the survival instinct. The microgenetic account of levels of awareness approximating the direction corresponding to forebrain evolution is also in agreement with Tulving's (1985) model of consciousness and memory. The "anoetic" (nonknowing) consciousness in Tulving's account corresponds to the procedural memory, which is pylogenetically an older form because it does not represent that which is not immediately present and in which sensation and action are locked in a single unit. In microgenetic theoretic terms, at this level, "there is no 'distance' between perception and action; both have an immediate, labile, or automatic quality" (Brown, 1977. pp. 15–16). This is similar to the sensory–motor intelligence, which Piaget (1961) places at the origin of all other higher forms of intelligence in ontogenetic development.

It is also worth mentioning in this context that the microgenetic conception of levels of processing and awareness makes a significant contribution in resolving the issues surrounding the imagery–perception equivalence debate (Farah, 1985, 1989; Kosslyn, 1987). The endogenous origin of cognition entails the primacy of categories and levels in the "exteriorization" of a percept or act. Thus, it account for the well-known similarity between visual imagery and visual perception—which has been a controversial topic in recent times in cognitive psychology. The microgenetic theory makes the equivalence between imagery and perception explicit when it postulates that "an image is a preparatory stage in the process leading to an object representation, and that the different types of images are manifestations of different levels of object representation" (Brown, 1985b, p. 90). On the representational similarity between visual imagery and perception, Farah (1989) observes that visual perception involves a series of representations and that imagery and perception share representations at multiple levels.

## Consciousness and Laterality

Before concluding this discussion, it may be pertinent to survey the role of conscious awareness in the microgenetic account of cognitive unfolding. In the microgenetic theory, consciousness has an emergent and developmental character, and consciousness is placed at the terminal end of the microgenetic continuum. In cognitive psychology, the Adaptive Control of Thought (ACT) model (Anderson, 1983) identifies consciousness with a temporary memory store referred to as *working memory,* which contains activated representations, active processing goals, and preexisting declarative knowledge structures activated by current inputs. Kihlstrom's (1987) definition of consciousness as the "experiential quality" that accompanies perceptual cognitive functions such as discriminative response to stimulation, perception, and other higher mental functions also suggests the emergent quality of consciousness. Degree or quality of consciousness varies with the level of microgenesis of a given mental function, and there is no sharp seperation between the contents of consciousness and consciousness itself.

According to the microgenetic theory, consciousness arises as a function of the elaboration of the featural processes in the left hemisphere of the brain. Consciousness and laterality have been studied by several investigators (e.g., Brown, 1977; Corballis, 1983; Eccles, 1979; Popper & Eccles, 1977). Eccles (1979) advocated the position that the left hemisphere is the seat of consciousness because of its capacity to mediate language. He argued that "the conscious self was liaison only with the dominant hemisphere" (p. 218). The dominance of the left hemisphere, Eccles reasoned, "derives from its verbal and ideational abilities and liaison to consciousness" (1979, p. 220). It is arguable whether we can deny consciousness to the right hemisphere on the grounds that it cannot process certain aspects of language and impute this capacity exclusively to the left hemisphere because of its unique capacity to process language. The decision to equate consciousness with left hemisphere processes now appears to be based on a metric rather than linguistic capability of the left hemisphere, as argued by Eccles (1979).

Bever (1980, 1983) presents a more plausible reason for considering the left hemisphere as the seat of consciousness. He argues that "the modern cognitive psychology now affords a theory of consciousness that satisfies the intuition that consciousness depends on relational processes. This motivates the prediction that the left hemisphere, the seat of relational activity is the usual seat of consciousness in normal people" (Bever, 1983. p. 20).

Libet's experimental demonstration of brain processes in conscious experience (Libet, 1965, 1987) and voluntary act (1985) further supports the microgenetic theoretic predictions concerning the temporal course in cognitive unfolding. A substantial amount of time—about 500 milliseconds—has been found to precede the conscious experience of a peripheral stimulation. In the case of volitional act, Libet (1985) found a readiness potential preceding the conscious intent to act by about 350 milliseconds. All these support the microgenetic contention that cognitive forms have an endogenous origin and that they approximate the object by the stage-wise constrainment by sensation.

Thus, ground has been cleared for ascertaining the material "reality" of consciousness and the role of the left cerebral hemisphere in its mediation. This leads to interesting "afterthoughts"—to borrow a metaphor from Harnad (1982). It appears now that consciousness is a by-product, a consequence, and free will, an illusion. Both Bever (1983) and Harnad (1982) provide provocative suggestions in this connection. According to Harnad (1982), consciousness is a "hind sight," a later outcome of a series of real-time neuronal processes. Bever (1983) captures the "afterthought" metaphor in his suggestion that the relational processes access the input and output of several modules of the mind and that a central mechanism determines the allocation of attentional resources to these modules. "The result of such decisions appears to be what we think of as consciousness. . . . In this sense, consciousness is an automatic consequence which resolves conflicting computational output of modules" (Bever, 1983, p. 33). According to Brown (1989), free will the agent oriented property associated with consciousness, then becomes an illusion that arises during the exteriorization of acts and percepts.

## Conclusion: Metatheoretic Implications of the Microgenetic Theory

One special feature of the microgenetic theory, not noted earlier, is the metatheoretic flavor inherent in its characterization of levels in microgenesis and its resemblance to the works of such theorists as Chomsky (1980), Piaget (1961, 1980), Marr (1978, 1980), and Marshall (1982). Microgenetic theory can lend itself to the elucidation of levels of theory construction as envisaged by Marr (1980), when he suggested that complex systems like a nervous system or a developing embryo can be studied and understood at several different levels. At the highest order of theory construction is the theory of computation (a theory of consciousness), and at the lowest level is the theory of mechanisms of implementation (a theory of neurophysiological or neurochemical processes of cells or cell assemblies). Marr's (1978, 1980) computational theory of vision exemplifies such a program. At the origin of vision is a primal sketch, which in Brown's microgenetic theory would constitute the primitive complex of affect and meaning access. In perceptual microgenesis, Brown posited three major levels: (1) the two-dimensional map of body space, (2) egocentric or viewer centered space, and (3) finally, three-dimensional object-centered space, corresponding to upper brain stem, limbic, and striate and prestriate brain mechanisms, respectively. The close parallel of this scheme to Marr's (1980) model is too obvious to require a further statement.

The argument that meaning is at the source of cognition is not new, but the significance of the microgenetic theory lies in making this concept at the core of its theoretical system. The close resemblance of the microgenetic theory with that of Piaget's and Chomsky's systems is also worth mentioning. Both Chomsky (1980) and Piaget (1980) agree on the primacy of meaning in cognition. Other structures like syntax or phonology may or may not share similarities with other cognitive domains, but implicit is the assumption that meaning is at the source of structure in any mental function—the semantic deep structure in Chomsky's (1980) system and the logical primitives in Piaget's (1961) system.

## *References*

Allen, K. (1983). Models of hemispheric specialization. *Psychological Bulletin*, *93*, 73–104.

Altman, J. (1978). Three levels of mentation and the hierarchic organization of the human brain. In E. Lenneberg & G.A. Miller (Eds.), *Psychology and biology of language and thought: Essays in honour of Eric Lenneberg* (pp. 87–109). New York: Academic Press.
Anderson, J.R. (1983). *The architecture of cognition*. Cambridge, MA: Harvard University Press.
Bever, T.G. (1980). Broca and Lashley were right: Cerebral dominance is an accident of growth. In D. Caplan & N. Chomsky (Eds.), *Biology and language*. Cambridge, MA: MIT Press.
Bever, T.G. (1983). Cerebral lateralization, cognitive asymmetry, and human consciousness. In E. Perecman (Ed.), *Cognitive processing in the right hemisphere* (pp. 19–39). New York: Academic Press.
Bradshaw, J.L., & Nettleton, N.C. (1983). *Human cerebral asymmetry*. Englewood Cliffs, NJ: Prentice-Hall.
Broadbent, D.M. (1958). *Perception and communication*. London: Pergamon.
Brown, J.W. (1977). *Mind, brain and consciousness*. New York: Academic Press.
Brown, J.W. (1983a). Rethinking the right hemisphere. In E. Perecman (Ed.), *Cognitive processing in the right hemisphere* (pp. 41–53). New York: Academic Press.
Brown, J.W. (1983b). The microstructure of perception: Physiology and patterns of breakdown. *Cognition and Brain Theory*, *6*, 145–184.
Brown, J.W. (1985a). Clinical evidence for the concept of levels in action and perception. *Journal of Neurolinguistics*, *1*, 79–87.
Brown, J.W. (1985b). Imagery and the microstructure of perception. *Journal of Neurolinguistics*, *1*, 89–141.
Brown, J.W. (1989). The nature of voluntary action. *Brain and Cognition*, *10*, 105–120.
Carr, T.H., Posner, M.I., Pollatsek, A., & Snyder, C.R.R. (1979). Orthography familiarity effects in word processing. *Journal of Experimental Psychology: General*, *108*, 389–414.
Chomsky, N. (1980). Cognitive structures and their development: A reply to Piaget. In M. Piattelli-Palmarini (Ed.), *Language and learning. The debate between Jean Piaget and Noam Chomsky* (pp. 35–52). London: Routledge & Kegan Paul.
Corballis, M.C. (1983). *Human laterality*. New York: Academic Press.
Corballis, M.C. (1989). Laterality and human evolution. *Psychological Review*, *96*, 492–505.
Cowan, N. (1988). Evolving conceptions of memory storage, selective attention and their mutual constraints within the human information processing system. *Psychological Bulletin*, *104*, 163–191.
Dixon, N.F. (1971). *Subliminal perception: The nature of a controversy*. London: McGraw-Hill.
Dixon, N.F. (1981). *Preconscious processing*. New York: John Wiley & Sons.
Eccles, J.C. (1979). *The understanding of the brain*. New York: McGraw-Hill.
Farah, M.J. (1985). Psychophysical evidence for a shared representational medium for mental images and percepts. *Journal of Experimental Psychology: General*, *114*, 91–103.
Farah, M.J. (1989). Mechanisms of imagery-perception interaction. *Journal of Experimental Psychology: Human Perception and Performance*, *15*, 203–211.

Fowler, C.A., Worford, G., Slader, R., & Tassinary, L. (1981). Lexical access with and without awareness. *Journal of Experimental Psychology: General, 110*, 341–362.

Groeger, J.A. (1984). Evidence of unconscious semantic processing from a forced error task. *Journal of Psychology, 75*, 305–314.

Harnad, S. (1982). Consciousness: An afterthought. *Cognition and Brain Theory, 5*, 29–47.

Harter, M.R., Aline, C., & Schroeder, C. (1982). Hemispheric differences in neural processing of stimulus location and type: Effects of selective attention on visual evoked potentials. *Neuropsychologia, 20*, 421–438.

Hellige, J.B., Cox, P.J., & Litvac, L. (1979). Information processing in the cerebral hemispheres: Selective hemisphere activation and capacity limitations. *Journal of Experimental Psychology: General, 108*, 251–279.

Hoffman, J.E. (1980). Interaction between global and local levels of a form. *Journal of Experimental Psychology: Human Perception and Performance, 6*, 222–234.

Holender, D. (1986). Semantic activation without conscious identification in dichotic listening, parafoveal vision, and visual masking: A survey and appraisal. *The Behavioral and Brain Sciences, 9*, 1–66.

Humphreys, G.W. (1981). Direct vs indirect tests of the information available from masked displays: What visual masking does and does not prevent. *British Journal of Psychology, 72*, 323–330.

Hunt, E., & Lansman, M. (1975). Cognitive theory applied to individual differences. In G.H. Bower (Ed.), *Handbook of learning and cognitive processes* (Vol. 1, pp. 81–110). Hillsdale, NJ: Lawrence Erlbaum.

Inhoff, A.W. (1982). Parafoveal perception: A further case against semantic preprocessing. *Journal of Experimental Psychology: Human Perception and Performance, 8*, 137–145.

Jones, B. (1982). The integrative action of the cerebral hemispheres. *Perception and Psychophysics, 32*, 423–433.

Kihlstrom, J.F. (1987). The cognitive unconscious. *Science, 237*, 1445–1452.

Konstandov, E.A., & Arzumanov, Y.L. (1986). The influence of subliminal emotional words on functional asymmetry. *International Journal of Psychophysiology, 4*, 143–147.

Kosslyn, S.M. (1987). Seeing and imagining in the cerebral hemispheres: A computational approach. *Psychological Review, 94*, 148–175.

Krueger, L. (1970). Visual comparison in a redundant display. *Cognitive Psychology, 1*, 341–357.

Kunst-Wilson, W.R., & Zajonc, R.B. (1980). Affective discrimination of stimuli that cannot be recognized. *Science, 207*, 557–558.

Lawrence, D.H. (1971). Two studies of visual search for word targets with controlled rates of presentation. *Perception and Psychophysics, 10*, 85–89.

Lewis, J.L. (1970). Semantic processing of unattended messages using dichotic listening. *Journal of Experimental psychology, 85*, 225–228.

Libet, B. (1965). Cortical activation in conscious and unconscious experience. *Perspectives in Biology and Medicine, 9*, 77–86.

Libet, B. (1985). Unconscious cerebral initiative and the role of conscious will in voluntary action. *The Behavioral and Brain Sciences, 8*, 529–560.

Libert, B. (1987). Consciousness: Conscious, subjective experience. In G. Adelman

(Ed.), *Encyclopedia of neurosciences* (Vol. 1, pp. 271–275). Boston: Birkhäuser.
Marcel, A.J. (1983). Conscious and unconscious reading: The effect of visual masking on word perception. *Cognitive Psychology, 15*, 177–238.
Marr, D. (1978). Representing and computing visual information. In P.H. Winston & R.H. Brown (Eds.), *Artificial intelligence: An MIT perspective* (pp. 17–80). Cambridge, MA: MIT Press.
Marr, D. (1980). Visual information processing: The structure and creation of visual representation. *Philosophical Transactions of the Royal Society of London, Series B, 290*, 199–218.
Marshall, J.C. (1982). Models of the mind in health and disease. In A.W. Ellis (Ed.), *Normality and pathology in cognitive functions* (pp. 1–18). New York: Academic Press.
Marzi, C.A., Stefano, M.D., Tassinary, G., & Crea, F. (1979). Iconic storage in the two hemispheres. *Journal of Experimental Psychology: Human Perception and Performance, 5*, 31–41.
McCarthy, G., & Donchin, E. (1978). Brain potentials associated with structural and functional visual matching. *Neuropsychologia, 16*, 571–585.
McCauley, C., Parmelee, C.M., Sperber, R.D., & Carr, H. (1980). Early extraction of meaning from pictures and its relation to conscious identification. *Journal of Experimental Psychology: Human Perception and Performance, 6*, 265–276.
Moscovitch, M. (1983). The linguistic and emotional functions of the normal right hemisphere. In E. Perecman (Ed.), *Cognitive processing in the right hemisphere* (pp. 57–82). New york: Academic Press.
Moscovitch, M., & Klein, D. (1980). Material specific interference for words and faces: Implications for models of capacity limitations, attention and laterality. *Journal of Experimental Psychology: Human Perception and Performance, 6*, 590–604.
Neisser, U. (1967). *Cognitive Psychology*. New York: Appleton-Century-Crofts.
Parasuraman, R., & Beatty, J. (1980). Brain events underlying detection and recognition of weak sensory signals. *Science, 210*, 80–83.
Piaget, J. (1961). *The psychology of intelligence*. London: Routledge & Kegan Paul.
Piaget, J. (1980). The psychogenesis of knowledge and its epistemological significance. In M. Piattelli-Palmarini (Ed.), *Language and learning. The debate between Jean Piaget and Noam Chomsky* (pp. 23–34). London: Routledge & Kegan Paul.
Popper, K.R., & Eccles, J.C. (1977). *The self and its brain.* New York: Springer-Verlag.
Ramachandran, V.S., & Anstis, S.M. (1986). The perception of apparent motion. *Scientific American, 254*, 102–109.
Ruggs, M.D., & Beaumont, J.G. (1978). Interhemispheric asymmetries in the visual evoked potential response: Effect of stimulus lateralization and task. *Biological Psychology, 6*, 283–292.
Schwartz, S., & Kirsner, K. (1982). Laterality effects in visual information processing: Hemispheric specialization or the orientation of attention. *Quarterly Journal of Experimental Psychology, 34A*, 61–77.
Seamon, J.G., Marsh, R.L., & Brody, N. (1984). Critical importance of exposure duration for affective discrimination of stimuli that are not recognized. *Journal of Experimental Psychology: Learning, Memory and Cognition, 10*, 465–469.

Sergent, J. (1982a). About face: Left-hemisphere involvement in processing physiognomies. *Journal of Experimental Psychology: Human Perception and Performance*, *8*, 1–14.
Sergent, J. (1982b). The cerebral balance of power: Confrontation or cooperation. *Journal of Experimental Psychology: Human Perception and Performance*, *8*, 253–272.
Sergent, J. (1983). The role of input in visual hemispheric asymmetries. *Psychological Bulletin*, *93*, 481–512.
Simion, F., Bagnara, S., Bisiacchi, P., Roncato, S., & Umilta, C. (1980). Laterality effects, levels of processing and stimulus properties. *Journal of Experimental Psychology: Human Perception and Performance*, *6*, 184–195.
Sperling, G. (1967). Successive approximations to a model for short term memory. *Acta Psychologica*, *27*, 285–292.
Stroop, J.R. (1935). Studies of interference in serial verbal reaction. *Journal of Experimental Psychology*, *18*, 643–661.
Treisman, A. (1964). Selective attention in man. *British Medical Bulletin*, *20*, 12–16.
Treisman, A. (1986). Features and objects in visual processing. *Scientific American*, *255*, 114–125.
Tulving, E. (1985). Memory and consciousness. *Canadian Psychology*, *26*, 1–12.

# 5
# Reflections on Perception and Action

Avraham Schweiger

Although action is traditionally distinguished from perception, it is generally recognized that the two are closely related, even in terms of their respective neuroanatomical substrates (e.g., Fuster, 1987). Despite this recognition, these two aspects of functioning in all organisms are often treated as separate. This separation is quite pervasive in many disciplines, most notably in psychology, where behaviorism held sway for many years with its "stimulus–response" distinction. Such a view permeates neuropsychology as well and is reinforced by the superficial dissociation between the two in brain-damaged patients. Thus we have "receptive" versus "expressive" aphasias, or transcortical "motor" versus transcortical "sensory" aphasias, even if the symptoms often overlap considerably. Even neuroanatomy seems to provide support for this dichotomy. For example, the division of the motor and sensory strips in the cortex, the distinction of the anterior from the posterior aspects of the spinal cord, carrying motor and sensory information, respectively, are just two of the many instances when neuroanatomy seems to provide the substrate for the action–perception dichotomy.

In this chapter I will attempt to outline the reasons for the apparent separation of action and perception and its functional role. Arguing for the unity of perception and action, I assume, much in the spirit of the "neurologized" microgenesis of Brown (e.g., 1987), that action (understood as a schema for potential movement, see following) and perception emerge from a unified underlying background, unfolding through neuronal substrates toward end products (the "figure"). This process is one of progressive specification, from diffused meaning (e.g., ongoing, functionally related processes, associated actions, perhaps affective material, etc., but all grossly underspecified), in which action and perception are not differentiated at all, to specific experience of either exteriorized, well-defined objects, and/or a sequence of coordinated output to motor systems resulting in purposeful action. This process, which occurs in a fraction of a second, is constrained throughout by environmental changes, which are experienced as well-defined objects *only at the end of the process*. In this framework, perception is bound up with and embodies action, in the sense that it develops out of acting on and manipulating objects early in the life of the organism (see following discussion). Likewise, action embodies perception, as it takes place in the context of perceived objects, body parts, and so on, and therefore it is also shaped by it. The two become distinct only at the late stages of the microgenetic process, probably associated closely with the functioning of the frontal lobes. This view of action–perception argues against the traditional view of perception as a passive process of registering "external information."

When an object is projected on the retina, rapid accommodative adjustments are made in the stimulated rods and cones, in terms of synthesis of pigments. So rapid is this adjustment that if the image is stabilized on the same retinal area, it will disappear in a matter of seconds (i.e., there is no more "stimulation"). This is just a case of habituation occurring universally in the nervous system. When such momentary "stimulations" are accompanied by assimilation into ongoing content of activity, so that unfolding waves from brain stem to cortex (described by Brown, 1983) incorporate them and are modified by them, the object will be perceived. In this microscopic scenario, then, the organism is not passively registering external information; rather, it constructs meaningful percepts with it. In this framework, it is impossible to separate "registration" of information from acting on it by the organism, because it is only the active reaction to environmental changes that results in the experience of external objects.

From a macroscopic perspective, to be emphasized here, action refers to the internal, abstract schema that precedes overt, large-scale motor output involving many muscle groups. However, whereas every overt movement is the result of realized action in the preceding sense, not every action is necessarily realized into overt movement. As will be discussed, action can be "aborted" before its realization into an actual motor sequence. The term *action* will be used here in the traditional, broad sense, which includes the actual motor output.

The notion that perception and action originate from the same cognitive structures is not new in psychology. It was Piaget who proposed that in the child, perception and action are not only unified but that perception of objects emerges out of action on them by the infant (Piaget, 1971). In fact, Piaget named the period spanning the first 2 years of life as the "sensory-motor" stage, to emphasize the adaptation of the infant to the environment through the combined effects of perception and action. More recently, Brown (e.g., 1987) elaborated this idea, as noted previously, casting perception and action in terms of the microgenetic approach and tracing their unfolding from a unified brain stem structures through neuronal substrates in the direction of phylogenetic and ontogenetic development to the cortex (cf. Brown, 1983). In this chapter, I will consider the issue of the uncoupling of action from perception in its psychological–functional and neuroanatomical context, while considering some data from brain-damaged patients. I propose here that during maturation, action becomes delayed, or inhibited, probably by frontal lobe systems, thereby allowing for symbolic consideration of consequences and alternatives. Therefore, the inhibition of action has an adaptive role by allowing abstract thinking (or "de-centering," as Piaget called the process by which a child can imagine objects and operate on them in their absence, i.e., purely in his/her "mind"), long-term planning, behaving socially to allow for communal life, and so on.

Considering the context of an organism adapting to its environment, it seems appropriate for action and perception to be unified. In this functionalist view, perceiving objects has an adaptive role: It is in the service of some action to satisfy a biological need. For example, the perception of a prey embodies in it the whole sequence of hunting and devouring it. In other words, the "meaning" of an object is in the actions associated with it, whether this object is food or something to avoid or chase. Of course, even this functional perception is constrained by biological and environmental parameters and is a result of interactions among them. It is only in humans (and perhaps to a very limited extent in some apes as well) that objects seem to be perceived apart from their associated action. In humans, perception developed and achieved an independent life of its own, culminating in the form of aesthetic experience: The appreciation of objects for their "beauty" alone, apart from any immediate survival function. (Even here, this experience involves more than merely the passive "registration" of an art object in the nervous system. In the process of accommodating to art objects, active participation is involved, as noted previously; see Brown, 1983.)

## Traditional Approaches to Perception

It is clear that purposeful action presupposes perception. The object, or context in which the action is to take place, must be perceived before, or at least together with, the planning and execution of an action. That is, in acting, the organism does so on something it perceives. But does perception likewise presuppose action? According to the traditional, 19th century psychological view, it does not. Thus, the role of perception through the senses is, in the Weberian–Fechnerian view (in Boring, 1950), to provide the organism with as veridical image of the environment as possible (be it visual, auditory, tactile, etc.). Consequently, perception is viewed as a passive act of registration: Transducing external energy into neuronal activity, which travels from sense organs to the appropriate analyzing centers in the cortex. In contrast, the studies of Piaget (see Piaget, 1971, for a summary) suggest that at the early stages of development, the infant develops what Piaget termed sensory-motor "schemata," or abstract cognitive representations of objects through his actions on them. Thus, through active manipulations of objects and the integration of all the associated experiences the infant has with objects (e.g., propioceptive, tactile, auditory, visual, gustatory, and olfactory), the abstract concept of well-defined objects emerges.

Much in the spirit of 19th century physiology, contemporary cognitive psychology strives to explore the nature of the mind's representation of the external world and the transformations it undergoes in the process from raw sensory data to a meaningful "picture" of the world. One of the main goals of this form of psychology is, then, to explain the algorithms used by the "mind" to "process" external stimuli in order to provide veridical "representation." In some sense, then, cognitive psychology admits to an active part of the brain en route from passive registration to meaningful representation, and therefore this whole endeavor is referred to as information "processing." This processing refers to presumed neuronal activities that correspond to the environmental stimuli (e.g., spoken or written language, lines representing objects, etc.) and that are shuttled from station to station in the brain and somehow analyzed, transformed, and perhaps matched against existing stored material, in order to provide the end product. The rules of such processing are said to be partially innate, as in the case of some linguistic processes (e.g., Chomsky, 1975) and partially learned through experience. It is noteworthy here that this contemporary view of perception embodies in it an internal action on the raw sensory data by the nervous system.

Unlike 19th century psychology, then, modern cognitive psychology no longer conceptualizes perception as the mere passive registration of objects out in the environment, although the first step in the perceptual process is still considered to be such registration by sense organs (e.g., Churchland, 1988). Despite this change from passive to active perception, however, cognitive psychologists have shown little concern for action as an integral part of perception, at least in the developmental stages of acquiring knowledge of the environment. Moreover, cognitive neuropsychology seems to pay little attention to either phylogenetic or ontogenetic processes and their roles in adult manifestations of brain functions and dysfunctions. This is understandable to some extent, given the problem of documenting developmental information in patients who present with brain damage as adults. On the other hand, perhaps a good part of the variations among individual symptomatologies, even when lesions are in homologous loci, can be accounted for by variations in individual developmental histories.

Fundamentally, the business of perceiving the world has changed little since the days of Laplacian determinism of 19th century physiology. Then and now, perception for the organism involves analyzing input from the environment to extract its true structure (objects) and meaning from it (is it food, danger, mate?), so that appropriate response can be made, if necessary.

Consider, as an example, a typical contemporary model of the process of reading (Ellis & Young, 1988; pp. 191–238). The process begins with visual analysis, followed by matching in the visual input lexicon, and from there, material goes to the "semantic system." This process incorporates all the traditional ingredients of perception: Written material (the stimulus) is first registered by the eyes and analyzed by identifying letters in words, encoding each letter for its position in the word (analyzing the units), then grouping those letters that belong together as part of the same word (putting the analyzed units together) (Ellis & Young, 1988, p. 224). The outcome of this perceptual analysis is then matched against existing storage of words (the so-called "visual input lexicon") to check if it is a real word and is finally sent to have meaning accessed and attached to it. Some arrows that point in the reverse direction are typically added to the model, for example, from the semantic system to the visual input lexicon and even back to the stage of visual analysis. These backward arrows are added to account, in an ad hoc fashion, for different symptoms exhibited by some patients with acquired dyslexia (Ellis & Young, 1988). Although these arrows are meant to add a "top-down" flavor to the process, they do nothing to change the general character of the process: Analyzing the units of the sensory input and putting them back together to come up with meaning.

The idea of top-down processing was necessitated by persistent phenomena indicating that what the organism perceives depends not merely on the physical energy reaching the sense organ as measured by the experimenter's instruments (known also as the proximal stimulus), but on myriad other factors, such as expectations, readiness, the context in which the stimulus is presented (including, e.g., the gender of the experimenter), to mention but a few examples. Thus, the whole concept of sensory sensitivity and threshold had to be modified eventually to incorporate the organism's bias to respond. This was done in the form of the signal detection theory and its receiver operating characteristics. All these modifications, however, left the basic perceptual process, as described previously, intact. Now material was being analyzed in the same passive way, except that some efferent activity was postulated which exerted some modifying influence on the process. A difficulty still remains here in accounting for the nature and control of the descending influence on the input, without resorting to some form of the homunculus problem: If, in the process of perceiving the environment veridically, some top-down influence causes modifications on the input, at times in a misleading way, who guides such descending influence, and to what purpose? If this is the way experience exerts its influence on perception, then without some purposeful control of this influence, can perception ever provide veridical information? And, if the purpose of perception is to provide a veridical picture of the world, what means are there for the organism to verify the output of the perceptual apparatus, at least at the earlier stages of development? It seems, then, that it is the very formulation of perception as a passive registration, divorced from some functional meaning for the organism and unrelated to action, that must be modified to circumvent these persistent problems.

## An Alternative View of Perception–Action

One approach to perception that avoids the problems mentioned previously is that offered by Piaget (e.g., 1971) and the microgenetic approach (e.g., Brown, 1977). These two approaches are complementary, the former approaching the problem from the phylogenetic–ontogenetic perspective; the latter, as its name suggests, analyzes the problem within a thin slice of time in the adult organism. The reader is referred to the numerous publications of J.W. Brown (e.g., 1977, 1983, 1987) for a detailed explanation of the microgenetic approach, which will not be discussed here extensively (see also Chapter 3 in this volume).

For Piaget (e.g., 1971), perception is a process of adaptation, and as such, its products reflect the characteristics of the organism, as much as those of the environment. Piaget studied cognitive development in children in great detail, noting that cognition emerges out of action the child performs on objects, as noted previously. This action can range from mouthing and sucking objects, to oculomotor accommodations, to manipulating objects in complex ways in one's thought, as is the case with solving logical problems. Piaget termed cognitive stages as the sensory-motor, preoperational, concrete, and formal operational stages, to underscore the active aspects of conceptual development. Every stage reflects different levels of acting, or operating on objects.

For the infant in the sensory-motor stage, then, there is simply no distinction between perception and action. The representations of objects are the outcome of adapting to them through action. As is the case in lower animals, for the infant, perceiving and "understanding" an object is acting on it. To the outside observer, for whom the object, say a feeding bottle, is an abstract concept and well-defined, it may seem that for the infant, seeing the bottle triggers sucking movements. Thus, imposing the adult's perspective on the infant, the wrong conclusion is arrived at: Perceiving the bottle precedes action on it. In effect, however, it is the assimilation of light patterns, corresponding to the bottle, into the schema of sucking which results in the perception of the bottle. In other words, the motor response here precedes the stimulus. It is through sucking that the object is recognized, that is, acquires meaning. Therefore, at a certain stage the infant overassimilates by sucking on any object put in his mouth. It is only with much experience (and disappointments) that the infant learns to inhibit sucking movements and save them only for appropriate objects.

At the preoperational stage (roughly between 2 and 7 years of age), action on objects becomes abstracted from them, in the sense that manipulating them becomes symbolized. The child no longer needs to perform the operations on the actual objects but on their symbolic representations (in the sense described above). This is also the stage when language becomes central to cognitive functioning. As noted earlier, language and thought become the arena for actions to take place, so they become uncoupled from immediate perception. One implication of Piaget's approach is that action is always embodied in the meaning of perceived objects; that is, in the nervous system, the "representation" of an object is bound up with associated actions, which form part of its meaning together with other characteristics (e.g., color, texture, form, etc.). Perhaps that is why aphasic patients can demonstrate the correct use of an object, while being unable to name it, or even to classify it into the correct category. In this sense, the operations on an object form an earlier layer in its meaning and tend to be spared following brain damage, when more recent layers (e.g., language) are impaired.

What follows from the preceding discussion is that cognitive psychology takes the end products of perception to be its "raw material," with which perceiving begins. In contrast, rather than conceiving of perception as beginning with the analysis of objects (visual or auditory) into their components, I propose here that the experience of well-defined objects is the achievement of the perceptual process, as opposed to being its input. This is also the view espoused by Werner (1948) and Brown (1983), and it is an extension of Piaget's approach to the ontogeny of perception and action. Whereas I referred to this view as an assumption, there is mounting evidence to support this approach (see the following discussion and, e.g., Brown, 1983, for a detailed discussion of this approach to perception).

Thus, for example, it has been shown that both normal subjects and brain-damaged patients can respond to the meaning of words that are not available to consciousness. For instance, Marcel (1983) has reported that normal subjects show semantic priming effects of words that they denied being aware of seeing. Likewise, Landis, Regard, and Serrat (1980) reported a patient with acquired dyslexia who could only read words in a letter-by-letter fashion. However, when this patient was shown words very rapidly so he could no longer read them letter by letter, he denied any knowledge of what the words were. But when asked to choose an object corresponding to the rapidly presented words from a multiple-choice array, even if he "did not know" what they were, the patient's performance exceeded chance levels of accuracy. Patients suffering from the syndrome known as deep dyslexia make semantic errors while reading words aloud. On the other hand, these patients cannot read individual letters, nor act on any phonological feature of words, and are said to access word meanings directly from the orthography (Ellis & Young, 1988). It seems, then, that deep dyslexic patients access meaning without having access to the more superficial (and, according to traditional processing order, before semantic) aspects of words, such as their phonology (see also Schweiger & Brown, 1988, for a discussion of this issue).

Returning to the example of reading, how can this process be characterized from the alternative perspective presented here? In the process of reading, the reader establishes a background of meaning, or a context, and continues to construct variations on this context through constraints of written text and internally imposed coherence simultaneously. Put differently, the words being scanned are perceived in terms of the established contextual meaning and the modification of it they impose. This is done by the complementary processes of assimilation (incorporating into existing structures) and accommodation (changing one's existing structures in accordance with environmental changes): Assimilating every new item and idea into existing context, while at the same time accommodating changes in the text by changing the context. Thus, when too many new words or new ideas are perceived in the text—that is, when the demand to accommodate exceeds the capacity of the reader to do so and assimilation is impossible (e.g., for lack of sufficient knowledge of the material being read)—the reader will not "understand" the text. Therefore, reading is not a process of assembling analyzed words together to come up with the correct meaning. Rather, it is a constructive process of creating a dynamic, internal state that is coherent and constrained moment to moment by created meaning of single words. The single word being evoked exerts its effect on the general meaning and dissipates into the next one, and so on. The subjective experience of this coherent meaning is one of understanding the text. That is why what remains in memory of reading a text is most often not the specific words but the meaning. In this sense, then, reading is not a passive process of registering material, but rather it requires active participation on the part of the reader.

## *Functional Considerations*

Given the close association between action and perception in animals and in human development, the following questions arise: (1) How can we conceptualize the apparent dichotomy between perception and action to the point of the emergence of aesthetic experience in adult humans? (2) What functions does this dichotomy serve? (3) What are the neuroanatomical substrates of this dichotomy, such that brain damage can impair it, resulting in disturbances of perception–action separation?

Considering the first question above from a phylogenetic perspective, we note that the evolution of nervous systems of species is marked, inter alia, by an increased period of development of the offsprings. This increased maturation period allows for learning of increasingly complex behaviors for adjusting to a larger range of environmental conditions. In other words, the delay of commitment to a given environment with specific, genetically determined patterns of behaviors allows an individual organism of a species to adapt to a larger range of environmental conditions (see Goldberg, 1987, for a review of evidence and a more detailed discussion of this issue).

Prolonging the period during which the nervous system is malleable to changes in response to external conditions or postponing the "critical period" improves adaptation and, thus, survivability.

Another characteristic that seems to emerge with the appearance of cortex, most highly elaborated in homo sapiens, is the delay of commitment to action. Although monkeys and, to a lesser extent, other animals such as pigeons (Grosch & Neuringer, 1981) are also capable of delaying motor response in some situations, entertaining consequences of and alternatives to one's actions before acting is characteristically human. Planning is a familiar form of the consideration of actions, sequencing them in the service of a goal, and so on. The use of symbols in general is also part of a general ability for abstraction—the distancing of behavior from the immediate action and perception of the present context. Indeed, I propose, extending Piaget's concept of cognition as an operation on objects in symbolic form, that thought processes, such as reflection and imagery, are precisely the delay of commitment to action, the content of which are the abstract, symbolic consideration of stimuli, actions, consequences and alternatives. From here, the road to a separation of perception and action is short: As the delay of acting increases, from minutes to hours, days, and longer, perception appears to take on a life of its own, divorced from the associated action.

With regard to the second point, the adaptive role of separating action from perception is far-reaching, and perhaps is best illustrated by some examples:

1. As noted previously, delayed action opens the road for considering alternatives and reflecting on the consequences of an action before its execution. This delay is essential for social functioning, when the individual must consider the consequences of his actions on others and avoid acting impulsively. In fact, impulsivity in action may be tolerated in young children, whose frontal lobes may still be undergoing myelinization, but is considered pathological in adults. Recent evidence indicates that children, who at a young age (around 4) delayed gratification longer in experimental situations developed into more cognitively and socially competent adolescents who achieved higher scholastic performance and were coping better with frustration and stress (Mischel, Shoda, & Rodriguez, 1989). This kind of evidence supports the notion of delayed action as being adaptive, by demonstrating the correlation between the capacity for delayed behavior in childhood and future academic and social success.

2. The ability to plan ahead and project actions into the future are necessary for the making of a civilization. Any intellectual act suggests the consideration of options in the abstract, that is, removed from their concrete context. Algebra is an example of such abstraction. Architectural construction, written language, and the arts all involve abstraction.

3. Overcoming fear—the urge to respond to an immediately perceived threat by some adaptive action (e.g., avoidance, flight, fight)—allows for

exploration of new possibilities. Here again, the essential element is the capacity to consider consequences beyond the immediate context, to consider alternative and long-term payoffs.

I turn now to the third question, concerning the neuroanatomical substrates of uncoupling action from perception. From the foregoing discussion, it may seem clear that the neuroanatomical structures traditionally associated with delayed action, planning, sequencing, and so on are those of the frontal lobes (e.g., Stuss & Benson, 1986, 1990). Moreover, damage to these anatomical areas results in a variety of symptoms characterized in terms of perseveration, disinhibition, loss of initiation (perhaps overinhibition), loss of abstract thinking, "stimulus boundedness," deficits in delayed responses, inappropriate social behavior and so on (see Brown, 1985, for a review). To a large extent, then, these symptoms involve the inability of the brain-damaged patient to inhibit a motor response that is associated with certain objects or situations but is inappropriate in the present context (Brown, 1985; Lhermitte, 1986).

One intriguing proposal, attempting to relate these "frontal lobes" symptoms to specific anatomical structures, was formulated by G. Goldberg (e.g., 1987). In his proposal, Goldberg postulates two motor systems in the frontal lobes. One is localized in the medial premotor areas (including the supplementary motor area) and is involved in forward-directed behaviors, independent of immediate context and based on planning. The other system, located at the lateral premotor areas of the frontal lobes, is involved in stimulus-bound activity and thus is responsive to environmental stimuli. According to Goldberg, lesions in either system result in specific, characteristic deficits, this being similar to Luria's two pathophysiological syndromes in patients with frontal lobe lesions (Goldberg, 1987; Luria, 1980). Thus, what emerges from all reviews, or theories, of frontal lobe functioning is the unifying theme of their involvement in the inhibition of output in one form or another. Moreover, a lesion to either frontal lobe does not typically impair either perception or action per se (Luria, 1980). I suggest it impairs the relationship between them, owing to the special role of the frontal lobes in the uncoupling of action from perception across different modalities. In addition, recall that abstract thinking is intimately related to the removal of overt action from immediate perception. As might be predicted from the foregoing, frontal lobe damage often impairs abstract skills.

From the preceding discussion, it is not clear how frontal lobe inhibition can be described in terms of microgenesis. The direction of frontal lobe influence seems to be the reverse of that proposed by Brown (1983), that is, "down" from cortex toward the brain stem. According to Brown's approach, however, perception and action traverse the frontal lobe structures on the way to primary cortical areas of sensory and motor functions (Brown, 1987). If this is the case, then the frontal lobes are in a strategic position en route to the final specification of objects in perception and the realization of action schemata into movement. In this position, the functioning of the frontal lobes may be exerted at the stage of perceptual specification when action associated with a percept is prevented from being realized into motor output. That is, the frontal lobes may serve as filters, suppressing action during the unfolding of perception, when this is called for functionally. Damage to the frontal lobes exposes the stage at which these lobes function in the unfolding process, namely, that of separating action from perception. The impairment results in the reemergence of the action–perception unity, which in the adult organism is regarded as pathological. Thus, the appearance of the grasp reflex in an adult may herald frontal lobe pathology, the impairment being in the separation and inhibition of grasping from tactile stimulation, both being unified in early ontogeny and microgeny.

Perseveration is another case in point; motor output associated with one context outlasts the context and becomes inappropriate. Patients with frontal lobe damage, for example, will perseverate on a task because the established context for one response compels them to continue that response even in the face of changed context. For example, if the patient is asked to write alternating *m* and *n*, he is likely to repeat the same letter twice in the absence of the suppressing influence of the frontal lobes. Once the context of writing n is established, normally functioning frontal lobes are needed to inhibit the repeated motor expression of this context. In short, contextually appropriate modulation of the realization of objects-related action requires intact frontal lobes.

It is noteworthy here that neuroanatomical studies demonstrate that the frontal lobes not only are late to develop during embryonic growth but also continue to myelinate possibly into the third decade of life (reviewed in Spreen, Tupper, Risser, Tuokko, & Edgell, 1984). Indeed, perseveration can be observed in young children in the early part of the preoperational stage. As suggested previously, it is a characteristic of late stages in cognitive development that abstract, symbolic thinking appears, with its reliance on delayed action and the ability to consider alternatives, consequences, and so on. Thus, there is additional evidence, from normal neuroanatomical development, supporting the role of the frontal lobes in the separation of action and perception.

## Conclusion

In this chapter, I presented a rather speculative discussion of perception–action relations in humans. The emphasis in this chapter was on the macroscopic level of ontogeny, which sets the stage for the adult functioning described, on the microscopic level, by the microgenetic approach. Many aspects of the relationship between ontogeny and microgenesis have not been worked out yet. For example, it is not clear through what mechanism specific interactions of the developing child with the environment establish the stability of perceived objects in the adult. In other words, it is necessary to spell out specifically the effects of early experience on microgenetic processes. This will help in identifying the effects of variations in ontogeny on individual differences in the manifestation of brain damage alluded to previously.

It is not enough just to say that the frontal lobes inhibit action. It is important to specify how such inhibition is guided. It was briefly noted here that such inhibition is functionally determined. This is not sufficient, as it delegates the problem to some teleological mechanism that is not specified. It does, however, set the requirement for such a mechanism to be a result of an adaptive process, rather than being some innate module, emerging out of chance mutation.

Although relatively little has been said in this chapter about the microgenetic approach, it is quite compatible with the view presented here. For example, in Brown's view (e.g., 1983), the experience of an object outside in the environment is the result of the unfolding of diffused meaning into a well-defined, exteriorized object. This process takes place, presumably, by neuronal activation traversing cerebral tissue from brain-stem structure to cortex. According to Brown, the exteriorized objects embody prior processes in them, such that brain damage at a particular level exposes the stage of the unfolding perception at the damaged level. During normal processes, these early stages are submerged in the final percept or action. This microgenetic view is echoed in the assertion, made in this chapter, that associated actions are embodied in perceived objects. The only difference is that Brown's approach focuses on the microgenetic level of object formation in perception, whereas in this chapter, the emphasis was on the ontogenetic level: the developmental aspects of action–perception relations.

The present focus on the uncoupling of action from perception leaves many unanswered questions. For instance, the issue of motor disorders and their relations to perception needs exploration within the framework presented here. Problems of apraxia, especially ideation apraxia, suggest that symbolic action on objects can be impaired while the perception of the objects remains intact, and occasionally, even naming of these objects is normal. I have studied an unpublished case of a patient with unilateral, upper extremity idiopathic dystonia, who presented with bilateral and bucofacial apraxia. The patient's cognitive and language skills were all intact. The picture presented by such patients suggests that concrete action may be realized into motor output devoid of earlier associated meaning. That is, unguided by contextual meaning, such as the one associated with the use of an object, the motor output reflects this absence by not being purposeful. But if all other cognitive skills are intact, why should such elementary meanings be absent? What is the role of the cerebellum in the schema of action presented here? How does the present view apply to language comprehension and production? Such questions and many more remain to be worked out, hopefully in a coherent framework that includes the whole range of cognition, as initiated by the microgenetic approach.

I will make one last point concerning aesthetic experience as it relates to the present chapter: Perceiving art objects requires active participation from the perceiver. It is such participation that results in the aesthetic experience being rewarding or frustrating. It is rewarding when the assimilation and accommodation demanded are balanced for a particular observer, in the sense that the observer has sufficient experience with related art objects, understanding of their context, and so on, while providing some novelty. To the uninitiated observer, an art object will require excessive accommodation with little assimilation, causing either frustration, boredom, or both.

## *References*

Baddeley, A. (1986). *Working memory*. Oxford, UK: Oxford University Press.

Boring, E.G. (1950). *The history of experimental psychology*. New York: Appleton-century-crofts.

Brown, J.W. (1977). *Mind, brain and consciousness*. New York: Academic Press.

Brown, J.W. (1983). The microstructure of perception: Physiology and patterns of breakdown. *Cognition and brain theory*, *6*(2), 145–184.

Brown, J.W. (1985). Frontal lobes and the microgenesis of action. *Journal of Neurolinguistics*, *1*(1), 31–77.

Brown, J.W. (1987). The microstructure of Action. In E. Perecman (Ed.), *The frontal lobes revisited*. New York: IRBN Press.

Chomsky, N. (1975). *Reflection on language*. New York: Pantheon Books.

Churchland, P.M. (1988). *Matter and consciousness* (Rev. Ed.). Cambridge, MA: M.I.T Press.

Ellis, A.W., & Young, A.W. (1988). *Human cognitive neuropsychology*. Hove, England: Lawrence Erlbaum.

Fuster, J.M. (1987). Single-unit studies of the prefrontal cortex. In E. Perecman (Ed.), *The frontal lobes revisited*. New York: IRBN Press.

Goldberg, G. (1987). From intent to action: Evolution and function of the premotor systems of the frontal lobes. In E. Perecman (Ed.), *The frontal lobes revisited*. New York: IRBN Press.

Grosch, J., & Neuringer, A. (1981). Self-control in pigeons under the Mischel paradigm. *Journal of Experimental Analysis of Behavior*, *35*, 3–21.

Landis, T., Regard, M., & Serrat, A. (1980). Iconic reading in a case of alexia without agraphia caused by a brain tumour: A tachistoscopic study. *Brain and Language*, *11*, 45–53.

Lhermitte, F. (1986). Human autonomy and the frontal lobes. Part II. Patient behavior in ocmplex and social situations: The "Environmental Dependency Syndrome." *Annals of Neurology*, *19*, 335–343.

Luria, A.R. (1980). *Higher cortical functions in man* (2nd ed.). New York: Basic Books.

Marcel, T. (1983). Conscious and unconscious perception. *Cognitive Psychology*, *15*, 197–237.
Mischel, W., Shoda, Y., & Rodriguez, M.L. (1989). Delay of gratification in children. *Science*, *244*, 933–938.
Piaget, J. (1971). *Biology and knowledge*. Chicago, IL: University of Chicago Press.
Schweiger, A., & Brown, J.W. (1988). Minds, models and modules. *Aphasiology*, *2*(6), 531–543.
Spreen, O., Tupper, D., Risser, A., Tuokko, H., & Edgell, D. (1984). *Human developmental neuropsychology*.
Stuss, D.T., & Benson, D.F. (1986). *The frontal lobes*. New York: Raven Press.
Stuss, D.T., & Benson, D.F. (1990). The frontal lobes and language. In E. Goldberg (Ed.), *Contemporary neuropsychology and the legacy of Luria*. Hillsdale, NJ: Lawrence Erlbaum.
Werner, H. (1948). *Comparative psychology of mental development* (2nd ed.) Chicago: Follett.

# 6
# Microgenesis: A Genesis From Prototheory to Neuropsychology

JOHN A. CEGALIS

## What Is the Nature of Perceptual Change in Microgenesis?

### *Stages of Microgenesis*

A primary question for any microgenetic theory is the question of the nature of nonimmediate changes in the percept over time. A second question is how to characterize, depict, or describe such changes. Most microgeneticists have used the construct of stages to describe qualitative changes in percept development. As Draguns (1984) pointed out, the construct of stage is both useful and problematic. The construct of stages provides a sense of orderliness, descriptive clarity, of conservation if you will, for our understanding of the nature of change. Yet the concept of stage may also blind us to subtler characteristics of processes that are subsumed in the coarser distinctions characterizing a stage.

Stages, in the least precise sense, are convenient descriptors of qualitative experiential changes at different points along a temporal continuum of percept construction. In a more precise sense, stages are descriptors of quantitative and qualitative changes that correspond to structural and, of significance to this volume, neurophysiological, neuroanatomical, and neuropsychological processes that result in transformations of perceptual content.

Unfortunately, many formulations of microgenetic changes have been vague, providing only generic descriptions of experiential changes in percepts over time. Graumann (1959), for example, distinguished changes that occur in four phases of one form of microgenetic development: (1) initial percept configurations are distorted in the direction of *Pragnantz*; (2) confusion with attention to details lacking integration into a meaningful whole; (3) partial integration of detail prevailing over attention to detail; (4) final perceptual configurations enabling recognition or reconstruction and the subjective feeling that the response fits the stimulus. Such descriptions are clearly pretheoretical rather than scientifically definitive of a stable phenomenon. To make matters worse, characteristics of stages may vary when microgenesis is studied by means of *merogenetic* as opposed to *hologenetic* methods.

Kragh and Smith (1970) devised an interesting schematic of stages of microgenesis. The model is summarized in Figure 6.1. In this model, preparatory phases (P-phases) result from successive stimulus presentations. Each P-phase is reconstructed in phenomenal representations, ultimately resulting in a final construction phase (C-phase) of the stimulus.

This model admirably incorporates assumptions about percept development in the context of the microgenetic experiment and the phenomenological method used to study this development. The model coincidentally provides a compelling analogue to microgenetic processes occurring in everyday experience—perceptual clarity and meaning may occur after a succession of exposures to a given situation.

Haber (1969) stated that while microgenetic theorists speak of stages, "they usually imply continuous processes of growth rather than qualitatively different operations being performed on the percept" (p. 3). Similarly, Brown (1977, 1988) postulated a process of continuous growth in the perceptual process. These positions do not accurately represent either the diversity of opinion among students of microgenesis or the results of several experimental efforts. Sander (1930), for example, stated that "emergent perceptual constructs are not imperfect versions of a final perception, but are characteristic metamorphoses with qualitative individuality, *Vorgestalten* (preformulations) due to structural causes not to constellation of stimuli." Certainly, Sander's use of the term *structural causes* refers in some sense to neuropsychological structures. Smith (1957), in elaborating preparatory and final stages of perception, contrasted an early mobilization of the organic (neuropsychological) system for multiprobable events and a later conformity of the percept to logic and to stimulus characteristics. Graumann (1959) described the process of unfolding of percepts, from nondifferentiation through certain stable structures, to complete integration, as a series of phases that do not proceed continuously or summatively, but often in a saltatory, discontinuous manner. He further reiterated Sander's contention that there may be two kinds of microgenesis: (1) a procession from undifferentiated wholes, to greater emphasis of detail, to integration of this detail and (2) from apprehension of details, to the apprehension of wholes, to changes within wholes. Linschoten (1959) contended that microgenetic processes take place in a saltatory and discontinuous fashion, leading toward a differentiated structuredness that depends on the stimulus.

Microgeneticists have been clear that there is no single form of percept development. The distinction between *merogenesis* and *hologenesis*, as a case in point, highlights the differences in the development of detail perception as opposed to the development of perceptual objects. A more accurate characterization based on experimental results is that microgenesis is

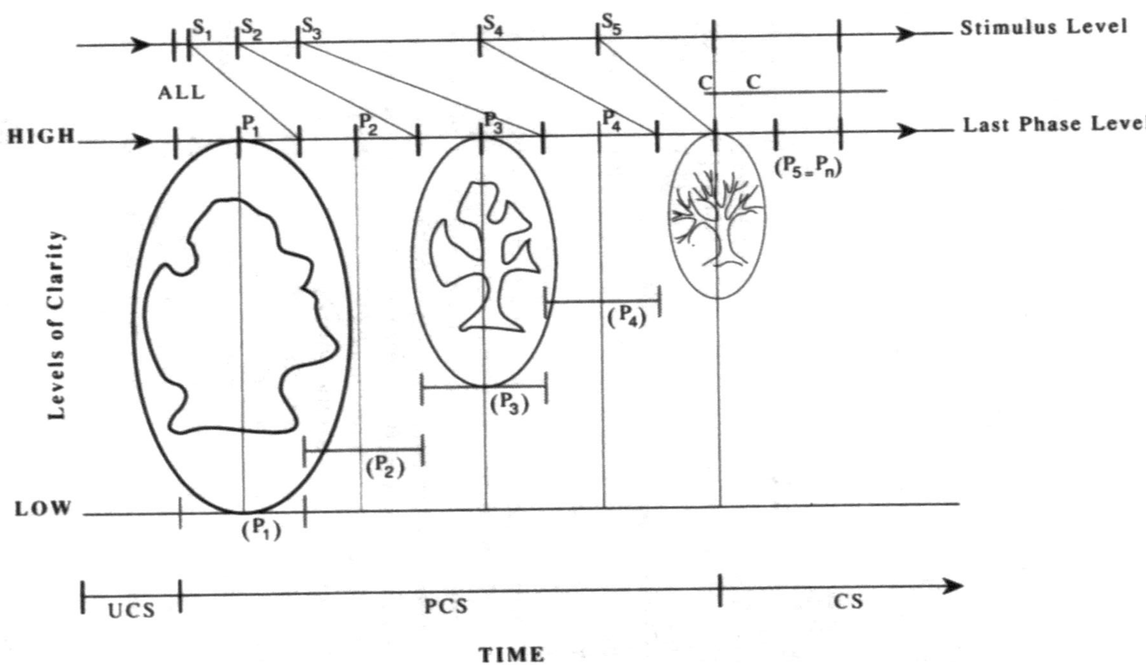


FIGURE 6.1. Schematic presentation of the microgenetic process in vivo preparatory (P) to construction (C) phases ($P_1 \ldots C$), as experimentally induced percept phase [($P_1$) . . ($P_N$)] by stimuli varying in duration ($S_1$–$S_5$) yielding increasing levels of perceptual clarity. The in vivo range of experience from absolute threshold (unconscious), to preconscious levels, to conscious levels of awareness. Note that it is assumed that experimental stimuli at successive levels result in experiences that are analogous to in vivo microgenetic processes with some (P) error attributed to overlap of succession P phase. (From "Transformations of Meanings During the Development of a Percept" in *Percept-Genetic Analysis* [p. 26] by U. Kragh and G.J.W. Smith, 1970, Lund: Gleerup. Copyright 1970 by Gleerup. Adapted by permission.)

a continuous developmental process of perception and thinking whose changes and forms of continuity may assume a variety of forms. The notion that certain percepts are the result of an abortion of the microgenetic sequence (Kantor & Herron, 1965) is a notorious example of problems resulting from assumptions about continuity and discontinuity in microgenesis. One definition of abortion in microgenesis is that a microgenetic process is truncated, such that content from earlier stages emerges into behavior or conscious experience, content that would otherwise undergo further microgenetic evolution toward a completed and integrated percept. Brown's recent (1988) microgenetic theory makes extensive use of the concept of abortion in his explanations of pathology. While the construct of microgenetic abortion is unnecessary to microgenetic theory, it can be used to partially explain autistic and other forms of psychopathological or neuropathological perceptual phenomena. Autistic logic, neologisms, "slips of the tongue," clang associations, for example, might be interpreted as examples of microgenetic abortions of discrete neuropsychological processes. On the other hand, microgenetic abortion may be an example of the effect of conflict or drive in microgenesis. Whereas neurological deficits may result in abnormal perceptgenesis, abnormal self-reports may result from pathological motivations or personality processes affecting the microdevelopment of meaning idiosyncratically through an intact structural medium. The explanatory power of this concept, then, comes at the expense of theoretical ambiguity.

Perhaps the most clear descriptive summary of the experience of microgenesis at different stages was provided by Flavell and Draguns. Their description is presented both because it characterizes the quality of early microgenetic work and because it provides a description of the phenomenon of microgenesis and descriptors of change that can be modeled by means of more sophisticated processing primitives and explicit algorithms allowing for scientific analysis.

> When a perceptual stimulus is presented under conditions of gradually increasing clarity, the initial perception is that of a diffuse, undifferentiated whole. In the next stage, figure and ground achieve some measure of differentiation, although the inner contents of the stimulus remain vague and amorphous. Then comes a phase in which contour and inner content achieve some distinctness and a tentative, labile configuration results. Finally, the process of Gestalt formation becomes complete with the addition of elaborations and modifications of the "skeletal Gestalt" (*Gestaltgerust*) achieved in the previous stage. (Flavell & Draguns, 1957, p. 198)

For our later analysis, Linschoten (1959) made several noteworthy remarks that may help to clarify Flavell and Draguns' exposition of microgenesis and the development of new experimental methodology for the study of neuropsychology. Linschoten essentially qualified the meaning of microgenesis, indicating the following: (1) Perception is not extended in microgenesis, rather, recognition is extended. (2) Recognition tends toward object-adequate structuring, whereas perception tends toward equilibrium or toward an optimal quality of configuration. (3) There is a competition between tendencies toward good form and a tendency toward recognition of the object. (4) In the preconfiguration stage, the *Vorgestalt* stage, perceptual tendencies prevail over recognition tendencies. (5) Not all perceptual processes are microgenetic. This important distinction essentially suggests a bifurcation in the perceptual process, a bifurcation that may be grossly described as one of figural representation and of meaning.

In this vein, Kreitler and Kreitler (1984) proposed that perception is a process of "meaning assignment." Clearly, this approach is consistent with the distinction between perception and recognition discussed by Linschoten (1959). In their study of perceptual microgenesis, Kreitler and Kreitler presented visual stimuli hologenetically. Subjects were asked to provide verbal descriptions of their perceptions after successive stimulus presentations; stimuli were degraded by varying exposure time, projection aperture, and focus. Verbal descriptions were then subjected to a detailed analysis of verbal meaning. The key constructs in this theory are *meaning value, meaning dimension, and referent*. Meaning value was defined as stimulus contents expressed verbally or through reconstructions, for example, "It looks bright." Meaning dimensions referred to general aspects of contents or the set of references to inputs, such as, sensory quality. Referents were said to denote any input differing in complexity, reality, and form. In this theory, the meaning of a given percept develops microgenetically in three stages. In the first stage of microgenesis, meaning values are assigned from among three meaning dimensions: sensory qualities (e.g., brightness), location (e.g., up, down), and quantity. Also, referents to these meaning values emerge, culminating in the attribution of a label. In the second phase, progressive differentiation of meaning values emerges from the referent label. Moreover, the referent becomes "particularized." In the third phase, the differentiation of meaning values is said to continue along the lines of a specific meaning dimension. The model, then, describes a hierarchy of meaning values branching along dimensions of meaning with a corresponding hierarchy of increasingly specific referents.

Froehlich (1984) has investigated several neurophysiological parameters of microgenesis. Their studies of the orienting reflex (OR) and of visual-evoked potentials (VEP) suggest that parallel physiological state changes appear to correspond to stages of microgenesis as reported in studies using traditional phenomenological whole-report techniques. In Froehlich's view, the OR creates an initial state of readiness for information processing. Later changes in OR and especially in VEP (habituation followed by activation) appear to represent changes to more complex stages of readiness.

Microgenetic theory and research have yielded a variety of hypotheses about the nature of changes that occur at proposed stages in the microgenetic evolution of a percept. The following summarizes several descriptive propositions characterizing discrete changes within stages of microgenesis:

1. Stages (or phases) of microgenetic perceptual development are described as qualitatively and quantitatively different at different microtime intervals (between absolute and differential thresholds) in terms of percept content, affective participation, and structural properties.
2. Microgenetic processes may vary in their directionality and in their end products. Percepts may be aborted in the course of microtime development, and the aborted products of this truncated development may emerge in consciousness or behavior.
3. Microgenesis, as a description of stimulus indeterminacies or stimulus representation, must be understood in terms of (1) the effect and contribution of past experience and (2) the context of personality structure and function.
4. The general quality of perceptual experience can be characterized as a progression from distorted and nonveridical to less distorted and more veridical.
5. Subjective experience can be characterized as proceeding from confusion to organized meaning and understanding.
6. Percept quality can be described as progressing from less clear to more clear.
7. Changes in the sense of subjective control over perception can be described as proceeding from alienation (egodystonic or dissociative) to percepts identified with a sense of belonging to the self, that is, nondissociated and self-controlled.
8. The affective experience accompanying early as opposed to later stages of perception can be characterized as a change from unpleasant high arousal to pleasant lower arousal.
9. The meaning of a percept and its verbalized referent can be said to undergo progressive differentiation and specification. When meaning is defined as verbal representation, the phenomenon of microgenesis can be quantified and given a rudimentary structural definition.

The stage descriptors provided by microgenetic theorists do not characterize microperceptual development in a manner accepted by many contemporary psychologists. Missing is a familiar sequence of stages crudely summarized as a process beginning with (1) a stored structural description of stimulus characteristics; (2) a later semantic representation of the structural memory; (3) a more distal phonological representation of the semantic representation. Rather, microgeneticists have typically been concerned with changes in the content of representations, especially as represented in whole-reports. In this connection, Catan's (1986) criticism of the use of microgenesis as a theory as opposed to microgenesis as a context for theory building is pertinent. Given that the results of some studies of microgenesis do not yield observations consistent with expected stages of microgenesis (e.g., Lastowski, 1976), the nature of changes becomes an open question. It is appropriate in this regard to view microgenetic techniques, stimulus-protracting techniques in Smith's (1983) words, as appropriate for discovering a stable phenomenon one might term *microgenesis*. In this sense, microgenesis is a testable assumption rather than a theory.

The prototheoretical quality of these stage descriptors is of a fundamentally different quality from the epistemic and logicomathematical stages described by Piaget (1957) in his ontogenetic theory of cognitive development. In contrast, an essential ingredient missing in theories of microgenetic development is the derivation of underlying structures characteristic of each proposed stage of microgenesis. Piaget's (1969) hypothesized isomorphism between the structures of perception and cognition can serve as one kind of model for future microgenetic research in the sense that theoretical and empirical confirmation of microgenetic constructs may strive to develop and test operations or heuristics that, when considered as a specific matrix at a given point in the temporal continuum, define qualitatively and quantitatively the nature of the transformations of a percept. The preliminary work of the Kreitlers (1984) and of Andersson (1984) are approaches to such a Piagetian model.

An important and an influential effort to describe early stages of visual perceptual information processing has been made by Marr (1982). After careful reassessment of the state of vision research and a painstaking analysis of the necessary assumptions for a theory of vision, Marr derived a five-state model that describes stages of perceptual development. These early stages of information processing are important enough to restate in Table 6.1, because they bear a remarkable similarity to the stages summarized by Flavell and Draguns (1957) and represent a remarkable contribution toward establishing the kind of structures, and operations comprising structures, demanded of any precise theory of development.

Marr (1982) assumed a metatheoretical purpose for vision—to derive a representation of shape. He specified the purpose of each stage, and of greatest significance, the mechanisms (primitives) critical to the development of each stage. Each stage in the proposed process requires a transformational mapping from one genre of representation to another. The significance of primitives at each stage is clear for the process of theory testing: A theory must provide testable primitives that are defined by specifying the precise mechanism that is required for a result rather than specifying that the mechanism is "like the process."

From this brief discussion of stages in microgenesis, it should be clear that there is no simple answer to the question. What is the nature of changes that occur in microgenesis? However, there is a recognition that the microdevelopment of perception must be studied at two general levels. First, visual perceptual representation undergoes microdevelopment, and indeed, the features of this process can be modeled and the constructs and

TABLE 6.1. A representation of Marr's (1982) theory of early visual information processing.[a]

| Representation | Purpose | Primitives |
|---|---|---|
| Image(s) | To represent intensity | Intensity value at each point in the image |
| Primal sketch | To provide information about the two-dimensional image, especially intensity changes and their geometrical distribution and organization | Zero-crossings<br>Blobs<br>Terminations and discontinuities<br>Edge segments<br>Virtual lines<br>Groups<br>Curvilinear organization<br>Boundaries |
| Two-dimensional sketch | To provide information about the orientation and rough depth of visible surfaces and contours of discontinuities in these quantities in a viewer-centered coordinate frame | Local surface orientation (the "needles" primitives)<br>Distance from the viewer<br>Discontinuities in depth<br>Discontinuities in surface orientation |
| Three-dimensional model representation | To describe shapes and their spatial organization in an object-centered coordinate frame, using modular hierarchical representation including volumetric primitives | Three-dimensional models arranged hierarchically, one based on a spatial configuration of a few sticks or axes, to which volume or surface-shaped primitives are attached |

[a] Including levels of stage representation, the purpose of each stage, and corresponding primitives used to derive each stage.

*Note.* Representational frame for deriving shape information from images. (From *Vision* [p. 37] by D. Marr, 1982, New York: W.H. Freeman. Copyright 1982 by W.H. Freeman. Adapted by permission.)

algorithms tested by computer simulation. However, given that the results of microgenetic research suggest several forms of geneses, we must be careful to temper our optimism for computer simulation and testing approaches to understanding the microgenesis of visual perception. Second, the meaning of visual perceptual representations appear to evolve microgenetically. Although meaning has been predominantly studied through analyses of verbal processes, the nature of "meaning" is sufficiently ubiquitous to require the investigation of other forms of meaning as well, for example, Westcott's (1967) analysis of intuition. Less clear, although nonetheless important, are parallel response processes, that is, affective and action schemata that also undergo temporal microdevelopment. The nature of the neuropsychological interface among these four processes and of the temporal synchrony or asynchrony in their respective microgeneses is, of course, a matter of intense contemporary theoretical and experimental effort.

## How Do Microgenetic Changes Occur?

### *Operations and Transformations Within Stages*

The proposition that percepts are subjective organizations of content from external and internal sources is fundamental to proponents of microgenesis. Within the temporal span from sensory registration to recognition and response, certain activities modify the initial registration. At issue are assumptions about the nature of these activities (operations, transformations, heuristics): What are the idiosyncratic or nomothetic characteristics of these activities, and what are the results of these activities?

No small part of the problem of defining the nature of the transformations that occur in microgenesis is the complexity of the task set by microgeneticists, that is, to understand the complex process of perceptual change at each microdevelopmental level. To highlight the complexity of the question of how to represent the nature of changes in microgenesis, consider a result accepted be a number of theories of microgenesis—that percepts become more clear toward later stages of microgenesis. A technique and methods that replicate this end point of microgenesis have even been imported into two well-known approaches to neuropsychological assessment (e.g., Christiansen, 1979). Yet, perceptual clarity has a number of potential meanings. Perceptual acuity, for example, represents one form of clarity. Certainly this form of clarity requires a minimum of conceptual operations. Haber and Hillman (1966), however, have demonstrated that mere repeated presentation of a stimulus can result in a growth in clarity. When subjects were presented targets that were below acuity thresholds, they were able to accurately discriminate targets when these targets were presented repeatedly. Their technique and results, however, do not provide a convincing distinction between the clarity one may call acuity and that which results from recognition or reconstruction. The data of Graham and Leibowitz (1972) further complicate the meaning of perceptual acuity. These authors have demonstrated that under posthypnotic suggestion and progressive relaxation, the acuity of severe myopes may improve without corrective lenses; this result obtains despite the lack of change in accommodation of the lens. In a carefully designed study, Graham and Leibowitz measured accommodation during an acuity task that required recognition of randomly presented Landolt "C" figures (standard figures for the measurement of visual acuity). As expected, accommodation to targets was poor for myopes. Subjects were then hypnotized or relaxed with the suggestion that their vision would improve. In fact, the results showed marked logarithmic improvement in acuity when subjects were hypnotized or relaxed. Measures of accommodation subsequent to hypnosis or relaxation were not significantly different from prerelaxation or prehypnosis levels. Of even greater import, several subjects reported flashes of "clear vision," despite the lack of change in accommodation!

Navon (1975), using an information-processing approach, executed several experiments designed to determine whether gross or fine detail took precedence in brief tachistoscopic presentations. Target stimuli consisted of large capital letters that were made up of smaller and different letters. Thus, for example, the target letter *H* consisted of two vertical columns and a horizontal row of *s*'s. Navon's results indicated that subjects typically perceived the larger letter with later recognition of the smaller constituent letters. Navon speculated that his results argued for a centripetal model of information processing. His model assumed that the "perceptual system treats *every* picture as if it was in a process of being focused or zoomed in, where at first it is relatively indistinct and then it gets clearer and sharper" (1975, p. 9). Navon's technique has been incorporated into a number of studies addressing pathological functioning such as agnosia (e.g., Farah, 1988). Kinchla and Wolfe (1979), however, demonstrated that there are limitations to the effect observed by Navon: Centripetal processing holds only under certain conditions related to the visual angle of the target. Suffice it to say that the issue of perceptual clarity is complex and that mere experiential descriptions of clarity are insufficient, if not misleading.

Given that there have been significant problems in defining stages of microgenesis, it should not be surprising that the specification of operations that occur within stages is even more problematic. Most proponents of microgenesis accept the general concept that percepts are constructed, that is, that percepts are active constructions and not passive copies of the sensed world. Beyond this general assumption, few microgeneticists have developed specific constructs to define the nature of the operations or transformations that contribute to the construction of the percepts. Although nothing akin to the primitives developed by Marr (1982) has been developed, I will discuss some representative approaches that offer perhaps the most clear expositions of microgenetic theories of the nature of operations and transformations in microgenesis.

In the context of studying personality–perception as a "unit-event over time," Kragh and Smith (1970) proposed a set of perceptual transformations delineated from the point of view of perception and dynamics. Three perceptual transformations were proposed including eliminations, cumulations, and emergences. To further clarify these transformations, Kragh and Smith distinguished between *perceptual organization*, that is, actual perceptual objects identified by the perceiver; *meaning*, as defined by the perceiver; and *structure*, a construct linking perception with personality. These distinctions might be construed as the subject's personal representations and organizations of the meaning of perception. The authors defined perceptual organization by the denotative and connotative features of language or by graphic reconstructions. Kragh and Smith further defined meanings as primary, when referring to features of the perceptual organization; secondary, when the referent is an association to percept organization; and tertiary, when the referent is a recollection, that is, a personalized memory referent. Kragh and Smith proposed that elimination, cumulation, and emergence transform perceptual organization, meaning, and structure. Elimination was defined as the disappearance of stimulus features with no observable effects. Cumulation was defined as the survival of stimulus features that become determinants of later stages. Emergence was defined as a descriptor of the apparent discontinuity from a preceding perceptual organization, meaning, or structure. From the point of view of dynamics, five sets of determinants were identified: (1) stimulus characteristics; (2) reconstruction; (3) prethreshold determinants; (4) cumulative and eliminative transformations of phases; and (5) emerging transformations with memory referents. Kragh and Smith indicated that the importance of stimulus characteristics increases throughout the microgenetic sequence. Of interest here, they described automatized microgenetic sequences as sequences in which there is near total reliance on stimulus characteristics. Similarly, in their discussion of reconstruction, Kragh and Smith referred to factors that influence communicated features of the perceptual experience, including set, such as experimenter-defined instructions, and defense mechanisms.

Kragh and Smith's (1970) theory thus presents a complex and comprehensive framework for a theory of microgenesis, outlining global characteristics of changes that occur by means of unspecified processes of differentiation, integration, and elimination. Omitting from our discussion details that are perhaps most relevant to the clinical psychologist, Kragh and Smith's emphasis on multifaceted determinants of perceptual responses is consistent with Linschoten's (1959) distinction between the microgenesis of perception and recognition. Both aspects are treated in their formulation. On the one hand, recognition is related to perceptual transformations. On the other hand, Smith and Kragh suggest a separate perceptual development whose microgenesis is influenced by proximal physical characteristics of the stimulus, the more distal state of the perceiver, and the most distal contribution of meaning and its microdevelopment.

As suggested earlier, Kreitler and Kreitler (1984) appear to have derived operations that are pertinent to a description of the genesis of recognition rather than perception. Perception, as a process of "meaning assignment," was characterized by the application of meaning values along meaning dimensions that are anchored to some referent. The Kreitlers proposed 21 meaning dimensions, each related to specific referents such as contextual allocation and classification; range of inclusion, function, purpose, or role; action(s), and potentialities for action. Meaning values and referents are related by forms and types of relations. Kreitler and Kreitler proposed four forms of relations between meaning values and referents: assertion, denial, conjunctive and disjunctive. Moreover, four types of relation between meaning values and referents characterize two kinds of meaning: lexical meanings that can be communicated and personal-subjective meaning. The four types of relation included attribution, comparison, exemplification-illustration, and metaphoric-symbolization. The Kreitlers described meaning as an open system in which the meaning of any referent may vary in terms of scope and complexity on a continuum from one meaning to nearly unlimited meanings. They further described meaning as a selectional system responsive to demand characteristics of referents and situational contexts as well as to features of personality and experience. Note that their system describes a complex active cognitive process in which the meaning of a given percept is categorized, anchored to a specific stimulus referent, and related to other stimulus or idiosyncratically defined content.

Froehlich and Laux (1969) have introduced concepts of readiness, selective attention, and information extraction to the process of microgenesis. Their introduction of attention as a variable in microgenesis is particularly noteworthy because it has been conspicuously absent in the work of microgeneticists. Unfortunately, their work, while suggestive of the presence of selective operations during early stages of microgenesis, does not clarify that nature of stage-specific selectivity, the mechanisms of selectivity, or its effect on the content or structure of perception.

In recent years, there has been a fortunate convergence of microgenetic and information-processing approaches to the study of perception. Despite general acceptance of the temporal nature of perceptual processing and development, the manner in which microgenetic and information processing theorists think about mediating activities can be polemic. A point of departure for understanding these polar views is the concept of operation. What is an operation from the point of view of information processing as opposed to microgenetic theories? The following from Haber (1969) is illuminating:

> Information processing analysis attempts to look for correlations between contents of the stimulus and contents of the responses measured at various times after the stimulation begins. By examining these correlations some notions can be gained of the properties of the flow of information on the nervous system, especially regarding the content of that information at any given point. . . . What is assumed is that if the appropriate operations could be devised, it should be possible to sample and examine the contents of stimulation at every point in time, and at every level in the nervous system. Comparing the stimulus and the perceiver's responses (be they description of his perceptual experience, or his detection, recognition, reaction-time, identification, or other discrete responses) would indicate the nature of the processing of that stimulus into perceptual experience and responses. (p. 2)

In this information-processing approach, then, operations assume the form of an experimental methodology involving a sampling of stimulus content, and a comparison of such samples with physical stimulus parameters and response processes. However, Haber's (1969) use of the term *operation* begs the question—is *operation* an experimenter-initiated manipulation of a stimulus parameter or an internal neuropsychological activity, an activity that in some manner transforms a stimulus? Smedslund's (1969b) remarks regarding such a definition and operational methodology provide a convenient contrast to Haber's position:

Complex inferences are necessary to diagnose even fairly simple processes. Mental processes have the status of constructs and are frequently operationally anchored, not to physically defined stimulus and response categories, but to the meanings of the subject's acts. The constructs and their anchorings are always tentative and subject to continuous revision. (p. 2)

In Haber's methodology, stimulus content is indicative of process change when such content is compared with stimulus content at several temporal points, by several sampling methods, in conjunction with changes among physical stimulus parameters. Smedslund's point is precisely that the stimulus content is unknown, hence, to measure a process in terms of an inferred correlation between response indicators and stimulus content is to measure an unknown in terms of an unknown. In a somewhat stronger posture, Smedslund (1969a) argued that the relationship between physical stimulus situations and meaning, and between actions and their intentions, "cannot be subsumed under any universally valid rule or principle" (p. 2). Experimenters, he argued, attempt to control the relationships by means of instructions. The experimental literature is replete with examples of the potency of the instructional variable in perceptual research, such as Leibowitz and Harvey (1967), who found extreme differences in size matching as a function of objective, apparent, and retinal instructions. The potency of this variable notwithstanding, one must consider whether classic psychophysical methods can ever provide adequate indices of process changes in perception.

Recognizing the importance of instructional variables, one may ask whether the comparison of stimulus content as described by Haber (1969) gives us a valid understanding of process changes in perception. Must we assume in the size constancy situation, for example, that three distinct processes of size perception occur? A more likely possibility involves the notion that response indices, as postperceptual processes, are more amenable to the conscious control of the subject; that is, the subject may select available contents to fit the demands of the experimental situation. That the subject is capable of providing retinal matches as opposed to apparent matches may imply an additional process of inhibiting the more adaptive tendency of responding in terms of apparent objects.

There are major difficulties in information processing approaches, and the converging operations strategy (Garner, Hake & Erickson, 1956) is by no means a panacea. The application of a number of discrete experimental procedures to a stable phenomenon does not of necessity recapitulate the process per se, or even the critical variables, which yield a given product of perception. In Dixon's (1971) words, "while the sum of converging operations may help us to define a concept, any change in the conditions by which this convergence is achieved, may equally well vitiate the procedure and lead us to an ever widening circle of alternative explanations" (p. 20). Often, converging operations involve the careful control of physical distal stimulus parameters of perception. Yet strict attention to physical parameters can also be misleading.

In contrast to Haber's (1969) rigid approach, other information-processing theorists have adroitly developed a variety of approaches to the study of mental chronometry. Navon's (1975) work is exemplary. Navon designed a series of studies to test a theory that is remarkably similar to some microgenetic theories. He hypothesized that the final percept is the result of "testing activity in the perceptual system." He reasoned that testing takes place by means of schemas. "The actual value of the output of a schema is determined by three factors: one, the agreement between the schema and the sensory data it is supposed to account for; two, the quality of the sensory input; three, the depth to which the schema was processed" (Navon, 1975, p. 2). The output of a schema is tested by means of a principal of "cursory verification," that is, "perception proceeds from global and gross analysis to more and more fine-grained analysis" (Navon, 1975, p. 9). The analysis in each level proceeds downward to a limited depth. Navon termed this process the principle of *cursory verification*. Of significance to our later considerations, Navon speculated that each level of processing is both "input driven" and "concept driven." Thus, his model provides for *top-down and bottom-up* development.

Marr's (1982) theory of perceptual information processing does not address problems of recognition or higher levels of meaning. More recent derivative information-processing theories have attempted to address these later stages of recognition. Some of these approaches, although emanating from information-processing theory, bear a striking resemblance to microgenetic theory (e.g., Biederman, 1987). Humphreys, Riddoch, and Quinlan (1989), using a variant of an earlier theory of parallel information processing, proposed a theory of cascade processes to explain picture identification. In this theory, Humphreys et al. propose a parallel microdevelopment of structural and semantic features in a picture-identification task. Thus, for example, a picture of an apple may activate its own and structural descriptions of similar objects with subsequent activation of semantic representations of an apple and the related objects. These contemporary efforts, with experimental operations derived from information-processing theory, explicate in a new direction the bifurcation in perception and recognition described by Linschoten (1959).

Microgenetic theorists have proposed several operations to describe gross changes that ostensibly occur within stages of microgenesis. Their approach to defining operations contrasts sharply with approaches developed within the information processing *Zeitgeist*. The following is a summary of several proposed operations that describe how percept changes occur:

1. Percepts are constructed, that is, transformed from sensory mapping to a representational mapping via active rather than passive processes.
2. Percepts undergo differentiation and later integration at later developmental stages.
3. Percepts may become abbreviated or aborted in the process of development. That is, development may not culminate in a final, "normalized" percept.
4. Several forms of transformations or operations have been suggested to explain the nature of changes within stages. These transformations include cumulation, eliminations, and emergences. These transformations, however, are descriptive of subject responses rather than testable operations that assume lawfulness by virtue of their structure and function. Other characteristics used to describe the nature of changes within stages include contraction, expansion, and clarification. These characteristics, also observable in whole reports of perceptual experience, specify post hoc the nature of specific changes in percepts, at different stages of microgenesis.

Microgeneticists have not come to grips with the notion of operations or transformations as comprising explicit structures. Using Piaget's theory as a model, *cognitive operations* are equivalent to reversible regulatory structures in an equilibrate system. Moreover, logical operations satisfy the conditions of combinativity, reversibility, associativity, identity, and analyticity. All operational structures evolve ontogenetically from a structure to a new structure. Piaget (1969) distinguished two classes of structures: logical and perceptual. He indicated that there is a *partial isomorphy* between these operational structures. As isomorphic structures, perceptual structures also undergo development, both ontogenetic and arguably microgenetic. Two essential aspects of experience comprise this development, the perception of object properties and the perception of relationships in a set of objects. Piaget also suggested specific perceptual mechanisms that may provide an entree to the derivation of microgenetic perceptual structures.

In keeping with the leitmotif distinguishing the microgeneses of perception and recognition, it is important to note at this juncture that few microgenetic theorists have carefully developed a means of distinguishing perception and thinking. Whereas Piaget (1969) indicated that the differences between perception and thinking were to be found in the processes, products, and fate of their products, he also developed constructs and tests of filiations between perception and thinking to support the hypothesis of their partial isomorphy.

At a cognitive level, operative transformations have been well documented by Piaget and his colleagues. At the level of perception, Piaget's development of the constructs of centration, decentration, and coupling appear to describe partially isomorphic transformational activities. It is premature, however, to suppose that Piaget's (1969) proposed perceptual operations are exclusive or exhaustive, or that the nature of changes in these activities is well understood ontogenetically. It is more likely that an understanding of clear links between microgenesis and orthogenesis will long be the least understood and last developed features in a comprehensive theory of microgenesis.

Operational methods or experimental manipulations can elicit only a limited aspect of microgenetic processes. Both constructive (inferential) and reconstructive (deductive) methods are necessary to approximate the complexity of this process. On the other hand, it is important to seek an understanding of microgenetic operations that can be tested and confirmed in a manner similar to that proposed by Marr (1982). To the extent that these operations are lawful, they will establish a structural basis to the nature of changes in microgenesis. To the extent that we have a well-developed structural model of cognitive and perceptual operations, we can test the limitations and differences in the isomorphy between perception and higher levels of cognition.

## What Is the Temporal Span of Microgenesis?

### *Unconscious, Preconscious, and Conscious Levels*

The definition of the span of microgenesis presented in the beginning of this chapter partially corresponds to a level of perceptual processing labeled *preconscious* and *unconscious*. Some have argued that microgenetic thought or perception is the nexus of a concept of the unconscious. Certainly, many of the phenomena attended to in the study of perceptual microgenesis are not phenomena typically associated with conscious experience.

Microgenetic treatments of the concept of unconscious differ from the approaches of most popular information-processing theorists. Kantor and Herron (1964), for example, discussed the development of perceptual control (selectivity) and efficiency, maintaining that conscious and unconscious mechanisms were integral to their development. These authors noted the similarity between early microgenetic states and primary process and made explicit the distinction between conscious–unconscious processes:

> That there is unconscious as well as conscious perception becomes a necessary postulate if the implications of perceptual control and microgenesis are followed. Both perceptual control and microgenesis involve levels of form discrimination some of which are inaccessible to consciousness. These subsurface, or unconscious form differentiations are characterized by varying degrees of structural and content entropy, and by the irrational inventory of fantasies traumata, thoughts, judgments, and memory which appear frankly in the range of human conduct. (p. 68)

Information theorists have generally ignored or avoided the question of unconscious determinants, especially those associated with affectivity, motivation, and personality referents.

Two approaches to defining the preconscious and unconscious portions of the span of microgenesis have predominated in contemporary microgenetic theory, the work of Kragh and Smith (1970) and that of Dixon. Kragh and Smith have explicitly discussed the demarcations between preconscious and conscious domains in a subtle yet persuasive discussion of focal versus marginal influences in behavior. Their preference for the study of marginal, nonstimulus-dominated influences in the study of perception–personality represents a classic process-oriented clinical psychological approach to the description of preconscious events and structural changes in the course of microgenesis.

Perhaps the most explicit treatment of the distinction between unconscious and conscious levels of processing in relation to microgenesis has been provided by Dixon (1983, 1984). Drawing from a host of research studies, Dixon (1984) concluded as follows:

> The sampling of events at these different [preconscious] stages has shown the effects of subliminal stimuli on figural synthesis, on autonomic responses, verbal associations, dreams, brain potentials, drive schemata in memory, reaction times, and sensory thresholds. (p. 225)

Dixon's work has melded microgenetic concepts and theory with comparable developments in the study of subliminal perception: "In short, the phenomena of subliminal perception have been to microgenetic theory as bricks and mortar are to a house" (1984, p. 225). In Dixon's view, stimuli that are not experienced in conscious awareness may nevertheless access long-term memory and may thereby affect the meaning of sensory input. Selectivity of sensory input can be initiated both by stimulus characteristics (via "bottom-up" processes) as well as through conscious processes such as volition. Moreover, preconscious responses to volition- and stimulus-initiated selectivity can interact with four sets of variables: (1) the need state; (2) idiosyncratic affective sensitivities or predispositions to stimulus characteristics; (3) information retained in long-term memory; (4) a neuropsychological state defined by arousal level, lesions, and hemisphericity.

In his distinction between conscious and preconscious processes, Dixon (1983) described conscious experience as an end result of multiple stages of preconscious processing in which the products of preprocessing reduce ambiguity. Preconscious processing included (1) monitoring of the sensory array, (2) feature analysis, and (3) emotional "appraisal" of stimulus characteristics. In this view, preconscious operations are both centripetal and centrifugal (bottom-up or top-down), interacting with long-term memory in the process of constructive representation. Moreover, in this view, need state and emotional appraisal may actually override "top-down" or "bottom-up" determinants of perception. Dixon's (1983) model for unconscious processing is presented in Figure 6.2.

Dixon's (1983) model is of great interest in the derivation of a scientific neuropsychology using microgenetic constructs and research techniques because the model incorporates information-processing constructs that allow for experimental test and verification.

Mainstream American psychologists have long shunned the study of unconscious or preconscious processes because of their historical association with psychoanalysis. However, the burgeoning interest in perceptual information processing (Posner, 1986) and explicit interest in "mental operations" among developmentalists and cognitive neuropsychologists has again heightened interest in this distinction. Freed from psychoanalytic interpretations that may require unacceptable metatheoretical assumptions about human and individual motivations, their goals and mechanisms, psychologists can legitimately ask nonreified yet nonetheless important questions about the effect and fate of stimulus content and memory that cannot be, or is not consciously experienced by the perceiver. Is this content lost? Does it have an effect on other percepts or percept meanings? Does it change the affective context of the percept? Dixon (1971) and others have repeatedly demonstrated that much stimulus content, while never reported or consciously experienced, nevertheless can be made available to, or demonstrable through subjective reports or other response processes; availability of content registered subliminally can be tested using a variety of indirect sampling techniques. The unexperienced and unavailable content can be demonstrated to have real effects on other perceptions, percept meanings, and physiological processes. Certainly, the study of preconscious information processing using microgenetic and information-processing methods yields results that are consistent with a multistage model of percept and meaning development.

The upper limits to the span of microgenesis have not been discussed because this chapter focuses primarily on the problem of perceptual microgenesis. The reader is referred to Draguns (1984) and Froehlich (1984), who have summarized other approaches to microgenesis, approaches that are more explicitly associated with higher level cognitive operations. As indicated by Draguns and earlier by Werner (1957), it is possible to study microgenesis in the range defined by Kragh and Smith (1964) as the "C" phase, over minutes, hours, weeks, years, and even centuries.

## Why and When Does Microgenesis Occur?

Two final questions will be asked of microgenetic theories: why and under what circumstances does microgenesis occur? These questions must be asked and answered because they form the basis of the scientific phenomenon in question. To my knowledge, only Draguns (1983) has squarely

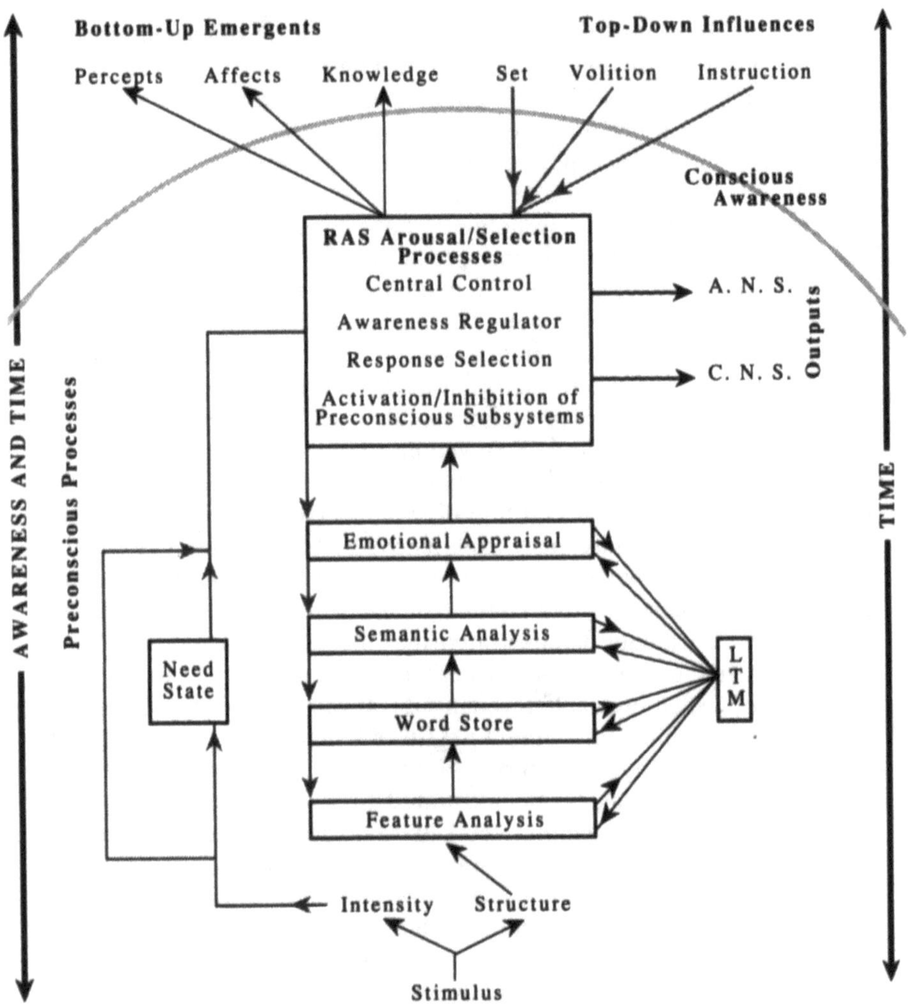


FIGURE 6.2. Dixon's 1983 model of conscious and preconscious systems participating in phenomenal representation. In this model, bottom-up emergents (percepts, affects, and knowledge) result from a set of selection processes (RAS, reticular activating system) that are influenced by and also influence linguistic subsystems. Bottom-up influences may be elicited by structural features of a stimulus. Top-down influences (excitatory and inhibitory) also affect substages of affective–linguistic arousal and may inhibit top-down determinants. Contact with long-term memory processes occurs at each stage of affective–linguistic processing. Stimulus intensity affects the subject's extant need state and ultimately arousal–attention systems. Psychosomatic resultants are outputs of arousal–selection processes. (From Conscious Experience System in "The Conscious-unconscious Interface: Contributions to an Understanding (p. 64) in *Archiv fur psychologie* by N.F. Dixon, 1983, Bonn: Bouvier Verlag Herbertgrundmann. Copyright 1983 by Bouvier Verlag Herbert Grundmann. Adapted by permission.)

addressed the former question. Draguns summarized three sets of factors that have been invoked to explain the occurrence of microgenesis. These factors might be characterized as follows: (1) genetic perceptual mechanisms of the human are adapted to seek identification and recognition; (2) motivations or drives (cognitive and physiological) impel activity toward identification and recognition; (3) demand characteristics in the experimental situation result in identification and recognition. Draguns's treatment of these factors focused extensively on cognitive motivations. I will not recapitulate Draguns's erudite discussion of these factors. Rather, I will focus on a position with the regard to the question "Why does microgenesis occur?" and on other perspectives that may provide some refinement to the proposed answers to this question.

A somewhat simplistic way out of this quandary is to establish a variety of situations in which the hypothesized phenomenon is reputed to occur. Microgenesis is most often reported in experimental situations in which the stimulus is degraded. That is, physical stimulus parameters are sufficiently weak or indefinite, thus, recognition is at best difficult. To summarize, microgenesis seems to occur in at least three such situations: (1) under conditions of stimulus impoverishment; (2) under conditions of stimulus novelty; (3) under conditions of stimulus ambiguity (Draguns, 1983).

## *Microgenesis Results From Conflict*

In the classic microgenetic experimental situation, microgenesis has been described as similar to "going beyond the information given" or "effort after meaning." Paradigmatically, a degraded stimulus (e.g., very brief stimulus exposure) is presented, and a subject is asked to respond to the stimulus (e.g., by verbal description). As summarized by Draguns, subjects' responses to such stimuli are typically schematized rather than rich in detail. In this case, responses to the degraded stimulus may represent: (1) verbal descriptions of the conscious experience of an unrecognized sensory event in which lack of organization is filled in by hypotheses (Linschoten, 1959); (2) partial recognition without associated content, such as Gendlin's (1962) "felt meaning"; (3) partial recognition with partial activation of associated content in Potzl's (1917/1960) sense; (4) a global physiological reaction to an unsymbolized experience (Froehlich & Laux, 1969). In my view, each of these processes occurring in the previously mentioned generic experimental situations described by Draguns (1983) create conflict, and conflict may be the underlying process driving microgenesis.

To understand conflict in the sense in which I am proposing it, consider two forms of microgenesis. First, a microgenetic experiment studying "forward" evolution of a percept or concept begins with the study of a poorly adapted (with reference to the stimulus or organic state characteristics) and poorly equilibrated state. The progressive addition of information (in the merogenetic sense) or increased opportunities to extract further information (in the hologenetic sense) essentially tests the limits of the degree to which the impermanent structure can be accommodated, hence assimilated. The meaning of conflict in this instance is the imperfect activation of a memory content or an action schema corresponding to a contemporaneous stimulus feature or internal transformational activity. The second form of microgenesis, microgenetic study of the "backward" evolution or transformation of a percept (Froehlich, 1984) or concept (i.e., progressive deterioration of a supraliminal stimulus or experimental subtraction of available information and the corresponding experience of change) essentially tests the limits of the adapted (equilibrated) perceptual structure, by testing the state of assimilation of the new percept or concept. The meaning of conflict in this instance is a mismatch between an assimilated percept and a newly emerging, unassimilated, or partially assimilated percept. For a given adapted perceptual structure, there is a greater or lesser assimilation to a current operational structure. Hence, percepts or concepts have more or less of the characteristics of transience or permanence depending on the degree to which they have been assimilated.

Microgenesis thus operates within the adaptive organization of perception and cognition. Conflict results from the failure of assimilation, thereby resulting in a change in existing structures. Given that stimulus influences and internal representational activities continuously compete for resources and completion, lack of completion and continuous use of resources both limit resources for other activities and may require new transformations or operations for completion. Imperfectly assimilated percepts require an accommodative activity that may result in the derivation of a new structure and a new perceptual representation, such as eye movements or a change in the focus of attention. Parenthetically, it is likely that percepts less totally assimilated would be characterized by more extended and less economic microgenetic sequences than percepts more totally assimilated. This statement must be qualified, however, (1) by the notion that the preceding statements only apply when the percept has affective or motivational investment or significance (cognitive or biogenic), that is, when the partially assimilated percept or concept "makes a difference" to a person as defined by past experience or current affective state; (2) by obvious limitations inherent in variables popularly termed *personality characteristics* or *styles*, such as conservative versus liberal response biases; and (3) by the possibilities of the emergence of aborted content.

In a discussion of information loss or retention (if indeed such is the case) Smith's (1954) remarks reinforce this line of reasoning and, coincidentally, confirm some of the remarks of Smedslund (1969a) quoted earlier in this chapter:

> A behavior event will become the immediate reflection of a physical-physiological process only if this process is conceived of as "reality" by the subject. As soon

as the individual's conception of reality is less "objective," less socialized, the response cannot and will not be a mere prolongation of stimulus (inside or outside). (Smith, 1954, p. 75)

Consistent with Dixon (1971), I must add that reality and importance need not be related to consciousness alone, and moreover, the reality alluded to by Smith need not be a verbally represented reality.

## *Limitations*

An inherent danger in many microgenetic theories is the assertion or implication that microgenesis occurs in any perceptual process. It should be clear that microgenesis cannot be equated with all processes of concern to students of perception and cognition. The danger in this assumption is precisely the danger of denying automatization of perceptual recognition processes. Microgenesis is likely to occur in conditions that are unfavorable to recognition, conditions in which stimulus properties or configurations render recognition difficult (e.g., stimulus impoverishment or embeddedness), or in situations in which recognition products are suppressed, denied, or distorted by postrecognition processes. Failure to limit the occurrence of microgenesis in theory is tantamount to the error of overemphasizing the effect of affective processes in perception, an error cogently elaborated by Klein (1970). Both information processing and microgenetic theorists suggest that perceptual as well as recognition processes are nonimmediate. Apparently, most microgeneticists are mainly concerned with the perceptual processes involving the attribution of meaning—in Fechner's (1860) sense, with defining the "apperceptive mass." Inasmuch as most microgenetic experiments typically deal with the conscious emergents of an exposure to a given stimulus, however brief, there remains a level of perceptual processing as yet unavailable to the most thorough microgenetic evaluation.

## *Why Does Microgenesis Occur?*

Draguns's (1983) discussion of why microgenesis occurs ended in what is perhaps the most important question for a further scientific evaluation of the proposed phenomenon: "What is the adaptive significance of microgenesis?" (p. 13). Draguns rightfully concluded that a meaningful answer to this question assumes that microgenesis actually occurs in the natural course of human experience, that the phenomenon is not simply an artifact of the methods used to study it. However, his direct answer to the question of the adaptive significance of microgenesis is really a question. In keeping with the notion that we need to articulate situations that ostensibly involve microgenesis, Draguns indicated that it would be helpful to establish the manner in which people cope and adapt to everyday circumstances. He then asked the question of what the adaptive significance might be to overestimating our knowledge and in acting on the assumption that we know more than we actually do. An answer to Draguns's question might be found, by inference, in the work of Piaget (1974) and Inhelder and Piaget (1958). A similar answer is reflected in decades of work on perceptual constancy. That is, an inherent feature of human perceptual and cognitive activity is a biogenic tendency to conserve. Because we conserve, we are able to extend our capabilities and adaptations to newer and more complex circumstances. Conservation, however, is a set of actions and an achievement of operations at a level removed from the stimulus and its simple representation. Conservation is not a passive noninteractive process.

Draguns (1983) discussed Linschoten's (1959) view of the likely assumptions of the subject in a microgenetic experiment. This view is related to what might be a significant problem for microgenesis. Draguns noted that changes in responses during microgenesis appear to derive from the assumption that the world is meaningful and orderly. This assumption, invoked in situations that are novel, unfamiliar, and unclear, is characterized in behavior that appears to be governed by structural or conjectural optimism. Conjectural optimism, however, is progressively tempered by conjectural realism as more information and structure become apparent. Linschoten's analysis is, of course, addressed to a cognitive level of perceptual representation although the principle may mirror lower level operations.

Finally, I would like to add a further dimension to this line of reasoning. Consistent with an earlier suggestion that microgenesis is driven by conflict, I would like to propose, after Piaget (1974), that perceptual microgenesis is subject to a dialectic between conservative and constructive operations (at the level of cognition) and operational isomorphs (at the level of perceptual representation). In this sense, stimulus representation, identification, and recognition serve not only to represent the world as it is but also as a foundation for the acquisition of new information and new meaning.

## *References*

Andersson, A.L. (1984). Toward a dialectical conception of the percept-genetic approach to perception personality. In W.D. Froehlich, G. Smith, J.G. Draguns, & U. Hentschel (Eds.), *Psychological processes in cognition and personality* (pp. 125–134). Washington, DC: Hemisphere.

Biederman, I. (1987). Recognition-by-components: A theory of human understanding. *Psychological Review, 94*, 115–147.

Brown, J. (1977). *Mind, brain and consciousness: The neuropsychology of cognition*. New York: Academic Press.

Brown, J. (1988). *The life of the mind: Selected papers*, Hillsdale, NJ: Lawrence Erlbaum.

Brown, J. (1989). *Essay on perception.* In J.W. Brown (Ed.), *Neuropsychology of visual perception* (pp. 234–256). Hillsdale, NJ: Lawrence Erlbaum.

Catán, L. (1986). The dynamic display of process: Historical development and contemporary uses of the microgenetic method. *Human Development, 29*, 252–263.

Christiansen, A.L. (1979). *Luria's neuropsychological investigation.* Copenhagen: Munksgaard.

Dixon, N.F. (1971). *Subliminal perception: The nature of a controversy.* New York: McGraw-Hill.

Dixon, N.F. (1981). *Preconscious processing.* Chichester, UK: Wiley.

Dixon, N.F. (1983). The conscious-unconscious interface: Contributions to an understanding. *Archiv fur Psychologie, 135*, 55–66.

Dixon, N.F. (1984). Subliminal perception and microgenesis. In W.D. Froehlich, G. Smith, J.G. Draguns, & U. Hentschel (Eds.), *Psychological processes in cognition and personality* (pp. 225–230). Washington, DC: Hemisphere.

Draguns, J.G. (1983). Why microgenesis? An inquiry on the motivational sources of going beyond the information given. *Archiv fur Psychologie, 135*, 5–16.

Draguns, J.G. (1984). Microgenesis by any other name. . . . In W.D. Froehlich, G. Smith, J.G. Draguns, & U. Hentschel (Eds.), *Psychological processes in cognition and personality* (pp. 3–18). Washington, DC: Hemisphere.

Farah, M.J. (1988). Is visual imagery really visual? Overlooked evidence from neuropsychology. *Psychological Review, 95*, 307–317.

Fechner, G.T. (1860). *Elemente der Psychophysik.* Leipzig: Breitkoph and Hartel.

Flavell, J.H., & Draguns, J.G. (1957). A microgenetic approach to perception and thought. *Psychological Bulletin, 54*, 197–217.

Froehlich, W.D. (1984). Microgenesis as a functional approach to information processing through search. In W.D. Froehlich, G. Smith, J.G. Draguns, & U. Hentschel (Eds.), *Psychological processes in cognition and personality* (pp. 19–52). Washington, DC: Hemisphere.

Froehlich, W.D., & Laux, L. (1969). Serielles Wahrnehmen, Aktualgenese, informationsintegration und orienttierungsreaktion: I. Aktualgenetisches modell und orientierungsreaktion. *Zeitschrift fur Experimentelle und Angewandte Psychologie, 16*, 250–277.

Garner, W.R., Hake, H.W., & Erickson, C.W. (1956). Operationalism and the concept of perception. *Psychological Review, 63*, 317–329.

Gendlin, E.T. (1962). *Experiencing and the creation of meaning: A philosophical and psychological approach to the subjective.* New York: Free Press of Glencoe.

Graham, C., & Leibowitz, H. (1972). The effect of hypnosis on visual acuity. *International Journal of Clinical and Experimental Hypnosis, 20*, 169–186.

Graumann, C.F. (1959). Aktualgenese: Die deskriptiven Grundlagen und theoretischen Wandlungen des aktualgenetischen Forschungsansatzes. *Zeitschrift fur Experimentelle und Angewandte Psychologie, 6*, 410–448.

Haber, R.N. (1969) (Ed.). *Information-processing approaches to visual perception.* New York: Holt.

Haber, R.N., & Hillman, E.R. (1966). The effect of repetition on the perception of single letters. *Perception & Psychophysics, 1*, 347–350.

Humphreys, G.W., Riddoch, M.J., & Quinlan, P.T. (1989). Cascade processes in picture identification. *Cognitive Neuropsychology, 5*(1), 67–103.

Inhelder, B., & Piaget, J. (1958). *The growth of logical thinking.* New York: Basic Books.

Kantor, R.E., & Herron, W.G. (1964). Perceptual learning in the reactive-process schizophrenia. *Journal of Projective Techniques and Personality Assessment, 29*, 58–70.

Kinchla, R.A., & Wolfe, J.M. (1979). The order of visual processing: "Top-down," "bottom-up," or "middle-out." *Perception & Psychophysics, 25*(3), 225–231.

Klein, G. (1970). *Perception, motives and personality*. New York: Alfred A. Knopf.

Kragh, U. (1955). *The actual-genetic model of perception-personality*. Lund, Sweden: Gleerup.

Kragh, U., & Smith, G.J.W. (1964). Accessorial and inclusive approaches to marginal perceptual phenomena. *Scandinavian Journal of Psychology, 5*, 80–90.

Kragh, U., & Smith, G.J.W. (1970). *Percept-genetic analysis*. Lund, Sweden: Gleerup.

Kreitler, S., & Kreitler, H. (1984). Meaning assignment in perception. In W.D. Froehlich, G. Smith, J.G. Draguns, & U. Hentschel (Eds.), *Psychological processes in cognition and personality* (pp. 173–192). Washington, DC: Hemisphere.

Leibowitz, H.W., & Harvey, L.O. (1967). Size matching as a function of instructions in a naturalistic environment. *Journal of Experimental Psychology, 74*, 378–382.

Linschoten, J. (1959). Aktualgenese und heuristiches prinzip. *Zeitschrift fur Experimentelle und Angewandte Psychologie, 6*, 449–473.

Marr, D. (1982). *Vision: A computational investigation into the human representation and processing of visual information*. New York: W.H. Freeman.

Navon, D. (1975). Global precedence in visual recognition. Unpublished doctoral dissertation, University of California, San Diego, CA.

Piaget, J. (1957). *Logic and psychology*. New York: Basic Books.

Piaget, J. (1969). *Mechanisms of perception*. New York: Basic Books.

Piaget, J. (1974). *Biology and Knowledge. An essay on the relations between organic regulations and cognitive processes*. Chicago: University of Chicago Press.

Potzl, O. (1960). The relationship between experimentally induced dream images and indirect vision. Monograph No. 7. *Psychological Issues, 2*, 41–120. (Original work published 1917).

Posner, M.I. (1986). *Chronometric explorations of mind*. New York: Oxford University Press.

Sander, F. (1930). Structures, totality of experience, and gestalt. In C. Murchison (Ed.), *Psychologies of 1930* (pp. 191–207). Worcester, MA: Clark University Press.

Smith, G.J.W. (1954). The place of physiological constructs in a genetic explanatory system. *Psychological Review, 61*, 73–76.

Smith, G.J.W. (1957). Perception—an event over time. *Psychological Review, 64*, 306–313.

Smith, G.J.W. (1983). Guest editor's preface. *Archiv fur Psychologie, 135*, 1–3.

Smedslund, J. (1969a). Meanings, implications and universals: Towards a psychology of man. *Scandinavian Journal of Psychology, 10*, 1–15.

Smedslund, J. (1969b). Psychological diagnostics. *Psychological Bulletin, 3*, 237–248.

Werner, H. (1957). The concept of development from a comparative and organismic point of view. In D.B. Harris (Ed.), *The concept of development* (pp. 125–148). Minneapolis: University of Minnesota Press.
Westcott, M. (1967). *Toward a psychology of intuition*. New York: Academic Press.

# 7
# The Microgenesis of Schizophrenic Symptoms

Ralph E. Hoffman

It is likely that no domain of mental life is immune to schizophrenia. Thought, affect, speech, perception, and belief are all altered by this disorder, frequently with disabling results. No social or racial group, moreover, is immune to acquiring schizophrenia. In a wide variety of countries and cultures, the prevalence of schizophrenia remains relatively constant at around .8% (Neale & Oltmanns, 1980). This enormous public health problem has triggered a broad research effort encompassing psychological, neurobiological, and cognitive perspectives. Despite these efforts, the etiology of schizophrenia remains unknown. To further complicate matters, genetic data now indicate that schizophrenia can result from different causes (Kennedy, et al., 1988).

Given these uncertainties, research strategies targeting particular signs and symptoms are warranted. It may be possible to identify a mechanism underlying a particular symptom even if different pathological processes can activate this mechanism, or if the ultimate cause of the disorder remains unknown.

A microgenetic perspective may facilitate our understanding of certain schizophrenic symptoms. I use the term *microgenetic* to characterize cognitive processes such as language production or perception that unfold in stages, generally within a second or a fraction of second (see Garrett, 1975; Marr, 1982). I will argue that a microgenetic analysis of complex mentation can be used to identify cognitive stages or processing levels when pathological disruptions occur in schizophrenia.

## Schizophrenia and the Experience of the Will

Many of the bizarre symptoms of schizophrenia correspond to alterations in the experience of the will (Bleuler, 1911/1950). Typical examples are those patients who complain that nonself forces, such as spacemen or a famous individual, control their actions, thoughts, or speech. This impoverishment of will also has its mirror opposite—those patients who believe that they possess special powers and abilities to influence the thoughts and actions of others.

These bizarre misattributions of willfulness are all the more puzzling given experimental data indicating that the reasoning abilities of schizophrenics are intact (Maher, 1974). What then causes the schizophrenic to so frequently draw false conclusions regarding the limits of his own will and/or the will of others?

One clue is that most of these patients harbor parallel false beliefs involving not control of actions but the efficacy of communication. A patient might note, for instance, that he receives messages in coded form over the television or from spacemen, or that he has telepathic abilities so that he can, whenever he wishes, communicate with Michael Jackson. False beliefs regarding the exertion of will and communication are referred to as *Schneiderian symptoms* (Schneider, 1957). Their frequent cooccurrence suggest that false beliefs about the domain of the will may be related to false beliefs about communication processes. In particular, the former may fall on a continuum with the latter and corresponds to a more extreme case: If I can communicate effectively to that spaceman (or he to me) then I can alter, in some significant way, his thoughts and actions (or he, mine).

Psychiatrists generally explain these phenomena in terms of a "loss of ego boundaries" or "inner/outer confusion." These terms, at best, describe aspects of the schizophrenic's irrationality while offering no new understanding of the cause(s) of such phenomena. Instead, I propose that decoding these symptoms requires an appreciation of an underlying truth for all of us—that in ordinary life we discover and reconfirm on a daily basis that by and large the only way to influence the will of other agents and for us to be influenced by others is via communication, especially, though not exclusively, via speech and language. In other words, various misattributitions of the will may be inferential products of misattributions concerning communication processes (Hoffman, 1986). This perspective assumes a two-stage process: (1) the schizophrenic person is prone to conclude that communication between himself and other agents is taking place when it, in actually, is not and (2) he believes that this communication can influence either his own decision-making processes, the decision-making processes of others, or both.

As argued above, stage 2 is quite reasonable and nonpathological. The question thus boils down to the etiology of the stage 1: Is some cognitive process active in schizophrenics patients that would cause them to believe that communication is occurring when it, in fact, is not? I will argue why the answer to this question is yes.

## Language Production Processes in Schizophrenia

It has long been appreciated that schizophrenic persons produce irregular utterances that are difficult for listeners to follow and understand (Bleuler,

1911/1950). These speech difficulties are diverse in nature. For instance, some schizophrenics seem to have difficulties in generating acceptable words. The results, neurolinguistically speaking, are paraphasias, for example:

[1] he is a *grassical* person (Hoffman & Sledge, 1984, p. 157)
[2] You have to have a *plausity* of amendments to go through for the children's code, and it's no mental disturbance of *puterience*, it is an *amorition* law. (Vetter, quoted in Chaika, 1982, p. 170)

Other schizophrenics produce paragrammatical sentences,

[3] After John Black has recovered in special neutral form of life the honest bring back to doctors agents. (Lorenz, quoted in Chaika, 1982, p. 172)

as well as higher order difficulties in combining phrases and sentences into coherent extended discourse:

[4] Interviewer: Tell me about [your experiences in] school?
Patient: School? Well there are schools of play and schools of fish, mostly you see fish school, people edumacating themselves themselves you see, sea is one thing and education is another. . . . (Hoffman, 1986, p. 507)

On the basis of examples such as these, Chaika (1974, 1977, 1982) argued that schizophrenics can demonstrate a kind of intermittent aphasia that cannot be distinguished from that produced by neurologically impaired speakers.

In an important paper, Fromkin (1975) responded to Chaika's hypothesis by noting that the speech of normal individuals is often deviant as well. The following are deviant "transformations" of speech produced by normal speakers

[5] soul hecond path (intended: whole second path)
[6] in a manner of speakingly (intended: in a manner of speaking)
(Fromkin, 1975, p. 502)

Chaika herself provides interesting examples of "nonproficient writing of an ostensibly normal college student":

[7] Generalizations have no place in terms of different opinions insofar as the discussion of heros or any other topic. (Chaika, 1977, p. 471)

She also provides an example of the verbiage of political speech making:

[8] In temperance due I don't see any reason why two men can't proceed as popular as ever both in themselves as a duocratic and as a democratic premise. (Laffal, quoted in Chaika, 1977, p. 471)

Segments such as these caused Fromkin (1975) to argue that language deviance produced by schizophrenics is not distinguishable from deviance produced by normal speakers and therefore should not classified as a type of neurological aphasia. Chaika (1977) responded to Fromkin by arguing that the speech errors produced by schizophrenics can be distinguished from those produced by schizophrenics because the latter are readily decipherable in terms of communicative intent while the former are not.

A case study of a schizophrenic speaker by Hoffman and Sledge (1984) attempted to shed light on the controversy. In spite of normal intelligence, he repeatedly generated quite distinctive speech errors, for instance:

[9] the communists who have a class-struggle creation (Hoffman & Sledge, 1984, p. 153)

Followed in a few seconds by the following:

[10] a creation class-struggles
(p. 153)

Examples 9 and 10 both reflected difficulties in generating the noun phrase, "creation [of a] class struggle[s]." These errors can be analyzed via a microgenetic perspective derived from an earlier study of normal speech errors reported by Garrett (1975).

Garrett's (1975) scheme requires dividing the vocabulary of English into two classes. The first class is referred to as "open-class" elements. This term refers to the nouns, verbs, adjectives and adverbs of the language; these are the words through which English and all languages expand and evolve. On the other hand, "closed class" elements are those words that do not change—they are grammatical words such as prepositions, conjunctions, articles, and so on. Garrett argues that an early stage of language production involves gathering open-class elements into groups that are associated with some propositional intent. At a later stage, individual elements belonging to these semantic "heaps" are sorted out into syntactic frames composed of closed class elements and "grammatical morphemes" such as *-ing* or *-ed* that attach themselves to open-class elements. Along these lines, Garrett argued that speech errors of the following type reflect errors in slotting open-class elements, which at an earlier stage have been grouped together, into a syntactic frame:

[11] Although *murder* is a form of *suicide*
(intended: suicide is a form of murder)
[12] McGovern favored *pushing busters*
(intended: busting pushers)
(1975, p. 149)

Thus, example 12 reflects an early microgenetic stage that groups together "McGovern," "favor," "push," and "bust." This is followed by a later stage where these elements are slotted in the syntactic frame:

subject–verb–*ed*—verb–*ing*–verb–*ers*

The error occurred when an exchange of open-class elements occurred at the last and next-to-last verb positions.

If this scheme characterizes the speech errors of ordinary sentence production, what is the nature of the linguistic disruption shown in samples 9 and 10? A reexamination of these examples suggests that the speaker successfully grouped together two open-class elements, *creation* and *class struggle*, before slotting into a syntactic frame. *Instead, the syntactic frame itself (*$noun_1$*-of-[article]-*$noun_2$*) seemed to be deficient.*

A problem with a single case study approach is that it is not clear whether the examples considered are generally produced by schizophrenic speakers or whether these deviant language constructions were idiosyncratic productions of this particular speaker. Consequently, my co-workers and I undertook a systematic study that examined grammatical deviance generated by different groups of speakers (Hoffman & Sledge, 1988). One group consisted of 11 schizophrenics, and the comparison group consisted of nine patients with psychiatric disorders other than schizophrenia. Both groups of patients had recently been hospitalized and therefore were acutely ill and were well matched in terms of age, gender, and educational level. Each patient in the study was requested to respond to a series of neutral queries such as, "Tell me about your experiences in school" (see example 4) or "Tell me about where you grew up." Two of the responses were randomly selected for careful transcription and analysis of grammatical deviance. For the purposes of this study, grammatical deviance was defined as words that did not belong to the English lexicon or combinations of words that violated syntax. Slang and variations attributable to local dialect were not scored as deviant. Of note is the fact that we did not choose normal subjects as a control group but rather other psychiatric patients; it was hoped that "nonspecific" factors tending to produce speech errors—anxiety, stress, fatigue, and soon—would be present in both groups and therefore would be at least partially controlled for.

We generated two types of scores for each patient. The first was the number of grammatically deviant segments produced relative to the total number of clauses produced. The second was an assessment, for each instance of deviance, as to the ambiguity of corresponding "target" or intention.

The major finding was that the mean number of instances of deviance was significantly greater in the schizophrenic group—even when the somewhat greater utterance lengths of schizophrenics were controlled for.

This finding was consistent with other recent studies demonstrating that schizophrenics showed an increased frequency of language deviance (Fraser, King, Thomas, & Kendell, 1986; Morice & Ingram, 1982). These earlier studies, however, did not analyze the type and severity of deviance. Our study attempted to address these issues. In terms of the type of error, there was a roughly equal number of inappropriate or poorly formed open-class words (nouns, verbs, adjectives, adverbs) among the two subject groups. Here are two examples:

[13] Fish *school* in their communities . . . ("school" inappropriately used as a verb; example from a schizophrenic patient) (Hoffman & Sledge, 1988, p. 97)
[14] The Israelis and the Arabs need to know that they are part of a strategic area and are *located* to world peace (possible target is important/critical; example from a manic patient) (Hoffman & Sledge, 1988, p. 97)

The schizophrenic patients, however, made many more errors involving grammatical morphemes (prepositions, conjunctions, suffixes, etc.). The following are two typical examples:

[15] That was a decent thing*s* to do (schizophrenic speaker) (Hoffman & Sledge, 1988, p. 97)
[16] We could be wheelchairs (intended: we could be *in* wheelchairs; schizophrenic speaker) (Hoffman & Sledge, 1988, p. 97)

Moreover, there was a strong trend in the direction of more ambiguous deviance within the schizophrenic corpus. Included among this group of errors was a relatively large number of "syntactic blends," where distinct syntactic structures are inappropriately combined. For example:

[17] bring me happier (intended: bring me happiness/make me happier; schizophrenic patient)

One such instance precipitated a "neologistic" word, whose intended meaning can be decoded from its context:

[18] I guess we went upstate somewhere I don't know *wirth* white people (the speaker, again schizophrenic, was a black woman recounting a childhood memory of attending a summer camp away from her native New York City; intended utterance seemed to be a blend of: I guess we went upstate somewhere—I don't know *where*/I guess we went upstate somewhere—I don't know—*with* white people) (Hoffman & Sledge, 1988, p. 98)

These data clearly showed that the frequency of these linguistic abnormalities among schizophrenic speakers in no way approached that of classically "aphasic" speakers. Moreover, in all cases, grammatical deviance was readily traceable to ordinary speech intentions; therefore, Chaika's (1977) criterion for differentiating the errors produced by normal versus schizophrenic speakers on the basis of their (un-)decodability did not apply.

What then are the mechanisms of the more sporadic, decodable forms of schizophrenic language deviance identified by our study? First, our data suggested that schizophrenic speakers produce errors in slotting open-class elements into a syntactic frame. Instead of difficulties in finding the right slots, however, (as in the case of normal slips described by Garrett, 1975), these speakers seemed to demonstrate difficulties in elaborating the syntactic frame itself; this finding supports our earlier case study (Hoffman & Sledge, 1984). Second, deviant blends of disparate syntactic structures, another common type of error among the schizophrenics, suggest a process where alternative syntactic frames competed for expression. Thus, microgenetically speaking, these two types of errors may reveal two distinct stages of language production that can be disrupted in schizophrenia, the former being the elaboration of a single syntactic frame, with the latter corresponding to the selection of one of many alternative syntactic frames.

Certain types of language irregularities generated by schizophrenic patients do not fit into the previously stated microgenetic model. The model as described reflects *combinatorial* processes, that is, operations that map clusters of elements (words, phrases, clauses, and sentences) into syntactically organized strings. Errors involving the generation of individual lexical elements don't seem to involve combinatorial processes. Typical examples, once again, include;

[1] he is a *grassical* person (Hoffman & Sledge, 1984, p. 157)
[2] You have to have a *plausity* of amendments to go through for the children's code, and it's no mental disturbance of *puterience*, it is an *amorition* law. (Vetter, quoted in Chaika, 1982, p. 170)
[19] people *edumacating* themselves (Hoffman, 1986, p. 507)

Some of these errors may still result from combinatorial difficulties. For instance, the context containing example 1 indicates that the speaker was discussing how educated and intelligent her boyfriend is. This suggests that an underlying conversational intention of the speaker was something like the following:

[1a] He is a person who studies/enjoys the Greek classics. (Hoffman & Sledge, 1984, pp. 157–158)

The speaker may have been unable to elaborate this complex syntactic structure but instead could only realize the simpler:

[1b] He is a [adjective] person.

In this case, the nominal phrase, "Greek classics" would have to pushed into the adjective position, resulting in,

[1c] He is a [Greek classical] person.

which then becomes condensed into a single word,

[1] He is a grassical person.

Thus, it may be that the generation of certain nonwords by schizophrenics may be triggered by a primary difficulty in elaborating complex syntactic structures. On the other hand, it is doubtful that all paraphasic constructions generated by schizophrenics (see again example 2) are due to syntactic problems but stem from some loosening of restraints governing the combination of morphemes into words.

In addition to disruptions in sentence production, other stages of language production are commonly disrupted in schizophrenic patients.

## Discourse Organization in Schizophrenia

In general, cognitive planning has become an important topic in artificial intelligence and cognitive science and seems to be a key determinant that permit the individual to experience his own actions as goal directed and intentional (Hoffman, 1986). Cognitive plans ensure that actions taken up in sequence cohere according to overarching goals and subgoals and are consistent with the individual's beliefs. Along these lines, research in psycholinguistics and computational linguistics indicates that normally a speaker generates a particular kind of discourse plan that reflects the gist or intention of what he will say (Allen & Perrault, 1980; Cohen & Perrault, 1979; Deese, 1978; Hobbes, 1979; Kintsch & Van Dijk, 1978; Van Dijk, 1980).

This discourse plan is transformed into lower level representations such as syntactic units, which form the basis of sentences and phonetic strings (Arbib, 1982; Garrett, 1975; Hoffman & Sledge, 1984). Without this initial stage of language processing, the speaker could not use multiple sentences or clauses in a coordinated fashion to express a single, coherent "message" and thereby attain communicative goals. These discourse-planning processes generally occur outside the conscious awareness of the individual, although, at times, the speaker may be consciously aware before speaking of two or three key words that will figure into the discourse product.

Deese (1978) has discussed a particular model of discourse planning whereby abstractly represented propositions that compose a communicative intention are arranged into a hierarchically organized data set. Topical propositions occupy high nodal positions in the tree. Structural subordination within the tree occurs if the truth of one proposition is presupposed in order to discern the pragmatic sense of a second (dependent) proposition. This model of discourse-level organizational processes was formalized by Hoffman (1986). The rudiments of the model can be stated as follows: A text (either written or spoken) is experienced as coherent if the presupposition relationship imposes a complete "partial ordering" of the constituent statements of the text. In formal terms, *partial ordering* breaks down into two axioms. (Hoffman, 1986, p. 507):

I. For all statement pairs, $s_1$ and $s_2$ belonging to some text T, either $s_1$ presupposes $s_2$, or $s_2$ presupposes $s_1$, or there exists a third statement, $s_3$ in T such that $s_3$ is presupposed by both $s_1$ and $s_2$.
II. If $s_1$ presupposes $s_2$, and $s_2$ presupposes $s_3$, then $s_1$ presupposes $s_3$, i.e., transitivity holds.

This definition of *partial ordering* produces a "frame" that organizes the text. This "frame" is analogous to the syntactic frame that organizes a sentence; however, the elements slotted into a discourse "frame" are whole statements rather than single words.

A well-organized, multisentence discourse structure or "frame" can be illustrated with a speech segment that was produced by a 54-year-old woman hospitalized for depression (Hoffman et al., 1986, p. 833):

[10] Interviewer: Can you describe where you live?
Patient: Yes, I live in Connecticut. We live in a fifty-year-old Tudor house. It's a house that's very much a home . . . ah . . . I live there with my husband and son. It's a home where people are drawn to feel comfortable, walk in, let's see . . . a home that is furnished comfortably—not expensive—a home that shows very much my personality.

The overall message of the above segment is fairly obvious—the woman is extolling the virtues of her house in terms of how it reflects on herself as a person. This resulting discourse structure is illustrated in Figure 7.1.

Deese (1978) first proposed that the disorganization of schizophrenic speech can be traced to a deviation of propositional structures from a strict tree form (see also discussions by Chaika, 1981, 1982, of the schizophrenic's failure to subordinate propositions to topic, or to adhere to a discourse macrostructure, a term from van Dijk, 1980). As a result, the processing requirements of these texts would be markedly increased for speakers, and the experience of "looseness" or incoherence would accompany encoding

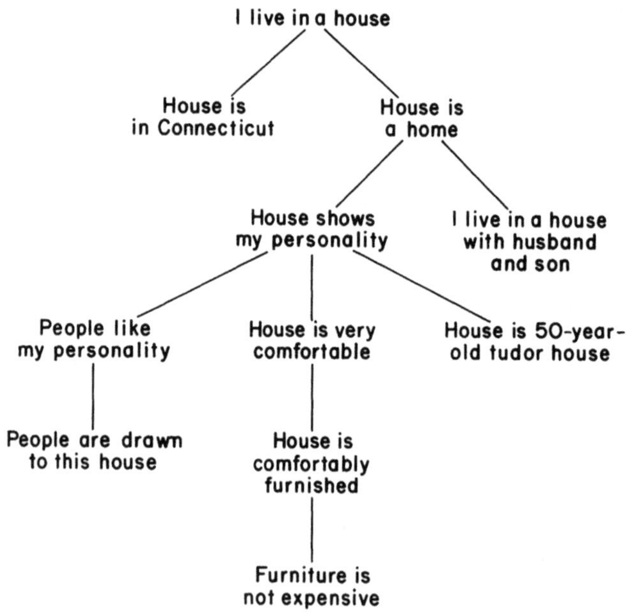


FIGURE 7.1. Hierarchical structure of coherent speech segment in which high level nodes connote main topic and subtopics. From "A Comparative Study of Manic Versus Schizophrenic Speech Disorganization" by R.E. Hoffman, S. Stopek, and N. Andreasen, 1986, *Archives of General Psychiatry*, *43*, p. 832. Copyright 1986 by the American Medical Association. Reprinted by permission.

efforts on the part of listeners. Using the formalization previously outlined for partial orderings, my colleagues and I devised a metric of textual deviance that reflects the degree with which the propositional structure of discourse departs from a strict tree form (Hoffman, Kirstein, Stopek, & Cicchetti, 1982). The simple presence–absence of nonhierachical discourse structure, blindly determined, differentiated schizophrenic versus nonschizophrenic speakers with 80% accuracy. Though a full description of the analysis is beyond the scope of this chapter, it can be illustrated with the following three schizophrenic speech segments (Hoffman, 1986, p. 507):

[21] Interviewer: Have you ever been out of New York?
Patient: No, I've never been no where—no where. . . . If I could go I would go . . . I feel like cashing in my welfare check now and just leaving . . . and I was gonna keep my—my two checks and save them and get an apartment. I wanna save them and just leave.
[22] Interviewer: Did you ever try to hurt yourself? (patient being asked about her suicidality after being admitted to a psychiatric hospital)
Patient: I cut myself once when I was in the kitchen trying to please David. I was scared for (sic) life because David didn't want me and if David didn't want me then no man would.
[23] Interviewer: Tell me about school?
Patient: School? Well there are schools of play and schools of fish, mostly you see fish school, people edumacating (sic) themselves, you see, sea is one thing and education is another. Fish is school in their community, that's why the community of man stands in the way of the community of the sea, and once they see the light of sunny sunshine then they well let it be . . .

For segment (21), the incoherence is due to the fact that "saving/keeping checks" has two different senses imposed by a shifting context—in the first case to provide money to leave New York and in the second case to provide money to stay. This corresponds to the deviant tree structure represented in Figure 7.2. Here the two separate chains of dependencies converge on the single saving–keeping money statement. As can be seen, presupposed statements corresponding to staying and leaving New York do not, in themselves, presuppose any third statement; hence this "upward branching" of presuppositional chains violates axiom I defining partial ordering.

Segment (22) also suggests a condensation of two disjoint messages. This is illustrated in Figure 7.3. The right-hand chain of statements describes a state of high stress of the type that might lead to suicidal behavior. This description substantiates the paragrammatical statement, "I was scared for life," which could be interpreted as "I was scared *of* life," or "I feared that my life was over." The left-hand hierarchy seemingly refers to an incident where the speaker accidently cuts herself. In this context, "I was scared for life" seems to refer to her reaction to seeing that she had accidentally cut herself. The result is a departure from a strict hierarchical ordering of statements, because statements such as "no man would want me" and

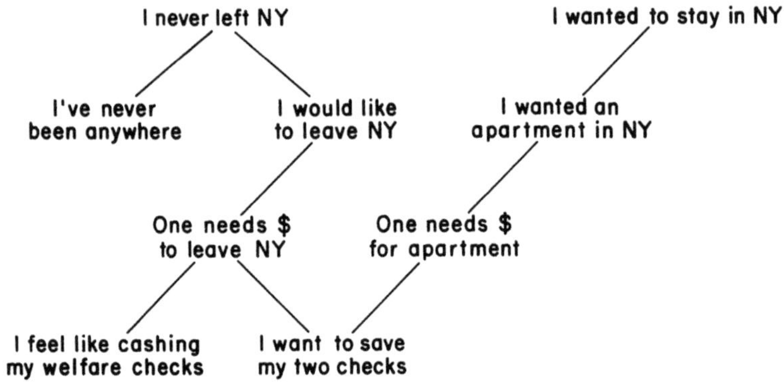


FIGURE 7.2. Hierarchical analysis of example 21. Two alternative presuppositional "chains" converge on the "I want to save/keep my checks" statements, imposing alternative readings. From "Verbal Hallacinations and Language Production Processes in Schizophrenia" by R.E. Hoffman, 1986, *Behavioral and Brain Sciences*, *9*, p. 507. Copyright 1986 by Cambridge University Press. Reprinted by permission.

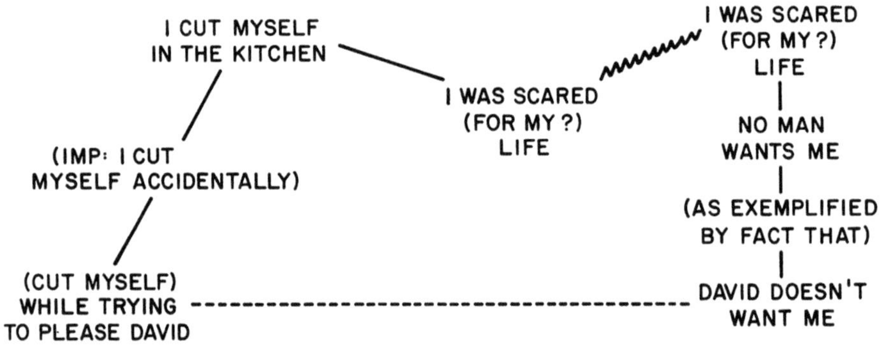


FIGURE 7.3. Hierarchical analysis of example 22. The jagged line connotes a break in presuppositional transitivity. On the one hand, "I was scared for life" seems to refer to a consequence of (accidentally) cutting one's self in the kitchen, presumably while preparing a meal. On the other hand, this statement corresponds to a general topic induced by the query about the patient's suicidal tendencies. As in example 21, a blending of two distinct communicative intentions can be appreciated. From "Verbal Hallucinations and Language Production Processes in Schizophrenia" by R.E. Hoffman, 1986, *Behavioral and Brain Sciences*, *9*, p. 507. Copyright 1986 by Cambridge University Press. Reprinted by permission.

"David doesn't want me" presuppose the "I was scared for life" statement and are referrable to the suicide theme but not the "I [accidentally] cut myself" statement. Thus, a break in transitivity of the presupposition relation (i.e., a violation of axiom II) occurs that is represented by a jagged line.

Segments (21) and (22), as mild discourse deviations, yield planning structures that condense disjoint messages corresponding to multiple statement hierarchies that deviate from any single communicative goal. On the other hand, segment (23) represents a practically total loss of hierarchical structure such that statements are juxtaposed primarily on the basis of word play and phonetic similarity.

Thus we can see a parallel when one compares problems in sentence construction among schizophrenics with their problems in generating multisentence discourse structure. In certain instances there was a partial degradation of structure: For sentence syntax, this was illustrated by examples 9, 10, 15 and 16, and for discourse structure this can be seen in example 23. On the other hand, schizophrenics, at both microgenetic levels, are also prone to produce blends of competing structures: At the level of sentence syntax, this was illustrated by 17 and 18 and at the level of discourse structure this was illustrated by 21 and 22.

Two comments can be made about this replication of error *pattern*. First, it is likely that the creation of structure (at either the sentence or discourse level) occurs, microgenetically speaking, before that stage when structures compete for expression. Thus, errors 9 and 10 occur at an earlier stage than 17 and 18, and the pathology underlying 23 occurs at an earlier stage in language production compared to 21 and 22. Second, whatever cognitive or neural pathology is active in altering language production in schizophrenia, it seems to be rather nonlocalized. Discourse planning—insofar as it involves "intentional" cognitive processes—probably occurs in prefrontal cortical areas closely associated with the supplementary motor area (Goldberg, 1985; MacNeilage, 1986), whereas syntax has classically been associated with the Broca'a area (Zurif & Blumstein, 1978). On the other hand, the fact that errors occurring at different levels demonstrate a common pattern suggests that the mechanisms whereby the neurocognitive pathology expresses itself at these different levels is similar.

Thus, a comprehensive microgenetic model of disruptions of language production in schizophrenia is suggested by these data. I will argue in the next section that this pattern of language disruption causes schizophrenics to have certain sorts of distorted experiences of communication processes which will lead to Schneiderian symptoms.

## Language Planning and the Will

Let us return to a question posed at the beginning of this chapter. How does the schizophrenic experience his own communication processes? I have argued that schizophrenics demonstrate difficulties in combining linguistic elements into larger structures. This results in two types of difficulties that are expressed at different microgenetic levels. The first consists in structural deficiencies, and the second consists in relatively well-formed structures that compete for expression. This pattern of deviance was noted to occur both at the level of sentence construction and when the speaker is attempting to combine multiple sentences into larger discourse structures. The latter corresponds to the formation of conversational intentions, that is, the crystalization of the "gist" of what the speaker has in mind to say.

Recall that the bulk of these combinatorial processes occur outside the speaker's awareness. We can choose, when speaking, to be aware of syntactic rules of sentence construction or, in a rough fashion, the interweaving of topics and subtopics of what we are preparing to say. In general, however, we are not consciously attending to these processes—by and large, we merely speak as we rely on our preconscious selection, combinatorial, and monitoring operations to yield acceptable utterances.

Recall also that, in general, the content of consciousness is quite "linear" or "one track." A simple example of this is the Necker cube (Rock, 1983). As we gaze at the Necker cube, we can appreciate that this figure offers two distinct perceptual "interpretations." However, at a given moment, we directly experience only one of those gastalts, followed, at a later time, by the other. Similarly, I would argue that, ordinarily, both the normal and schizophrenic speaker are able to be aware of only a single gestalt or message as they speak.

Try now to imagine what it is like to have one thing in mind to say, and instead, produce discourse that says something quite different. The closest most of us have come to this experience is when we generate slips of the tongue and other speech errors of the sort discussed earlier in the chapter. These errors generally seem motivated primarily by fatigue, phonetic similarity of exhanged elements, and the like. The error itself does not often express it own "message," unless, of course, one is undergoing a Freudian psychoanalysis and has received special training in interpreting the "meaning" of slips in terms of, for instance, Oedipal wishes. You may be surprised, irritated, or amused by the slip, but ordinarily it does not clearly say to you something that is distinct from what you had mind to say. But now suppose that, instead of a slip involving a word or two, the speech product included one or more sentences that not only were were inconsistent with what you had in mind (as in the case of ordinary speech errors), but expressed its own fully elaborated, coherent "message," a message that you did not have any prior awareness of.

This is precisely the experience that is predicted if the schizophrenic suffers from the *second* type of microgenetic language disturbance, that is a failure in (unconsciously) sorting out competing discourse intentions. This in turn produces a potential disparity between the "message" that is consciously registered in the mind as the intended speech act and what ends up expressed by a competing discourse plan.

An illuminating condition in neurology has been identified by Goldberg (1985). The supplementary motor area, as mentioned before, seems to be involved in higher level planning of sequential actions. Lesions involving this area of the cortex produce a very interesting syndrome in which the upper extremities, if unattended to, will wander out of control and seem to behave in a goal-directed fashion. For instance, the hand may attempt to unbutton the person's shirt. Individuals with this lesion, without prior psychiatric history, end up concluding that their hands are controlled by another person. It seems that the deciding factor in the creation of this "delusion" is that the hand movements were not random but purposeful, seeming to have their own "goals."

I believe that the schizophrenic suffers from a similar plight—in this case it is not his hand movements that seem purposeful, but his language productions that seem to have their own goal or expressive intention; similar to patients with supplementary motor area lesions, the results are experienced as being caused from nonself agents. This is an expectable inference insofar as discourse expressing messages that one did not have in mind to say is ordinarily produced by other speakers.

When a discourse-planning defect productive of multiple competing messages is operative, the schizophrenic will be prone to produce instances of extended speech expressing a message that he did not have in mind to say. Consequently, he may draw the conclusion that these manifestations derive from nonself-forces. In short, the schizophrenic is thrust into a realm of experience where the origin of speech intentions is thrown into question; it may be that the only confirmation that he is the one who is originator of the speech act is the proprioceptive experience of his own vocal musculature while he is speaking. He is likely to develop a variety of misconstrued beliefs (which to us seem bizarre, but to him quite reasonable) about the effectiveness of his own will and the willfulness of others.

These propensities may not simply apply to overt speech production but to covert, "inner" speech as well. Verbal images as "discourse to one's self" are a frequent component of human consciousness (Hoffman, 1986; Sokolov 1972; Vygotsky, 1962); there is good evidence that this talking to one self derives from the same processes as overt speech production, although certain phonetic and syntactic determines may be less fully elaborated (Vygotsky, 1962). If schizophrenics suffered from a failure in sorting out competing discourse plans, this failure, then, would also be expressed in their own inner speech. Under these conditions, the experience of inner speech, in essence, of one's own thought, could be extremely disconcerting if one experienced the intention behind the thought as alien. Once again, this would reinforce certain miconstrued beliefs as to the effects of an "alien will" that is operating on the self.

Particularly vivid manifestations of this type of language pathology are the verbal hallucinations or "voices" heard by schizophrenics. These patients often report hearing the voice of another individual who is either not present or if he is present isn't actually speaking to him. These experiences are highly prevalent among schizophenics and probably are the result of competing, discordant discourse plans. In essence, the microgenesis of this symptom would consist in the expression of a discourse plan that clashes with respect to the conscious discourse plan, thereby altering the experience of intentionality associated with the expression of that plan as inner speech, which in turn caused the unintended segment of inner speech to be experienced as if it were derived from another speaker, that is, that it had an external origin. An earlier study of a large group of schizophrenics, some of whom reported hearing "voices" and some of whom did not, demonstrated that the severity of the disturbance in discourse planning predicted which schizophrenics heard "voices" (Hoffman, 1986); those with more severe disturbances heard "voices." The hypothesized relationship between discourse planning disturbances and verbal hallucinations has received additional support more recently. My colleagues at Yale and I have developed a type of "language therapy" that is designed to enhance the ability of speakers to generate coherent, goal-directed discourse and to avoid blending together competing discourse "messages." Although still in an early phase of development, these therapeutic techniques—which are based on certain speech therapy techniques used with aphasic patients—have been used with two schizophrenic patients. In both cases, these efforts resulted in significant improvements in the patients' ability to produce coherent discourse and, at the same time, caused almost total elimination of the experience of verbal hallucinations. This inverse correlation of discourse-planning abilities and verbal hallucinations over time is precisely what is predicted by the aforementioned microgenetic model.

What about the reverse situation, namely, that the schizophrenic himself believes that he can magically communicate with others? While I do not have empirical data that directly examine this problem, I believe that our discussion provides a very reasonable explanation for this class of symptoms. The explanation can be proposed on the basis of the following three claims:

1. While the earlier discussion in this chapter deals primarily with language production, there is good reason to believe that pathological processes that effect language production also effect language comprehension (Ojemann, 1983; Zurif & Blumstein, 1978). If schizophrenics have difficulty generating and selecting alternative syntax structures and discourse plans, then it is likely that it will be harder for them to generate syntactic and discourse structures implicit in the speech of another.

2. A growing body of evidence indicates that the noise and indeterminacy of normal speech makes speech comprehension dependent on higher order expectations on the part of the listener about what the speaker is saying (McClelland & Elman, 1986). Although hypotheses about what the speaker might be saying are generated preconsciously by the listener, they are often required to "disambiguate" speech input.

3. The indeterminacies of ordinary speech spoken at normal rates,

coupled with probable difficulties that schizophrenic listeners have in generating syntactic and discourse structure implicit in speech inputs, make it highly likely that these patients will be less able to discern the gist of what a speaker is actually saying. This is supported by a study of subjective experiences of schizophrenics indicating that they frequently have considerable difficulty comprehending the speech of others (Freedman, 1974; Freedman & Chapman, 1973).

While the schizophrenic is "tracking" an utterance produced by another, his speech perception apparatus is attempting to generate a corresponding discourse plan—with the proper delineation of communication goals, topics, and subtopics—implicit in the speech of the other. Let us now assume that a schizophrenic is suffering from a discourse-planning deficit of the second type, that is, multiple, disparate competing discourse can be activated simultaneously. If claim 1 is the case, that is, the production of discourse structures involves the same processes and the detection of discourse structures implicit in external speech, then it is likely that the speech-perception processes for this patient will not only produce a trial representation of some discourse plan consistent with the phonological input of the external utterance but also will produce competing alternative discourse plans that derive solely from the the schizophrenic himself. Because the schizophrenic already has difficulties in processing external speech, he will be overly dependent on his own expectations and preconceptions to generate hypotheses about what the speaker is saying. Insofar as hypotheses and expectations can cause even normal individuals to misperceive speech sounds (McClelland & Elman, 1986), it is likely the schizophrenic will be prone to "hear" words and phrases that reflect his own ideas rather than what the other person actually said. He would then conclude that he was controlling what the other person was saying. In essence, he believes that the other speaker is saying what he, the schizophrenic, is thinking, because what the schizophrenic is thinking is the overriding context that "disambiguates" the intrinsic uncertainties of external speech and compensates for his own difficulties in structuring his speech input. The expectable result is that the schizophrenic would conclude that he can control what other people are thinking and saying.

Although this leg of my explanatory model remains untested, it is entirely consistent with my previous research (Hoffman et al., 1982, 1986; Hoffman & Sledge, 1984, 1988) of language disorders in schizophrenia. Overall, the model of schizophrenic symptoms presented here does not unpack the ultimate etiology of schizophrenia (see Hoffman, & Dobscha, 1989, and Hoffman et al., 1991, for one such hypothesis); however, it does take a first step in rendering comprehensible many of its most bizarre symptoms. It is, moreover, consistent with a growing body of research indicating dominant hemisphere difficulties in schizophrenia (for review, see Hoffman, 1986). Hopefully, the future will bring a greater convergence of cognitive, linguistic, and biological studies of this disorder.

## References


Allen J.F., & Perrault, C.R. (1980). Analyzing intention in utterances. *Artificial Intelligence, 15*, 143–178.

Arbib, M.A. (1982). From artificial intelligence to neurolinguistics. In M.A. Arbib, D. Caplan, & J.C. Marshall (Eds.), *Neural models of language* (pp. 77–94). New York: Academic Press.

Bleuler, E. (1950). *Dementia praecox or the group of schizophrenias*. International University Press. (Original work published 1911)

Chaika, E. (1974). A linguist looks at "schizophrenic" language. *Brain and Language, 1*, 257–276.

Chaika, E. (1977). Schizophrenic speech, slips of the tongue, and jargonaphasia: A reply to Fromkin and to Lecours and Vanier-Clement. *Brain and Language, 4*, 464–475.

Chaika, E. (1981). How shall a discourse be understood? *Discourse Processes, 4*, 71–88.

Chaika, E. (1982). A unified explanation for the diverse structural deviations reported for adult schizophrenis with disrupted speech. *Journal of Communication Disorders, 15*, 167–189.

Cohen, P.R., & Perrault, C.R. (1979). Elements of a plan-based theory of speech acts. *Cognitive Science, 3*, 177–212.

Deese, J. (1978). Thought into speech. *American Scientist, 66*, 314–321.

Fraser, W.I., King, K.M., Thomas, P., & Kendell, R.E. (1986). The diagnosis of schizophrenia by language analysis. *British Journal of Psychiatry, 148*, 275–278.

Freedman, B.J. (1974). The subjective experience of perceptual and cognitive disturbances in schizophrenia. *Archives of General Psychiatry, 30*, 333–339.

Freedman, B.J., & Chapman, L.J. (1973). Early subjective experience in schizophrenic episodes. *Journal of Abnormal Psychology, 82*, 46–54.

Fromkin, V.A. (1975). A linguist looks at "A linguist looks at schizophrenic language." *Brain and Language, 2*, 498–503.

Garrett, M.F. (1975). The analysis of sentence production. In G. Bowers (Ed.), *The Psychology of Learning and Motivation* (Vol. 9, pp. 131–177). New York: Academic Press.

Goldberg, G. (1985). Supplementary motor area: Review and hypotheses. *behavioral and Brain Sciences, 8*, 567–588.

Herbert, R.K., & Waltensperger, K.Z. (1980). Schizophrasia: Case study of a paranoid schizophrenic's language. *Applied Psycholinguistics, 1*, 81–93.

Hobbes, J. (1979). Conversation as planned behavior. In *Proceedings of the 6th International Joint Conference on Articicial Intelligence*, Tokyo.

Hoffman, R.E. (1986). Verbal hallucinations and language production processes in schizophrenia. *Behavioral and Brain Sciences, 9*, 503–517.

Hoffman, R.E., Buchsbaum, M.S., Escobar, M., Makuch, R.W., Nuechterlein, K., & Guich, S.M. (1991). EEG coherence of prefrontal areas in normal and schizophrenic males during perceptual activation. *Journal of Neuropsychiatry and Clinical Neurosciences*, in press.

Hoffman, R.E., & Dobscha, S.K. (1989). Cortical Pruning and the development of schizophrenia: A computer model. *Schizophrenia Bulletin, 15*, 477–489.

Hoffman, R.E., Kirstein, L., Stopek, S., & Cicchetti, D.V. (1982). Apprehending schizophrenic discourse: A structural analysis of the listener's task. *Brain and Language, 15*, 207–233.

Hoffman, R.E., & Sledge, W. (1984). A microgenetic model of paragrammatisms produced by a schizophrenic speaker. *Brain and Language*, *21*, 147–173.
Hoffman, R.E., & Sledge, W. (1988). An analysis of grammatical deviance occurring in spontaneous schizophrenic speech. *Journal of neurolinguistics*, *3*, 89–101.
Hoffman, R.E., Stopek, S., & Andreasen, N. (1986). A comparative study of manic versus schizophrenic speech disorganization. *Archives of General Psychiatry*, *43*, 831–838.
Kennedy, J.L., Giuffra, L.A., Moises, H.W., Cavalli-Sforza, L.L., Pakstis, A.J., Kidd, J.R., Castiglione, C.M., Sjogren, B., Wetterberg, L., & Kidd, K.K. (1988). Evidence against linkage of schizophrenia to markers on chromosome 5 in a northern Swedish pedigree. *Nature*, *336*, 167–170.
Kintsch, W., & Van Dijk. T.A. (1978). Toward a model of text comprehension and production. *Psychological Review*, *85*, 363–394.
MacNeilage, P.F. (1986). Bimanual coordination and the beginning of speech. In B. Lindblom & R. Zetterstrom (Eds.), *Precursors of early speech* (pp. 189–201). Oslo: Stockton Press.
McClelland, M., & Elman, J.L. (1986). Interactive processes in speech perception: The TRACE Model. In *Parallel Distributed Processing* (Vol. 2, pp. 58–121). Cambridge, MA: MIT Press.
Maher, B.A. (1974). Delusional thinking and perceptual disorder. *Journal of Individual Psychology*, *30*, 98–113.
Marr, D. (1982). *Vision: A computational investigation into the human representation and processing of visual information*. New York: W.H. Freeman.
Morice, R.D., & Ingram, J.C. (1982). Language analysis in schizophrenia: Diagnostic implications. *Australian and New Zealand Journal of Psychiatry*, *16*, 11–21.
Neale, J.M., & Oltmanns, T.F. (1980). *Schizophrenia*, New York: John Wiley & Sons.
Ojemann, G.A. (1983). Brain organization for language from the perspective of electrical stimulation mapping. *Behavioral and Brain Sciences*, *2*, 189–230.
Rock, I. (1983). *The logic of perception*. Cambridge, MA: MIT Press.
Schneider, K. (1957). Pramäre und secundäre symptome bei Schizophrenie. *Fortschritte der Neurologie, Psychiatrie und Ihrer Grenzgebeite*, *25*, 487–490.
Sokolov, A.N. (1972). Inner speech and thought. New York: Plenum Press.
van Dijk, T. (1980). *Macrostructures: An interdisciplinar study of global structures in discourse, interaction, and cognition*. Hillsdale, NJ: Lawrence Erlbaum.
Vygotsky, L.S. (1962). *Thought and language*. (E. Hanfmann & G. Vakar, Eds. & Trans.). Cambridge, MA: MIT Press.
Zurif, E.B., & Blumstein, S.E. (1978). Language and the brain. In M. Hale, J. Bresnan, & G.A. Miller (Eds.), *Linguistic theory and psychological reality* (pp. 229–245). Cambridge, MA: MIT Press.

# 8
# The Psycholinguistics of Microgenesis: The Nature of Paraphasia

HUGH W. BUCKINGHAM

The aim of the present chapter is to suggest that numerous significant correlations and connections exist between microgenetic theory and psycholinguistic theory and that Caplan perhaps overstated his case when he wrote that, "In Brown's case, the model of sentence production he proposed has no clear connection with any models proposed by psychologists working on normal language production" (1987, p. 138). If I am successful in what I am about to say, then Caplan's quotation will have been tempered somewhat.

The psycholinguistic model that I will use in this chapter to compare with microgenesis is that of Merrill Garrett. It is a model of sentence production and has been constructed on the basis of data from slips of the tongue (Garrett, 1975, 1976, 1980a, 1980b, 1990). Garrett has also shown how his model can be extended to characterize the breakdowns in aphasia (Garrett, 1982, 1984, 1988). Analyses of slips of the tongue and their use in the construction of models of normal language production have a healthy and vigorous status in psycholinguistics (Cutler, 1981; Fromkin, 1973, 1980). Slips of the tongue have also played a role in the search for evidence for linguistic theory (Fromkin, 1971; Stemberger, 1983), and researchers have long observed the correlation between the slips of normals and many of the errors made by aphasics (Buckingham, 1980; Cutler & Fay, 1978; Lenneberg, 1960).

The structure of the present chapter is as follows. First, I will briefly outline the components of Garrett's model; I will assume the reader is familiar with the microgenetic model (for a recent and brief review of Brown's model, see Braun, 1989). I will then make some general comments on parallel versus hierarchic models and on the relations between evolutionary reasoning and psycholinguistic reasoning. I will then attempt to map Garrett's levels and computations on the structure of the microgenetic model. I will subsequently go into more detail concerning the functional characterizations of paraphasias that stem from psycholinguistic inquiry and at each point will interrelate these with the functional characterizations that come from microgenetic models. Finally, I will treat message level pragmatics and the construction of intonational contours as they have been considered in the psycholinguistic and pragmatic literature, and I will try to place the phenomena involved into the overall picture of microgenesis.

## The Garrett Model: A Hierarchy

As can be seen in Figure 8.1, Garrett's (e.g., 1984) model is hierarchical in structure. I will now turn to a brief description of the computational processes that underlie the various representational levels in that system.

The message level representation is formed through diverse inferential processes, which serve as the "proximal" cause of sentence production. These inferential processes reflect (are constructed on) the speaker's current perceptual and affective stages and on his general knowledge of the world. That is, the message level representation will express what the speaker is committed to at the time of utterance. The conceptual formulation of the message level includes speech act encodings, which is to say that at this level the system determines whether what is said is a representative, a directive, a declaration, a commissive, or an expressive (Searle, 1969). Conversational implicatures (Grice, 1975) are appreciated at the message

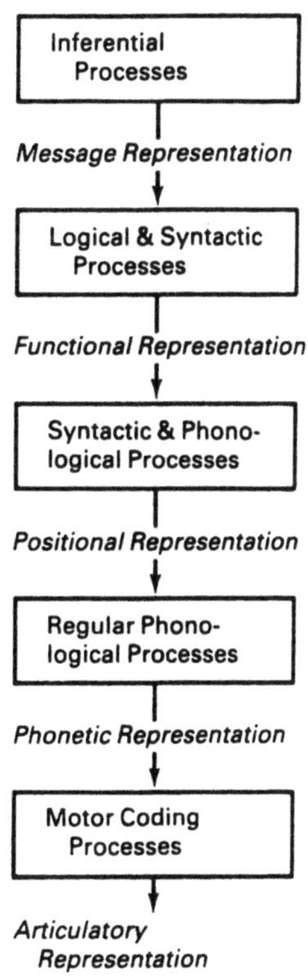


FIGURE 8.1. A schematic diagram of Merrill Garrett's model for sentence production. From "The Organization of Processing Structure for Language Production: Applications to Aphasic Speech" by M.F. Garrett in D. Kaplan, A.R. Lecours, and A. Smith (Eds.), *Biological Perspectives on Language*, 1984 Cambridge, MA: MIT Press. Copyright 1984 by MIT Press. Reprinted by permission.

level, and if, for example, an ironic or sarcastic or metaphorical tone is to drive the sentence production, that tone is formulated at the message level. This, of course, means that somewhere in the inferential processing the speaker acts on the so-called "cooperative" principle (Grice, 1975), whereby speakers can operate on the assumption that hearers "read between the lines" and can draw implicatures when conversational maxims are flouted. Message-level formulation also, and very importantly, includes the speaker's consideration of what will be "new" information for the audience and what will already be known to the audience, either through the immediate context (physical or linguistic) or though schematic knowledge in long-term memory. These processes also include the formulation of emphasis on some entity or event, which may already be known to the hearer. As will be discussed later, many of these processes are interlocked with the establishment of sentential intonation patterns. In sum, it appears that most of the so-called pragmatic information is constructed at the message level.

Various logical and syntactic processes subsequently operate on the message level in the construction of the functional level. The next few levels can be seen in more detail in Figure 8.2. Here, the computations involve the determination of the functional level structures and an assignment of lexical items to the functional structures. The lexical items that are selected and assigned positions at the functional level are appreciated in terms of their meanings only. At this level, form is not involved in lexical selection. The syntax here is logical and does not reflect utterance order—it is purely relational and is not unlike an atomic predicate–argument structure or a deep case structure (in the sense of Fillmore, 1968).

To be sure, the computations that map the functional level on the positional level are the most numerous and in many ways the most heterogeneous and intricate. It is at this level that utterance order is brought into play through the determination of surface-order planning frames, chunked into phrase-sized units that make up a clause. There are reasons to believe that in general the matrix establishing processes at this level construct at most one clause at a time. The planning frames come with intonation contours specified, and the slots are marked for the positioning of closed class morphemes, both free and bound. Lexical items (the contentives) are selected on the basis of their representative form and are assigned to their respective matrix slot.

Somewhere during the process of assigning the contentives to these slots, their segmental units are sequentially ordered for the utterance by mechanisms that operate on phoneme-sized units in syllabic patterns. One might rightfully ask why we need a second ordering, because presumably there is some order to the representative form that has already been accessed. Garrett (1988) argues that the positional level matrix frames are initially linked with functional level structures; recall that the lexical items there have not been evoked with respect to segmental information. At the

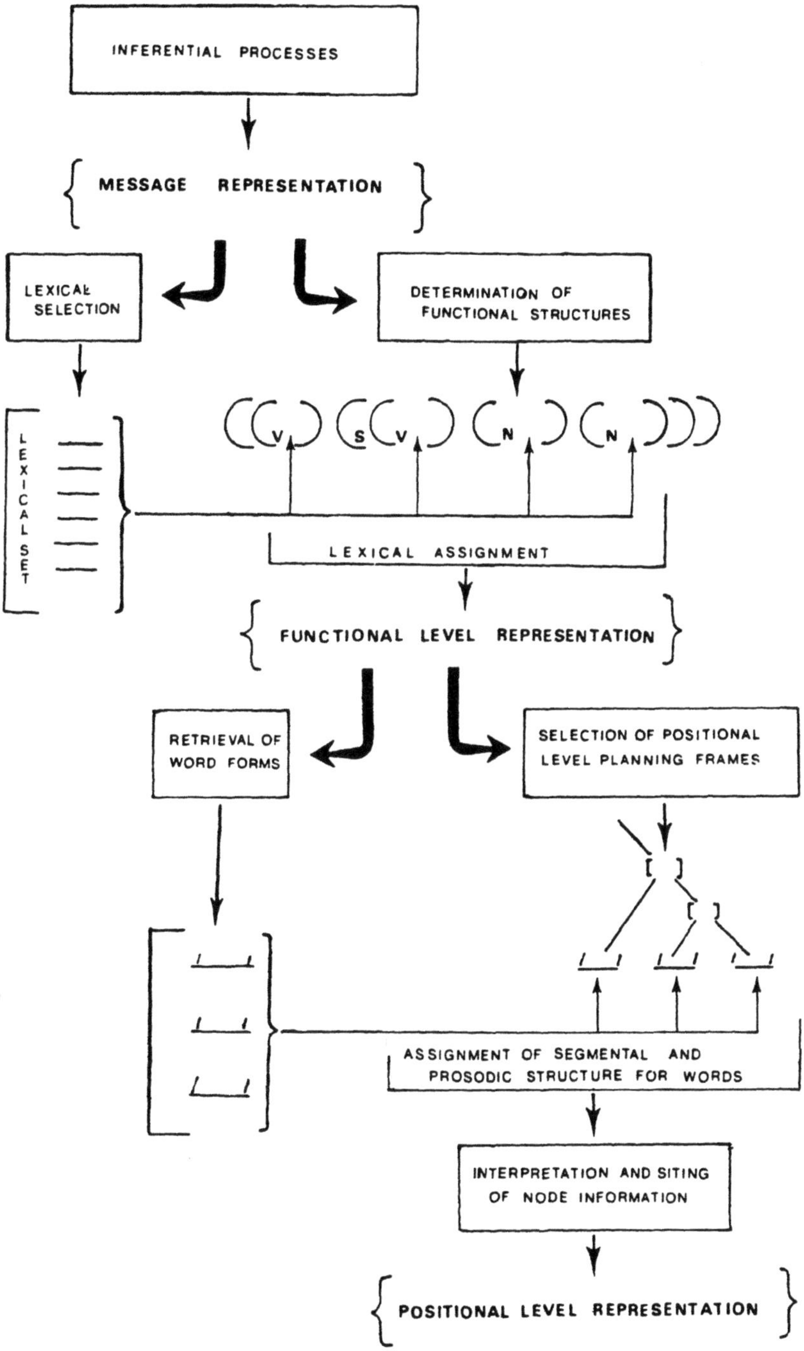


FIGURE 8.2. Successive assignment of lexical content to phrasal structures. From "The Organization of Processing Structure for Language Production: Applications to Aphasic Speech" by M.F. Garrett in D. Kaplan, A.R. Lecours, and A. Smith (Eds.), *Biological Perspectives on Language*, 1984 Cambridge, MA: MIT Press. Copyright 1984 by MIT Press. Reprinted by permission.

interface between these two levels, then, the segmental composition of the content words must be added or copied on awaiting syllabic templates, which can subsequently feed into motor–articulatory processes. This is essentially the argument of Shattuck-Hufnagel (1979) and of Keller (1987). The mechanism that orders the segments of the lexical items actually is conceived of as "copying" the segments on a productive order. That mechanism stems from the investigations of Stephanie Shattuck-Hufnagel (1979, 1983, 1987), and I have in several publications (Buckingham, 1980, 1983, 1985, 1987) suggested that they properly fit as additional computations that operate at the positional level in Garrett's model. Others have followed suit (e.g., Kohn, 1984, 1985, 1988, 1989; Schwartz, 1987). In a buffer memory system, the sequential orderer (Shattuck-Hufnagel's term is the *scan copier*) operates as it scans the lexical forms in the string (about the length of Garrett's phrasal frames). After a segment is copied on its productive order slot, it will be erased from the buffer by a mechanism that Shattuck-Hufnagel refers to as the "checkoff monitor." Although I cannot go into any detail at this point, I have (Buckingham, 1987, 1990a) suggested that well-motivated phonological constraints operate to condition the operations of both the scan copier and the checkoff monitor, ensuring that the vast majority of segmental errors conform to the morphotactic structures of the language in question. Finally, and still at the level of phonological readying, I should add that Brian Butterworth (1979) has suggested that in case any speaker is unable to retrieve lexical forms and, consequently, to impart any order to their segments by such operations as scan copying, a sort of backup system can produce phonological material to fill in the gap. Garrett (1982) has claimed that this would account for various types of glossolalia and other sorts of "nonce" forms, while Perecman and Brown (1981) and more recently Perecman (1989) suggest its use, or something like it, in order to account for what they call phonemic jargon. Again, I have placed this "random generator" of Butterworth within the computations that lead into the positional level representations (Buckingham, 1985, 1987). (I have gone into the preceding detail with these positional level phonological computations, because they will come up again later in my treatment of paraphasia within the microgenetic model.)

Finally, once the phrasal frames have been lexically determined, the functor morphemes (bound affixes and free forms) are assigned to their respective frame slots. In a very important sense, the computations that place content words in frame slots and the computations that place function words and affixes in the frames are distinct and separate sets of operations. In sum, the utterance order is more directly reflected in the positional level representation.

At the ensuing stage, the so-called "regular phonological processes" map the positional level on the phonetic level of representation. These processes are typically characterized as the "allophonic" rules of the language, the input to which are the phonemic-level segments of the positional level. According to Garrett (1980b), these computations are post-positional level. Therefore, any speech error (be it aphasic or a slip of the tongue) that involves derailments of positional level processes will be "accommodated" by the processes operating between the positional and the phonetic level. That is, if at the positional level, phonemes erroneously move to new phonological positions, their phonetic form will accommodate to that new position and likewise for morphemic units. An unaspirated *p* in the word *apple*, if it is erroneously scan copied onto the empty onset slot (which is empty because *apple* is a vowel-initial word), will be aspirated, because syllable-initial voiceless oral stops in stressed syllables are aspirated (e.g., *papple*). The process that imparts aspiration to voiceless oral stops in this phonological position is a "regular phonological process" and properly belongs to the set of computations at the phonetic level. Similarly, when morphemes shift in errors assumed to be at the positional level, their allomorphic realization is accommodated by these processes as well. For example, when the third-person singular, present-tense morpheme {−s} in "it certainly run*s* out fast" shifts one word to the right to "it certainly run out*s* fast," the shifted morpheme {−s} will be accommodated, and its proper allomorphic shape [s] (because it now comes after a /t/) will be produced. Had it not moved, the allomorph would have been [z], which is how the morpheme {−s} would be realized after an /n/.

The phonetic level of representation is then mapped onto articulatory representations by the "motor-coding processes" that account for all low-level coarticulatory specifications. Finally, the articulatory level of representations are mapped to the vocal tract articulators through actual motor commands to the musculature. In a natural way, this model claims that the lower in the system one is, the closer to articulatory reality one is. This, then, concludes the outline of the levels and processes that make up Garrett's model. Levelt (1989) provides an in-depth treatment of precisely this sort of production hierarchy from top (intention) to bottom (articulation).

Before discussing some specific correlations between the Garrett model and that of microgenesis, I will comment on Garrett's model in general and mention some very basic ways in which the two systems relate to each other. First, the model just presented is most definitely hiearchical in structure. As such, it may be claimed (and the claim is most often emphasized by its detractors, e.g., Stemberger, 1985) that the computations operate in strict serial fashion and that no interaction is allowed to work up and down the levels. The microgenetic model, as well, is hierarchic; the hierarchy following evolutionary, neuroanatomical phylogenetic growth of the language system up the neuraxis from bilateral depths to left, lateralized focal neocortex. Garrett's hierarchy is functional but hinges on a real-time sequence to productive operations. The brain, of course, is not involved. The sequential (and thus serial) nature of the operations falls in with the logic of the statements that describe what is going on. For example, the accommodation processes are quite properly viewed as having to "wait" for errors to occur at the positional level, because until those derailments take place, the proper input to the regular phonological processes cannot be specified. Likewise, it makes little sense to conceive of scan copying phonemic segments of lexical items if those segments are not in some sense first appreciated or apprehended on the basis of their forms.

Both the microgenetic model and Garrett's model, however, should not be considered as *strictly* hierarchical and serial. Note that the microgenetic view involves at the outset both serial processing and parallel processing. Within each axis (anterior and posterior), the system operates hierarchically, but both axes work in parallel as the processing moves upward and leftward. The parallel synchrony is assured through white fiber connections between the anterior and posterior systems as they operate. There is nothing inherent in Garrett's model to prevent a "cascade" type of processing, whereby lower level computations may initiate before *all* of the higher level processing is finished. That is, there may be more interaction in Garrett's system than one may imagine (see Buckingham, 1987, for a discussion of this point). This interpretation has been appreciated by many psycholinguists, the most recent being Giovanni B. Flores d'Arcais (1988, p. 114), who writes:

> Notice that the notion of interaction is not incompatible with the idea of specific processing at a given level. The question is whether interaction is restricted to the output of the processing level or is necessary for the processing at a given level.

Viewed this way, in Garrett's model certainly could include interaction involving the outputs of the computations at each level. In a sense, it would also be preferrable to have no interaction among the distinct sets of computations so that they could run on in a modular fashion: very fast and reflex-like, subject to their own operational principles, and in a sense, cognitively impenetrable. There is no reason why the *computations* at the functional level need to penetrate those at the positional level, for instance. Output interaction, however, is quite another issue.

The models of both Garrett and Brown appear capable of incorporating at least some degree of feedback. The reciprocity (not simply unidirectionality) in the neural connectivity of the microgenetic model (see Deacon, 1989, for a detailed account of connective complexities in anatomical structure and their consequences for microgenetic theory) could allow for feedback, while Garrett's model does not necessarily rule out feedback from lower outputs back to higher outputs.

In sum, then, both Garrett (e.g., 1988) and Brown (e.g., 1988) have constructed hierarchical models, which at the same time allow for various degrees of interaction, and cascading or parallel processing. Garrett's set of outputs, as distinct from the modular computations, and its possible cascading operation allow for this. The neuroanatomical connectivity of white fiber relay systems assures Brown's model of a great deal of non-gradiental interaction: corticothalamocortical, corticocortical, and corticostriatopallidothalamocortical loops, and so on. Functionally, and in terms of theoretical artificial intelligence, both these hierarchical systems of processes could be simulated on a von Neumann machine (serial/digital).

I have often claimed that Garrett's model fits the dictates of modern cognitive psychology in Fodor's (1983) terms (Buckingham, 1986). Fodor (1983, p. 29) claims:

> Contemporary cognitive theory takes it for granted that the paradigmatic psychological process is a sequence of transformations of mental representations and that the paradigmatic cognitive system is one which effects such transformations.

Consequently, Garrett's system could be simulated by a von Neumann machine with strictly serial processing of precisely locatable binary symbols. Boden (1989, p. 4) writes:

> Such concepts and associated theories may be termed formalist, since they assume that *computation* and *representation* necessarily involve symbol-manipulation defined in terms of formal rules.

Boden further describes parallel distributed processing (PDP) systems and models of the mind but ends up claiming that, in principle, all connectionist models can be simulated on a von Neumann machine (see also the essay by Hawthorne (1989) for comments to the same effect). To this extent, serial and PDP models share computational properties.

## Mapping Psycholinguistics to Microgenesis

In what follows, I will claim that the correlations I draw between psycholinguistics and microgenesis are all the more striking, because the development of the two models by Garrett (e.g., 1988) and Brown (e.g., 1988) has been carried out quite independently, and those models have been constructed from very different data bases: Garrett, with slips of the tongue; Brown, with aphasia and other neurogenic syndromes. Garrett's model is purely functional, while Brown's model specifies functions *plus* their presumed neuroanatomical substrates. Although Caplan (1987, p. 102) is certainly correct in his criticism that Brown often omits the necessary linguistic detail regarding functional characterizations, I believe one can in many instances roughly correlate the functions specified by Garrett, which themselves often leave the functional linguistic complexities unspecified, with those posited in Brown's microgenetic model.

In a very general, and quite obvious sense, one could begin to map Garrett's model on the microgenetic scheme by turning it on its head. That is, the higher levels and computations in the Garrett model generally are deeper in the cortex and essentially bilateral in Brown's model. As one goes down the model of Garrett, microgenetically, it can be said that one travels higher up the anterior–posterior neuraxis and toward the dominant hemisphere. In the dominant hemisphere, as one moves lower in Garrett's scheme, one gradually moves from generalized neocortex to more focal neocortex. After one arrives at the lowest levels in the Garrett model, which compute motor–articulatory functions, microgenetically, one is strongly lateralized to left, focal neocortex in the dominant hemisphere. To be sure, one must do some rearranging of Garrett's model at this point to square it with microgenesis.

To begin with, absolutely nothing in the purely functional Garrett model would divide the computational duties into posterior and anterior neocortical systems of the dominant and nondominant hemispheres. Here, we must split up the Garrett levels and computations into posterior and anterior regions. By the time the processing arrives at the positional level of function, we will have arrived at generalized neocortex in the left dominant hemisphere according to the microgenetic model. Therefore, positional level functions are left lateralized but must subsequently be divided as to temporoparietal or frontal function. For example, an integral part of the phrasal frame skeleton that is evoked at the positional level is the intonational contour, which is superimposed above the frame. According to microgenetic theory, formation of the linear scheme and sentence intonation are placed in generalized neocortical frontal regions and clearly separated from the posterior processes that are more involved in the selection and syntactic placement of the content words into the slots of the frames. Function words are more tightly alligned to the frame evocation, and therefore are assigned to the frontal lobe. Nothing at all in the Garrett model prohibits the separation of these various positional level computations into anterior and posterior functions of the brain for the simple reason that Garrett's model is not motivated by neuroanatomical factors. Again, it is purely functional. The idea, of course, in Garrett's scheme is that the whole operation is carried out in real time, but the physiology is left completely open. Although the positional level computations are tightly interlocked, they operate as independent sets of manipulations. Even though the positional level computations are parceled out into anterior and posterior systems in the brain, their functional interaction is physiologically assured through the white fiber connections. In this fashion, Brown's system is at once hierarchical, parallel, and nongradiental, in the sense of Goldberg (1989). The hierarchy is instantiated through the operations as they move from the depths to focal neocortex, while the parallelism is assured through the long white fiber system that hooks the anterior and posterior systems in a lattice-like structure. The positional level in the Garrett model is a pivotal one, and it contains many of the crucial phonological, morphological, and syntactic processes. In terms of the model of microgenesis, the various processes will map on either anterior or posterior systems in the brain. Thus, it would not be strange at all to see patients with anterior lesions or posterior lesions, or both, who reveal computational breakdowns at the positional level of function in Garrett model. In fact, it would be precisely what one would expect on a nongradiental view.

Microgenetic systems that comprise posterior–anterior lobe functional interaction appear to instantiate a nongradiental design, that does not necessarily have much functional–neuroanatomical isomorphism. A gradiental approach (Goldberg, 1989) to brain-function relations would prefer a design with a high degree of consistency between the spatial and functional properties of the cortex. With this sort of design, any two cortical regions will be functionally proximate only if they are spatially close. By showing that tightly related psycholinguistic functions in the Garrett model are neuroanatomically separate in Brown's model, I have demonstrated the essential nongradiental character of the microgenetic model. Goldberg (1989, p. 509) argues that the preferred system is gradient:

> A mosaic-interactive design of cortical organization is rather impractical, since it implies intensive interactions between neuroanatomically distant regions.

Goldberg (1989, p. 509), however, states:

> The adaptive wisdom of the brain . . . can be expected to follow the principle of spatial economy, which means adherence to the principle of functional-neuroanatomical isomorphism, and a continuous organization.

For the moment, at least, Brown and Goldberg appear to be at odds.

## Functional Characterizations of Paraphasia: Microgenesis Versus Psycholinguistics

### *Lexical Phenomena*

Close affinities exist between Garrett's scheme and microgenesis as they account for lexical and segmental language derailments. To begin with, both models clearly separate a level at which one appreciates the semantic underpinnings of lexical items with no recourse to phonological form. This level is functionally dissociated from the level at which words are appreciated in terms of their sound shapes. Few, if any, psycholinguistic models fail to distinguish what may be termed a first "lexical lookup" from a second "lexical lookup." For Garrett, the first lookup is exclusively meaning based and is computed at the functional level, while the second lexical lookup is computed among the processes that operate at the positional level. Again, and by independent inquiry, Brown makes what for all intents and purposes turns out to be the same claim (e.g., Brown, 1977, p. 36; Brown, 1982, p. 455). What I believe is significant is that distinct kinds of data led both these researchers to the same notion: Garrett, from slip data; Brown from aphasia. In addition, Brown's positing of two lexical lookups (semantic and phonological) is part of a more general claim that "language develops in the mind of a speaker like an object in perception." (Brown, 1982, p. 455). Brown's point is that before an object is fully perceived, the mind appreciates its meaning, that is, meaning before full form. This overriding principle obtains for language as well.

> Words develop out of a stage of meaning relations and strive toward referential adequacy. . . . These mechanisms correspond with systems of word meaning relationships in the preliminary stages of lexical selection. The representation of an object in perception and the representation of a word in a language are ordered by a common process. In perception, this leads from a stage of symbolic relations to one of form representation; in language, from a semantic operation to a phonological one. (Brown, 1982, pp. 455–456.)

The two models, however, differ somewhat. Brown (1977, 1982), for example, stresses the distinctions between "associative" semantic bonds among words and "categorical" bonds. So, for instance, somewhat bizarre lexical substitutions seen with bilateral lesions of the limbic connected medial temporal regions have been reported: "smoker" for *pipe*, "telescope" for *glasses*, and so on. Categorical bonds are involved with the more typical semantic field errors reported in the literature, items such as "chair" for *table*, and the like. Garrett, on the other hand, proposes a direct connection between the meaning appreciated word and the phonologically based appreciation in the form of a "linking address." This will ensure that the two lexical components match up ultimately and that the form selected will be that of the item previously appreciated by meaning only..

## *Segmental Phenomena*

At the segmental level, as well, striking parallels between Garrett (1984, 1988) and Brown (1977, 1988) are found. In general, most psycholinguistic models of production stipulate, in one way or another, that segmental manipulation takes place at the point where lexical items are being accessed on the basis of their shapes, those lexical items being the contentives. Most psycholinguistic models as well as microgenesis claim that functors are not selected by the same computations that select contentives. Furthermore, most agree that when functors are accessed for placement into planning frames, they are accessed as whole units and manipulated as such. Fromkin (1971) posits a stage whereby the phonological material of words is accessed from the semantic representation. At this level, the phonemic units are then selected and ordered for utterance preparation. Obviously, breakdowns here give rise to the myriad of segmental slips of the tongue that Fromkin analyzes. Although for Garrett, the linking address alluded to carries the phonological information for a semantically selected word;

nevertheless, after that form is selected, it must somehow be placed into a working buffer so that other selection and sequencing mechanisms can work on the structure of the word such that it is readied for production order. Shattuck-Hufnagel (1987), as well, claims that her "scan copier" operates on full phonological representative forms that have been placed into the working buffer. In addition, Caplan (1987, p. 227) has written:

For instance, the fact that phonemic paraphasias occurring in sentences affect mainly content words shows that they may arise at the stage of inserting the sounds of content words into sentences.

I suggested this myself, again drawing parallels between the stage at which phonemic paraphasias arise and the stage at which segmental slips of the tongue arise, combining the model of Garrett with the additional segmental ordering mechanisms that had just been proposed by Shattuck-Hufnagel (Buckingham, 1980). Recently, I should add, many have emphasized this stage of "phonemic string construction" as uniquely involved in the phonemic paraphasic derailments of conduction aphasia (see especially Kohn, 1984, 1985, 1988, 1989; Nespoulous, Joanette, Beland, Caplan, & Lecours, 1984; Buckingham, 1986).

Again, microgenetic models of language production lead to strikingly similar conclusions. Brown (1977, p. 39) writes:

[Phonemic disorders] point to a stage in the production of language at which the intended word, although it has been properly selected, does not achieve correct phonemic realization. . . . The disturbance primarily affects the content words.

For Brown, form selection and segmental manipulation are secondary to the computations that appreciate lexical items on the basis of their meanings.

Brown (1980) has been criticized (e.g., Caplan, 1987) for not being more precise regarding the linguistic complexities of the processes he addresses. For example, quite a number of distinct operations can derail in the processes involved in readying phonological segments for ultimate utterance order, many of which are captured through the mechanisms of the scan copier and the checkoff monitor.

The error may involve anticipation with or without addition of a segment and perseveration with or without addition of a segment. When the anticipated phoneme is actually added to the inventory of the lexical segments, a previously unfilled phonological slot would then be filled. With no addition, a substitution would be involved, but the source would be clear. Anticipated phonemes may or may not be deleted from their "home" environments. When they are not deleted from their original positions, of course, a "doublet" will have been formed (Buckingham, 1987, 1990a). The same latitude exists for errors of a perseverative nature. Rather significant syllable conditions serve to constrain phonological derailments. Syllable slot is usually sacrosanct. That is, except for intrasyllabic switches, syllable onsets move to onset positions, while codas move to other coda positions. In addition, the sonority principle of syllable structure (see Buckingham, 1987, 1990a) crucially constrains the nature of phonological derailments, this principle interlocking in interesting ways with the scan copier and checkoff operations. Brown, a neurologist, can certainly be forgiven for failing to carve out the complex edges involved in phonological processing.

The "linearization" problem (Levelt, 1989) deals with the issue of imparting serial order to strings of elements, which in their deep-seated encoding origins have no order. As Brown sees it (personal communication, 1989), serial ordering in its essence is tightly bound to the nature of psychological time (see Chapter 3). At the deeper levels of microgenesis, the segmental representation of lexical items, as with other kinds of objects and images, have no temporal order. Time and order are in some way inextricably fastened and exist at the deeper levels of Brown's model in some sort of simultaneity. For Brown, time order is established in depth-to-surface microgeny, and as part and parcel of time-order establishment, segmental ordering unfolds. To date, however, Brown has said very little about the intriguing relationship between processes of linguistic serial ordering and the nature of psychological time.

Garrett's early investigations and his initial depictions of his model also left out most of the details of phonological manipulation. It was the work of Shattuck-Hufnagel that began to concentrate seriously on the microstructure of segmental ordering, and in several publications I have tried to square her mechanisms with the overall model of Garrett (Buckingham, 1980, 1983, 1985, 1986, 1987), adapting and embedding them at Garrett's positional level (see Garrett, 1988, for further discussion). In any event, Brown and Garrett have much in common as concerns the stage at which the phonological *form* of contentives is appreciated and subjected to segmental copying—a stage that is clearly subsequent to semantic appreciation.

I should point out here that Kohn (e.g., 1988, 1989) makes a distinction between a phonological error (Wernicke's aphasia) and a phonemic error (conduction aphasia). By this she means that Wernicke's aphasics have a more severe problem accessing the phonological shape in order to submit that shape to the operations of mechanisms like the scan copier. In other words, Wernicke's aphasics have "deficient information about target phonemes" (Kohn, 1988, p. 110) as they exist in the underlying representative shape, and so, reasons Kohn, that representative string cannot be easily sought and placed into the operating buffer. For Kohn, to successfully reach the level of constructing phonemic strings, the lexical form in its representative shape must be retrieved and placed in the working memory so that scan-copying operations and the like can work on it, readying the segments for ultimate utterance order. It is the conduction aphasics who have more success in retrieving the representative lexical string for placement into the buffer. Only at this point does the conduction aphasic begin to have trouble, and consequently the conduction's phonemic paraphasias, according to Kohn, are more readily characterized as breakdowns with the Shattuck-Hufnagel–type (1979) mechanisms of selection and sequential ordering.

Kohn (1988) offers several pieces of evidence that seem to support this distinction between phonological (Wernicke's) and phonemic (conduction) errors. On naming, Wernicke's aphasics' errors exhibit fewer of the target phonemes than do those of conductions. Quite often, the phonemic substitution errors of Wernicke's aphasics appear to be more random, differing from presumed targets by many more than one distinctive feature. The Wernicke's patients have a hazier image (so to speak) of the underlying representative string, and therefore their errors will often have more randomly scrambled target phonemes. One wonders, however, just what is doing the scrambling if not something very much like a scan copier! A very important observation here is that the Wernicke's errors tend to disagree more than do the errors of the conduction aphasics in number of syllables. That is, the target word may have two syllables, while the error may have four or five. Conduction errors appear to agree more often in number of syllables with their targets. Another observation that Kohn claims supports this distinction is that Wernicke's aphasics tend to produce more neologisms. I have argued (e.g., Buckingham & Kertesz, 1974, 1976) that neologisms quite often appear to adumbrate a more or less complete lexical form-access breakdown. Of course, to account for the phonological material that nevertheless *was* produced by the patient, I had to make recourse to either perseverative/anticipatory processing of the material in the immediate context of the utterance or to some sort of random generator (Buckingham, 1981; Butterworth, 1979) that could produce phonological material when nothing was forthcoming from the lexicon.

The only problem here, of course, is that neologistic forms have been observed in certain cases of conduction aphasia (Benson et al., 1973). Case 2, in that clinicopathological study, presented with a severe naming disturbance, " . . . most of the errors being caused by literal paraphasic contamination, often so excessive as to be considered neologistic" (Benson et al., 1973, p. 343). If this patient was truly a conduction case, then this would be a problem for Kohn (1988). There is some reason, however, to doubt that Case 2 was anything like a true conduction aphasic. First, he had many verbal paraphasias, and his lesion involved the entire cortical region of Wernicke's area and the subcortical white matter subjacent to Wernicke's area. His naming was not helped by cuing, which it should have been, as will be discussed if the patient was a typical conduction aphasic. Evidently, what made the authors claim that this patients was a conduction type hinged on their observation that "Comprehension was tested repeatedly, by many examiners, and was always found normal" (Benson et al., 1973, p. 343). The gnawing possibility, however, of a right hemisphere function for comprehension in this patient certainly exists, because the authors point out that he did have one daughter who was strongly left-handed. This observation should have been followed up by the authors, because that left open the possibility that Case 2 was a Wernicke's aphasia but with comprehension mediated in the nondominant hemisphere. Unless the authors can rule this out, they cannot be sure that Case 2 was a true conduction aphasic, and consequently the neologisms would be those of a Wernicke's aphasic.

It has also been observed that Wernicke's errors do not reveal "Tip of the tongue" (TOT) information in their errors. This, of course, relates to the previous observation that for Wernicke's, there is much less agreement on number of syllables between errors and targets. Nor do Wernicke's aphasics appreciate phonemic cuing from the examiner. One other important difference between these two types of paraphasic disorders is the behavior of Wernicke's aphasics and conductions in *conduit d'aproche* situations (see also Joanette, Keller, & Lecours, 1980). It is more often the case that when patient with Wernicke's aphasia make several attempts to produce a target, their attempts get further from the targets as they proceed, while conduction aphasics seem to get closer to the target representative shape with their attempts. The claim, of course, is that the conduction aphasics have a better hold of the target item and can keep it more clearly in mind as they try to produce it correctly across several attempts. The study of the *conduit d'aproche* can be quite revealing in this respect. In sum, there is no doubt that different aphasics may reveal greater or lesser degrees of initial form appreciation (which will, in any case, be subsequent to semantic appreciation) of the underlying representative lexical string of phonemes and that this disparity will correlate with different types (both qualitative and quantitative) of segmental paraphasic productions.

## *The Two-Stage Error*

The sequential separation of the two lexical lookups allows for the characterization of the so-called "two-stage error." It is a logical consequence of both the Garrett (e.g., 1980a) and the Brown (e.g., 1972, 1977) models that there could be a semantic selection error, which subsequently undergoes a phonemic error as well. The idea is an old one, going back at least to the work of Arnold Pick—work that no doubt influenced Brown's thinking early on (note that Brown in 1973 published his own translation of Pick's 1931/1973 book *Aphasia*). Although the two-stage error type would not of necessity produce a neologism, most forms undergoing this combination likely would appear neologistic to the hearer if for no other reason than that the word that was placed into the buffer for scan copying was an error itself and likely to be somewhat out of context to begin with (this is more fully discussed in Buckingham & Kertesz, 1976). One small scan-copy error could therefore be enough to render the actual target word unrecognizable. The two-stage error, however, can only be further analyzed within the context of the elusive nature of the neologistic paraphasia.

## *The Elusive Neologism*

To begin with, Brown (e.g., 1977) generally admits of two basic interpretations for neologistic production. In mild cases, he claims:

> The neologism probably consists of a normal underlying word frame that is distorted to the point of unintelligibility by phonemic paraphasia.

This has come to be known as the "conduction" theory of neologism (see Kertesz & Benson, 1970, and a commentary on that paper in Buckingham, 1977). In the Garrett model, this account of the neologism would place the breakdown with the scan copier and the like, because the error nevertheless "consists of a normal underlying word frame." Presumably, a normal underlying word frame would at least make it to the operating buffer for subsequent segmental selection and sequential ordering. A problem, however, would occur for Kohn's (1988, 1989) scheme that was outlined previously. Her model seems to disallow neologisms as coming from the level of string construction, but we are forced to that position in following Brown's reasoning—and that of many others, I might add. For the same reason, Kohn seems to be claiming that we will not get neologisms with conduction aphasics. She could, however, easily incorporate the explanation in her model by simply allowing for some cases for which severe disruption at the level of string construction would yield unrecognizable and bizarre forms.

The two-stage error is the second principal interpretation of the neologism for Brown. Almost 20 years ago, Brown (1972, p. 62) wrote that "neologistic jargon is a phonemic distortion of severe verbal paraphasia." More recently, Brown (1977, p. 43) has cautiously written:

> Although the position of neologistic jargon in the aphasias is uncertain [indeed!], there is evidence that, at least in the most florid cases, it may represent a combination of semantic jargon and phonemic aphasia [by which Brown meant "conduction aphasia"]. In such cases, semantic paraphasias would be produced that would not achieve correct phonemic realization, the result being a phonemic distortion superimposed on a semantic paraphasia.

Other contemporary aphasiologists have held this view as well (Lecours & Lhermitte, 1972; Luria, 1970). Again, the seeds of this notion can be glimpsed at least as far back as Pick (1931/1973). There, Pick provided quite modern descriptions of verbal paraphasia and of phonemic paraphasia (which he termed, as did many in the past, *literal paraphasia*). As mentioned, Pick was well aware of the relationships of aphasia and slips of the tongue and referred directly to the work of Meringer and Mayer (1895/1978). For Pick, literal paraphasias, as well as slips of the tongue, could be characterized as "anteception" (anticipation, a right-to-left misordering), "metaception" (metathesis or exchange), "postception" (a left-to-right misordering, not considered perseveration), and "paraception" (substitution). To these Pick added, "contamination" (possibly blending) and perseveration. For Pick, "disinhibition" was the overriding cortical abnormality that lead to perseverations—both verbal and phonemic. On the two-stage possibility, Pick (1931/1973, p. 57) writes:

> The not infrequent mixture of verbal and literal paraphasia presumably corresponds to the simultaneous occurrence of disinhibition in both stages in question.

The problem with disinhibition for Pick (1931/1973) works differently for verbal paraphasias and literal paraphasias. For verbal paraphasia, the normal network links among related words are somehow "loosened up." The disrupted coherence among the lexical associations is not strong enough to normally suppress (disinhibit) other words that are evoked by semantic sphere links, thus leading to the ultimate production of the verbal paraphasia. Literal paraphasia stems from a disruption of the normal guiding role of acoustic information that is involved in the selection and sequential ordering of phonemes. The combination of verbal and literal paraphasia for Pick, therefore, represents a serious breakdown that leads to jargon aphasia.

Recovery patterns are often cited as support for the two-stage error characterization for neologisms. The use of reasoning on the basis of recovery patterns goes at least as far back as Pick (1931/1973). First, it is claimed that verbal paraphasia indicates some sort of "amnestic" syndrome, that is, anomia. Then it is claimed that in later stages of recovery, once the phonemic paraphasic component of the neology has subsided, the amnestic syndrome is revealed, initially, perhaps, with unencumbered lexical substitution errors but then eventually with only the vestiges of the halting and hesitating speech of an anomic. This is the picture we see in Pick (1931/1973) and in Kertesz and Benson (1970). The point is that arguments from recovery phenomena stem at least as far back as Pick. In sum, the models from psycholinguistics and microgenesis are easily motivated to handle the two-stage error and thus the neologism thereby produced. In fact, Pick's work can easily be classified as early psycholinguistics, although Pick is rarely cited in the current psycholinguistic literature on language production. This affinity between Pick and Brown further highlights the points of contact among microgenetic and psycholinguistic models of language production.

## *The Random Generator*

The issue of the elusive nature of the neologism requires further comment on the nature of a random generating device that can place phonological material into the language-productive process when the phonological material of lexical representations cannot be accessed at all.

After it appeared that some neologisms may not have been spun off some underlying target, the question then became, "What is the origin of the phonological material that constituted the neologism?" What reason was there to suspect that some neologisms might not reel off a target word through phonemic paraphasia? First, Kertesz and I (Buckingham & Kertesz, 1976) noticed that a qualitative break in paraphasic forms appeared to occur in neologistic jargon aphasia: those bizarre productions that appeared to have no relation at all to any conceivable target (given the context) and those phonemic paraphasias for which targets were relatively easy to discern. This led us to suspect that a qualitatively different component might be at work, producing many of the bizarre looking neologisms (now referred to as "abstruse," Lecours, 1982, p. 235). The notion of some sort of distinct error mechanism for the abstruse neologism often fails to be considered, and in many cases, this is because certain researchers, unwittingly or not, seem to be under the impression that the bizarre neologism and the phonemic paraphasia simply rest on a continuum of severity. For example, those who hold to the previously mentioned "conduction theory" of neologisms are likely to claim that neologisms arise from numerous phonemic paraphasias, while "literal" paraphasias arise from only a few. The difference, therefore, would be merely quantitative. Butterworth (1979) found an important qualitative difference between the bizarre neologisms and the simple phonemic paraphasia (which he, somewhat unfortunately I believe, referred to as a "target-related neologism"). The difference he observed was that immediately preceding the production of the abstruse neologism, the patient exhibited significant pause or hesitation, as if he were searching the lexicon for the representative shape of some target word. After approximately 250/ms or more, the neologism was produced, presumably after an unsuccessful search. He observed no pauses before the phonemic paraphasias or, for that matter, before semantic paraphasias. Butterworth, therefore, postulated that a random generator was capable of producing the material that made up the neologism.

I (Buckingham, 1987, 1990b) reviewed the evidence for postulating a mechanism of this sort and suggested that Butterworth did not necessarily claim that this mechanism was some mysterious cognitive component that was set up as a result of the lesion, but rather that it was simply a metaphorical description for what otherwise was simply the knowledge speakers have of their phonological inventories and the syllabic structural conditions that are obeyed when units of those inventories are concatenated—knowledge that is separated from the lexical inventory of the language and therefore knowledge that can be called on in one or another instance, when lexical forms cannot be accessed or are not specifically needed. Glossolalic behavior, the occasional production of a nonsense form on request, and the production of "nonce" forms have been suggested as other productions of the random generator (Garrett, 1982, p. 72) I further claimed (Buckingham, 1987) that the phonemic jargon described by Perecman and Brown (1981, 1985) and, more recently, Perecman (1989) may very well emanate from this sort of productive mechanism, which nevertheless must be dissociatable from the stock of lexical representations of the language and therefore can be called into action independently of the lexicon. Perecman and Brown (1981) go so far as to say that phonemic jargon allows one to study the sound structure that is provided from "a linguistic network" where there is no systematic correspondence among sounds and meanings. My claim is that their "linguistic network" is instantiated by the random generator. (Please consult Buckingham [1987, 1990b] for more detailed discussion concerning the evidence for a random generator.)

In some recent work, I have shown where the random generator might fit into the production model of Garrett (Buckingham, 1985, 1986, 1987). In these studies, I suggested that this mechanism is best understood to operate at the positional level, where it would fit among the second lexical lookup processes that provide the representative phonological shapes of words to the buffer. When a patient fails to access a word from the lexicon at the second lexical lookup, the random generator would be able to supply material at that point, and the production process could proceed. Some additional evidence suggests that the random generator provides its material to the buffer and that from there on the scan copier and checkoff monitor work as usual. Neologisms must have their segments sequentially ordered as well, and the neologism must obey the phonotactics and other syllable properties of the language in question. This is best left to Shattuck-Hufnagel's (1979) mechanisms. Note, too, that there can be typical segmental ordering errors on neologistic material as well, so that, as reported in Buckingham (1987), an initial neologism such as *frabeiber* can subsequently show up as *fabreiber*, with the /r/ transposed.

Although, for the reasons stated, Brown's model of microgenesis needs recourse to a phonological productive system such as the random generator, it is not clear yet in his system where such a mechanism would fit. Nor is it clear precisely where it would operate in his microgenetic scheme. It would necessarily be at a segment-producing level, but it is not clear that the lexical and semantic levels would have been traversed in the normal scheme that Brown proposes. In the microgenetic system, the semantic system usually has been traversed, and the phonological shape (in its abstract form) usually has been accessed before phoneme units can be manipulated. The random generator, however, seems to be able to swing into action at different points in the production. For neologisms in neologistic jargon, the claim would be that the patient has indeed traversed lexical lookup 1, because in many cases (again, see Buckingham, 1987, for details), although a neologism is produced, the patient apparently often has the meaning in mind. For Brown's phonemic jargon, on the other hand, it does not appear that the patient has traversed the semantic level (i.e., lexical lookup 1). In any event, more work needs to be done to establish where and how a random generator could interact in a microgenetic model of language production.

Finally, I will turn to a little-explored area in Brown's microgenetic model—message-level pragmatics and sentential intonational contours.

## Message Level: Intonational Links

Subsequent to the pioneering work of the British linguist M.A.K. Halliday (e.g., Halliday, 1970), it has been known that a very important aspect of a speaker's message-level planning is the computation of what is called the "information structure." This structure is divided up into what the speaker considers to be the given information, which the hearer should already know or be readily able to access, and the new information, which will be new to the hearer—otherwise there would be no information in the message. As Halliday claims (1970, p. 162), "In English, information structure is expressed by intonation." According to Halliday's scheme, speakers must include in every tone group (most often coextensive with the clause) a unit of new information, phonologically marked by the tonic pitch movement. On Halliday's account, the establishment of what is given and what is new is determined by the speaker. Although not in complete accord with any one of them, Yule (1980) summarizes various definitions of "given." (1) The given is offered as recoverable by what has been presented earlier in the linguistic text or by what is in the situation of the discourse. (2) The given information is in a sense a point of contact between the speaker and the hearer. (3) Given information is most often that which the speaker can assume to be present in the hearer's consciousness at the time of speaking. In terms of psychology and artificial intelligence, (4) given information serves as an "address" directing the listener to the memorial location where the new information is to be integrated and stored. Although it is often the case that material in the preceding discourse will have established given information, this does not necessarily have to be the case. As Yule (1980, p. 284) writes, "The speaker's decision regarding what he treats as given is made as he proceeds to speak and need not be determined by what has already been said in the discourse." Above all, however, what is to be given and what is to be new is a "product of the speaker's intentions" (Yule, 1980, p. 284).

It is invariably the case that the new information structure is marked by either high pitch (high Fo) or by a major movement of pitch (usually in the direction of low to high). Yule (1980), however, points out that although new information correlates with high pitch or with extended pitch movement, so do such items as contrast, emphasis, redirection of the hearer back to a topic previously mentioned, or, for whatever reason, focus on certain given elements. It cannot be denied, however, that the perceptual prominence of high pitch or major pitch movement will better ensure that hearers "get the message." Acoustic prominence of this sort is communicatively advantageous, because the major points of information that the speaker wishes to impart to the hearer will thereby be perceptually enhanced, consequently increasing the likelihood that information can be transmitted.

Having now established message-level–intonational links, let us consider the microgenetic model. Deep in the cingulate gyri (bilateral limbic cortex) of both hemispheres, a sort of primitive, oscillatory–rhythmic pattern is generated. For Brown (1982, p. 453), "The most primitive level in this structure is that of a 'motor envelope.'" It links vocalization with general body motility and is related to respiratory rhythms. This deep, bilateral rhythmic base frequency feeds into the generalized neocortical level at the next stage of microgenesis, where it unfolds into the actual speech rhythm or intonational pattern (Brown, 1982, p. 454). We witness here the microgenesis of "the rhythms of dialog" (Brown, 1990, p. 204). In contradistinction to the bilateral, limbic "motor envelope," we now have the generalized neocortical intonational contour (Brown, 1988, p. 58). Therefore, at this intermediate microgenetic stage in the anterior system, intonational patterns arise. There has been some confusion in the literature as to just where Brown places the computation of sentential intonational contours (e.g., Caplan, 1987, p. 102; Caplan, 1988, p. 245). The frontal neocortical region is the anterior way station between the primitive oscillatory motor envelope and the focal neocortical level of sound sequencing, and it is here rather than in the bilateral cingulate gyrus that Brown locates sentential intonation. More recently, Brown (1988, p. 298) writes, "This deep rhythmic structure is derived through left generalized (premotor) cortex to an oscillator elaborating the speech melody." Therefore, sentential intonational contours are more directly tied to the "speech melody" than to the "motor envelope" out of which they develop.

Brown (e.g., 1988) gives little, if any, attention to message-level pragmatics, either functionally or neuroanatomically, but apparently, the conversational pragmatics would have to be tightly linked to Fo manipulation, if we are to account for the previously mentioned phenomena of information structure, high pitch, and major pitch movement. It is not known yet *how* they are linked in Brown's model or in any other model for that matter.

At the outset, these two linguistic functions appear to be strange bedfellows: high-level semantics and suprasegmental phonology. Nevertheless, in the microgenetic view, sensory posterior systems link to motor–phonological anterior systems through white fiber tracts, thereby allowing "seemingly disparate performances" to share a common basis. He makes this point while contrasting speech perception (sensory) and inner speech (motor), but in general the argument holds for most of the anterior–posterior-linked performances (Brown, 1982, p. 461). This point would have to be considered if the message-level function is determined to belong to the posterior system.

At this point, however, it is not clear where Brown would place message-level function. In general, the posterior regions are semantic for Brown, but his emphasis is usually restricted to lexical semantic systems. Again, he says little if anything concerning what has been referred to here as given–new information structure.

Two problems therefore must be solved. First, is the message-level system that handles given–new pragmatic information and that therefore controls intonational contours to be located within the anterior or posterior axis in Brown's (1988) model? Second, is the message-level function deep and bilateral, or is it more likely to be localized in the intermediate level of the generalized neocortex? Crosson, Novack, and Trenerry (1988) and Crosson (1985) claim that language formulation is a function of the anterior cortical language zones (inferior frontal, opercular, and insular). High-level language planning and formulation, however, could be the product of much larger ranges of frontal cortex, which, of course, has massive connections with subcortical structures. Damasio (1985) has shown that damage to the dorsolateral region of the frontal lobe most often impairs high-level cognitive abilities, such as extracting meaning from ongoing experience, planning elaborate verbal responses to complex questions, and planning future actions in general. Further, he points out that the impairments are more dramatic and more permanent with bilateral lesions. If message-level planning could rightfully be considered to be a part of these higher level cognitive systems, then one could place them among frontal lobe functions, and they could interact with the establishment of the "speech melody" there.

Concerning the production of intonational patterns, there seems to be some evidence that would conflict with Brown. Note first, that in the microgenetic model, intonational patterns arise from the deep, primitive, and bilaterally produced "motor envelope" but only unfold as a meaningful linguistic structure at the generalized neocortical level. This, in turn, implies that the function is left lateralized. Foldi, Cicone, and Gardner (1983) report that right-hemisphere–damaged patients show impaired production contours. They note that these patients often reveal "flat" intonational contours or intonation "lacking in emotion." This production abnormality might be linked with other studies reported in Foldi et al. (1983), which indicate various types of pragmatic breakdowns in nondominant-hemisphere–damaged patients (also see Joanette, Goulet, Ska, & Nespoulous, 1986). Right-hemisphere–damaged patients reveal problems with appreciating indirect and nonliteral language, with inferring, and with processing humor and various emotional nuances. Gardner, Brownell, Wapner, and Michelow (1983, p. 173) write as follows:

Although less intimately involved with the traditional building blocks of language, the right hemisphere seems pivotal in the processing of extra- or paralinguistic facets of language—facets which contemporary students of language would designate as part of pragmatics or the discourse function of language.

It would certainly not be unreasonable to expect that these same patients would have difficulties keeping the hearer's point of view clearly in mind, which would subsequently lead to a failure to manipulate the information structure of their messages such that the given and new material would be correctly packaged for the hearer. In any event, the fact that so many pragmatic level functions seem to be vulnerable to right-hemisphere damage may indicate that these kinds of abilities would be deep and bilateral in the sense of Brown's microgenesis. The "flattened" intonational contours of the right-hemisphere–damaged population (see also Behrens, 1989) may also argue that crucial aspects of Fo control may still be under the influence of lower, anterior "motor envelope" function. In fact, Brown (1983, p. 41) "rethinks" many right-hemisphere syndromes along the lines of microgenetic theory and claims:

> . . . can all be explained by a theory of perception in which the parietal lobe (presumably deep in the lobe—HWB) of the right *and left hemisphere* (underlining mine—HWB) forms a *unitary* system indicating a preliminary stage in perception.

So, in microgenesis, message-level pragmatic control of Fo would be deep and bilateral and probably in the posterior system—hooked as it were with the anterior processing of rhymicity in its phonological makeup.

Another complicating factor is that Wernicke's aphasics have been demonstrated to exhibit inappropriate alteration of intonational patterns (Danly, Cooper, & Shapiro, 1983). Their Fo declinations ranged over much shorter syntactic domains than normals. These patients presented with an inability to maintain a single Fo pattern over normally integrated syntactic constituents. It appeared that the intonational abnormalities correlated with difficulty in processing syntactic structures. So, perhaps the Wernicke's problem with Fo is secondary and is a consequence of disrupted syntactic computation. Broca's aphasics, on the other hand (Danly & Shapiro, 1982), actually had better control of intonational patterns than had originally been thought. They exhibited some degree of abnormality, however. Sentence-final Fo fall was normal, and general Fo declination was normal over simple sentences but was absent over larger and more complicated syntactic domains. So, for patients with Broca's aphasia as well as for those with Wernicke's aphasia, the intonational disruptions may have been deriviative. In any event, it should be obvious that correct intonational production must pass several functional levels before reaching the end stage. Ultimately, however, a viable model is needed that will allow meaningful links at some stage between message-level pragmatics and intonational contour manipulation. Brown will have to figure out how they interact microgenetically, while Garrett will have to figure how his message level ultimately controls the intonational pattern, evoked as it is subsequently at the positional level and attached to the overall phrasal frame.

## Conclusions

At the outset of this chapter, I challenged Caplan's (1987, p. 138) overly pessimistic characterization of Brown's (1977, 1980, 1982) microgenetic model as it may or may not connect with psychological models of language production. According to Caplan, microgenesis has no clear connection with any of those models. It was the express purpose of this chapter to show that there are more points of contact between Brown and the psychologists than Caplan claims. The psychologist I treated was Merrill Garrett (e.g., 1988, 1990) and although his work and that of Brown were carried out independently of each other, each arrived at similar points and issues.

First, both Garrett's and Brown's model are at once serial and parallel. Both models are hierarchical, but both may actually work more in parallel to an extent not appreciated on cursory examination. As Brown's microgenetic system works its way up from the depths of the nervous system in a clear hierarchy based on evolutionary reasoning, its anterior and posterior systems run in parallel fashion, each level communicating with the other through white fiber tracts. Garrett's model is set out in purely hierarchical fashion, with stratified representational levels mapped by sets of computational processes. The levels range from deep semantic to surface peripheral articulatory muscular contractions. The system, however, certainly could run in a cascading fashion, with operations at subsequent lower levels initiating before all operations at the higher level are finished. Furthermore, feedback through a system such as Garrett's is possible, so long as that feedback is between the *outputs* of the various levels. For instance, if there is a phonological error at the positional level, it would not be unreasonable that that level could check back to the semantic–lexical level to make sure that the error was, in fact, at least a viable word in the language. Parallel distributed processing proponents always point to the number of errors that are produced at the phonological level but that nevertheless are still words in the language (e.g., Dell, 1988). Eschewing low-level word status checking "filters," they argue that a production model therefore needs phonological back to lexical–semantic feedback to ensure that the error is nevertheless a word in the dictionary of the speaker's language. The feedback capabilities of Garrett's model allow for this possibility and in the same way demonstrate the parallel aspect to that model.

Brown's microgenetic model and Garrett's sentence production model both propose two stages of lexical access, one that operates first and appreciates the meaning only and the other that operates on the actual phonological form of the word. That is to say, both models involve a "semantic to phonological flow" (Brown, 1988, p. 121), where "word meaning [is] extracted prior to phonology "(Brown, 1988, p. 121). The establishment of the two lexical lookups, with the semantic access occurring before the phonological access, was arrived at totally independently, through independent inquiry and reasoning and with different sorts of data bases. Again, Garrett considered errors from slips of the tongue, while Brown's data came from the clinic, largely from the speech of aphasic patients. I pointed out as well that since the work of Meringer and Mayer, there have been many points of commonality between neurologists and psychologists as concerns the use of aphasic data and data from slips of the tongue. Arnold Pick (1931/1973), as well, played an early and crucial role in influencing Brown, thereby bringing Brown's work clearly into the realm of psychology.

Another commonality between microgenesis and Garrett is the precise juncture in the production process where phonological segments are manipulated through the processes of selection and sequencing. Both postulate that segmental errors (whether slips or paraphasias) occur at the point where the phonological shape is accessed—Kohn's (1989) location of "string construction." Granted, neither investigators went very deeply into the linguistic complexities of segmental selection and ordering, but both clearly would claim that the computations that accomplish these operations should be placed at the same point in the production scheme.

An additional similarity among these models is a strict separation between the phonetic and the phonological. For Garrett, this separation is instantiated through distinct representative levels and computations. Note that in his model there are two sets of what he calls "phonological processes." The higher level (more or less at the phonemic or morphophonemic level) segmental computations feed into the positional level, while the lower forms of segmental computations such as those that establish the accommodations required for allophonic and allomorphic realization are processed at the phonetic level. For Brown, the two levels of operations are kept apart by assigning the phonological operations to the posterior system and the more motoric phonetic operations to the anterior system. Both place the phonological operations at some point before the phonetic operations, obviously because slips of the tongue as well as phonemic paraphasias ultimately need to be accommodated by lower level operations to ensure that changed or moved phonemes and morphemes receive their expected phonetic realizations in terms of allophones or allomorphs, respectively.

In the final section, I pointed out that both Garrett and Brown reserve a place for sentential intonation contours, anterior generalized neocortex for Brown and positional level phrasal frame construction for Garrett. Although Garrett has a clear level for message planning and Brown does not, Garrett says relatively little about the message level, characterizing it through logical reasoning concerning a speaker's current perceptual and affective states and his general knowledge of the world rather than through reasoning based on the nature of errors from slips of the tongue. Garrett, however, says nothing about Halliday's (e.g., 1970) information structure and the puzzle of how the given–new contract would be formulated at the message level, much less how that information would control the establishment of the intonation contour superimposed on the phrasal frame at the positional level. This lacuna appears in Brown's model as well. However, it would be of no little theoretical importance for microgenesis to investigate the neurolinguistic link between message formulation and sentential intonation (Brown's "speech melody") that arises out of the anterior system.

Finally, the comparisons that I have attempted to draw in this chapter have vividly demonstrated that the well-motivated functional analyses of Garrett (e.g., 1990) from slip data in normals, which propose that certain processes operate together at the same level (functional), do not require that these functions be located in spatial proximity in the nervous system. Quite often, investigators get into the murky quagmires of category mistakes when arguing that functionally linked operations must somehow be near one another in the brain. Somehow, and at some point, they would need to interact, but the functions themselves need not be grouped together in, say, the same cerebral lobe. Accordingly, Brown's model (e.g., 1988) would not be gradiental. Garrett's positional level operations are a good case in point, because although they comprise a set of functionally intertwined computations located in the same functional space (i.e., between the functional and the positional levels) in the model, in Brown's microgenetic model, various of those functions are parceled out into anterior and posterior cerebral systems. Functor morpheme manipulation, phrasal frame evocation, and intonational setting are anterior functions in Brown's model, while the second lexical lookup and phonological selection and sequencing are posterior cortical functions. They exist together functionally in Garrett's model. This situation, however, is not at all paradoxical; in fact, one should expect it to be the case, so long as one does not take the gradiental approach to neuroanatomical functional organization.

## References

Behrens, S.J. (1989). Characterizing sentence intonation in a right hemisphere-damaged population. *Brain and Language*, *37*, 181–200.

Benson, D.F., Sheremata, W.A., Bouchard, R., Segarra, J.M., Price, D., & Geschwind, N. (1973). Conduction aphasia: A clinicopathological study. *Archives of Neurology*, *28*, 339–346.

Boden, M.A. (1989). *Artificial intelligence in psychology*. Cambridge, MA: MIT Press.

Braun, C.M.J. (1989). Microgenetic theory: An inspiration for cognitive neuroscience? A review of *The life of the mind* by Jason W. Brown, M.D. *Brain and Cognition*, *11*, 139–143.

Brown, J.W. (1972). *Aphasia, apraxia and agnosia*. Springfield, IL: Charles C. Thomas.

Brown, J.W. (1977). *Mind, brain, and consciousness*. New York: Academic Press.

Brown, J.W. (1980). Brain structure and language production: A dynamic view. In D. Caplan (Ed.), *Biological studies of mental processes* (pp. 287–300). Cambridge, MA: MIT Press.

Brown, J.W. (1982). Hierarchy and evolution in neurolinguistics. In M.A. Arbib, D. Caplan, & J.C. Marshall (Eds.), *Neural models of language processes* (pp. 447–467). New York: Academic Press.

Brown, J.W. (1983). Rethinking the right hemisphere. In E. Perecman (Ed.), *Cognitive processing in the right hemisphere* (pp. 41–53). New York: Academic Press.

Brown, J.W. (1988). *The life of the mind*. Hillsdale, NJ: Lawrence Erlbaum.

Brown, J.W. (1990). Preliminaries for a theory of mind. In E. Goldberg (Ed.), *Contemporary neuropsychology and the legacy of Luria* (pp. 195–210). Hillsdale, NJ: Lawrence Erlbaum.

Buckingham, H.W. (1977). The conduction theory and neologistic jargon. *Language and Speech*, *20*, 174–184.

Buckingham, H.W. (1980). On correlating aphasic errors with slips of the tongue. *Applied Psycholinguistics*, *1*, 199–220.

Buckingham, H.W. (1981). Where do neologisms come from? In J.W. Brown (Ed.), *Jargonaphasia* (pp. 39–62). New York: Academic Press.

Buckingham, H.W. (1983). apraxia of language vs. apraxia of speech. In R.A. Magill (Ed.), *Memory and control of action* (pp. 275–292). Amsterdam: North-Holland.

Buckingham, H.W. (1985). Perseveration in aphasia. In S. Newman & R. Epstein (Eds.), *Current perspectives in dysphasia* (pp. 113–154). Edinburgh: Churchill Livingstone.

Buckingham, H.W. (1986). The scan-copier mechanism and the positional level of language production: Evidence from phonemic paraphasia. *Cognitive Science*, *10*, 195–217.

Buckingham, H.W. (1987). Phonemic paraphasias and psycholinguistic production models for neologistic jargon: A review. *Aphasiology*, *1*, 381–400.

Buckingham, H.W. (1990a). The principle of sonority, doublet creation, and the checkoff monitor. In J.-L. Nespoulous & P. Villiard (Eds.), *Morphology, phonology and aphasia* (193–205). New York: Springer-Verlag.

Buckingham, H.W. (1990b). Abstruse neologisms, retrieval deficits and the random generator. *Journal of Neurolinguistics*, *5*, 215–235.

Buckingham, H.W., & Kertesz, A. (1974). A linguistic analysis of fluent aphasia. *Brain and Language*, *1*, 43–62.

Buckingham, H.W., & Kertesz, A. (1976). *Neologistic jargon aphasia*. Amsterdam: Swets & Zeitlinger.

Butterworth, B. (1979). Hesitation and the production of verbal paraphasias and neologisms in jargon aphasia. *Brain and Language*, *18*, 133–161.

Caplan, D. (1987). *Neurolinguistics and linguistic aphasiology*. New York: Cambridge University Press.

Caplan, D. (1988). The biological basis for language. In F.J. Newmeyer (Ed.), *Linguistics: The Cambridge survey: Vol. 3. Language: Psychological and biological aspects* (pp. 237–255). New York: Cambridge University Press.

Crosson, B. (1985). Subcortical functions in language: A working model. *Brain and Language*, *25*, 257–292.

Crosson, B., Novack, T.A., & Trenerry, M.R. (1988). Subcortical language mechanisms: Window on a new frontier. In H.A. Whitaker (Ed.), *Phonological processes and brain mechanisms* (pp. 24–58). New York: Springer-Verlag.

Cutler, A. (Ed.). (1981). Slips of the tongue and language production [Special issue]. *Linguistics*, *19–7/8* (245/246). Berlin: Mouton Publishers.

Cutler, A., & Fay, D. (Eds.). (1978). Introduction. In R. Meringer & C. Mayer, *Versprechen und Verlesen* (pp. ix–xi). Amsterdam: John Benjamins.

Damasio, A. (1985). The frontal lobes. In K.M. Heilman & E. Valenstein (Eds.), *Clinical neuropsychology* (2nd ed., New York: Oxford University Press.

Danly, M., Cooper, W.E., & Shapiro B., (1983). Fundamental frequency, language processing, and linguistic structure in Wernicke's aphasia. *Brain and Language*, *19*, 1–24.

Danly, M., & Shapiro, B. (1982). Speech prosody in Broca's aphasia. *Brain and Language*, *16*, 171–190.

Deacon, T.W. (1989). Holism and associationism in neuropsychology: An anatomical synthesis. In E. Perecman (Ed.), *Integrating theory and practice in clinical neuropsychology* (pp. 1–47). Hillsdale, NJ: Lawrence Erlbaum.

Dell, G.S. (1988). The retrieval of phonological forms in production: Tests of predictions from a connectionistic model. *Journal of Memory and Language*, *27*, 124–142.

Fillmore, C.J. (1968). The case for case. In E. Bach & R.T. Harms (Eds.), *Universals in linguistic theory* (pp. 1–88). New York: Holt.

Flores d'Arcais, G.B. (1988). Language perception. In F.J. Newmeyer (Ed.), *Linguistics: The Cambridge survey: Vol. 3. Language: Psychological and biological aspects* (pp. 97–123). New York: Cambridge University Press.

Fodor, J.A. (1983). *The modularity of mind*. Cambridge, MA: MIT Press.

Foldi, N.S., Cicone, M., & Gardner, H. (1983). Pragmatic aspects of communication in brain-damaged patients. In S.J. Segalowitz (Ed.), *Language functions and brain organization* (pp. 51–86). New York: Academic Press.

Fromkin, V.A. (1971). The non-anomalous nature of anomalous utterances. *Language*, *47*, 27–52.

Fromkin, V.A. (Ed.) (1973). *Speech errors as linguistic evidence*. The Hague, The Netherlands: Mouton.

Fromkin, V.A. (Ed.) (1980). *Errors in linguistic performance: Slips of the tongue, ear, pen, and hand*. New York: Academic Press.

Gardner, H., Brownell, H.H., Wapner, W., & Michelow, D. (1983). Missing the point: The role of the right hemisphere in the processing of complex linguistic materials. In E. Perecman (Ed.), *Cognitive processing in the right hemisphere* (169–191). New York: Academic Press.

Garrett, M.F. (1975). The analysis of sentence production. In B. Gorden (Ed.), *The psychology of learning and motivation* (pp. 133–177). New York: Academic Press.

Garrett, M.F. (1976). Syntactic processes in sentence production. In R.J. Wales & E. Walker (Eds.), *New approaches to language mechanisms* (pp. 231–256). Amsterdam: North-Holland.

Garrett, M.F. (1980a). Levels of processing in sentence production. In B. Butterworth (Ed.), *Sentence production 1: Speech and talk* (pp. 177–220). London: Academic Press.

Garrett, M.F. (1980b) The limits of accommodation: Arguments for independent processing levels in sentence production. In V.A. Fromkin (Ed.), *Errors in linguistic performance: Slips of the tongue, ear, pen, and hand* (pp. 263–271). New York: Academic Press.

Garrett, M.F. (1982). Production of speech: Observations from normal and pathological language use. In A.W. Ellis (Ed.), *Normality and pathology in cognitive functions* (pp. 19–76). London: Academic Press.

Garrett, M.F. (1984). The organization of processing structure for language production: Applications to aphasic speech. In D. Caplan, A.R. Lecours, & A. Smith (Eds.), *Biological perspectives on language* (pp. 172–193). Cambridge, MA: MIT Press.

Garrett, M.F. (1988). Processes in language production. In F.J. Newmeyer (Ed.), *Linguistics: The Cambridge survey: Vol. 3. Language: Psychological and biological aspects* (pp. 69–96). New York: Cambridge University Press.

Garrett, M.F. (1990). Sentence processing. In D.N. Osherson & H. Lasnik (Eds.), *An invitation to cognitive science: Language* (Vol. 1, pp. 133–175). Cambridge, MA: MIT Press.

Goldberg, E. (1989). Gradiental approach to neocortical functional organization. *Journal of Clinical and Experimental Neuropsychology*, *11*, 489–517.

Grice, H.P. (1975). Logic and conversation. In P. Cole & J.L. Morgan (Eds.), *Syntax and semantics: Vol. 9. Pragmatics* (pp. 41–58). New York: Academic Press.

Halliday, M.A.K. (1970). Language structure and language function. In J. Lyons (Ed.), *New horizons in linguistics* (pp. 140–165). Middlesex, England: Penguin Books.

Hawthorne, J. (1989). On the compatibility of connectionist and classical models. *Philosophical Psychology*, *2*, 5–15.

Joanette, Y., Goulet, P., Ska, B., & Nespoulous, J.-L. (1986). Informative content of narrative discourse in right-brain-damaged right-handers. *Brain and Language*, *29*, 81–105.

Joanette, Y., Keller, E., & Lecours, A.R. (1980). Sequence of phonemic approximations in aphasia. *Brain and Language*, *11*, 30–44.

Keller, E. (1987). The cortical representation of motor processes of speech. In E. Keller & M. Gopnik (Eds.), *Motor and sensory processes of language* (pp. 125–162). Hillsdale, NJ: Lawrence Erlbaum.

Kertesz, A., & Benson, D.F. (1970). Neologistic jargon: A clinicopathological study. *Cortex*, *6*, 362–386.

Kohn, S.E. (1984). The nature of the phonological disorder in conduction aphasia. *Brain and Language*, *23*, 97–115.

Kohn, S.E. (1985). *Phonological breakdown in aphasia*. Unpublished doctoral dissertation, Tufts University, Medford, MA.

Kohn, S.E. (1988). Phonological production deficits in aphasia. In H.A. Whitaker (Ed.), *Phonological processes and brain mechanisms* (pp. 93–117). New York: Springer-Verlag.

Kohn, S.E. (1989). The nature of the phonemic string deficit in conduction aphasia. *Aphasiology*, *3*, 209–239.

Lecours, A.R. (1982). On neologisms. In J. Mehler, E.C.T. Walker, & M.F. Garrett (Eds.), *Perspectives on mental representation* (pp. 217–247). Hillsdale, NJ: Lawrence Erlbaum.

Lecours, A.R., & Lhermitte, F. (1972). Recherches sur le language des aphasiques: 4. Analyse d'un corpus de neologismes; notion de paraphasie monemique. *Encephale*, *61*, 295–315.

Lenneberg, E.H. (1960). A review of speech and brain mechanisms by W. Penfield and L. Roberts. *Language*, *36*, 97–112.

Levelt, W.J.M. (1989). *Speaking: From intention to articulation*. Cambridge, MA: MIT Press.

Luria, A.R. (1970). *Traumatic aphasia*. The Hague, The Netherlands: Mouton.

Meringer, R., & Mayer C. (1978). *Versprechen und verlesen, eine psychologisch-linguistische Studie*. Stuttgart: Goschense Verlagsbuchhandlung. Amsterdam: John Benjamins. (Original work published 1895)

Nespoulous, J.-L., Joanette, Y., Beland, R., Caplan, D., & Lecours, A.R. (1984). Phonological disturbance in aphasia: Is there a "markedness effect" in aphasic phonemic errors? In F.C. Rose (Ed.), *Advances in aphasiology*: *Vol. 2. Progress in aphasiology*. London: Raven Press.

Perecman, E. (1989). Bilingualism and Jargonaphasia: Is there connection? *Brain and Language*, *36*, 49–61.

Perecman, E., & Brown, J.W. (1981). Phonemic jargon: A case report. In J.W. Brown (Ed.), *Jargonaphasia* (pp. 177–257). New York: Academic Press.

Perecman, E., & Brown, J.W. (1985). Ukeleles, condessors, and fosetch. *Language Sciences*, *7*, 177–214.

Pick, A, (1931/1973). *Aphasia*. (J.W. Brown, Trans. & Ed.). Springfield, IL: Charles C. Thomas. (Original work published 1931)

Schwartz, M.F. (1987). Patterns of speech production deficit within and across aphasia syndromes: Application of a psycholinguistic model. In M. Coltheart, G. Sartori, & R. Job (Eds.), *The cognitive neuropsychology of language*, (pp. 163–199). London: Lawrence Erlbaum.

Searle, J. (1969). *Speech acts*. Cambridge, UK: Cambridge University Press.

Shattuck-Hufnagel, S. (1979). Speech errors as evidence for a serial ordering mechanism in speech production. In W.E. Cooper & E.C.T. Walker (Eds)., *Sentence processing*: *Psycholinguistic studies presented to M.F. Garrett* (pp. 295–342). Hillsdale, NJ: Lawrence Erlbaum.

Shattuck-Hufnagel, S. (1983). Sublexical units and suprasegmental structure in speech production planning. In P.F. MacNeilage (Ed.), *The production of speech* (pp. 109–136). New York: Springer-Verlag.

Shattuck-Hufnagel, S. (1987). The role of word-onset consonants in speech production planning: New evidence from speech error patterns. In E. Keller & M. Gopnik (Eds.), *Motor and sensory processes of language* (pp. 17–51). Hillsdale, NJ: Lawrence Erlbaum.

Stemberger, J.P. (1983). *Speech errors and theoretical phonology: A review*. Unpublished manuscript, Indiana University Linguistics Club, Bloomington, IN.

Stemberger, J.P. (1985). An interactive activation model of language production. In A.W. Ellis (Ed.), *Progress in the psychology of language* (Vol. 1, pp. 143–186). London: Lawrence Erlbaum.

Yule, G. (1980). Intonation and givenness in spoken discourse. *Studies in Language*, *4*, 271–286.

# 9
# The Role of Neuromotor Activation in the Facilitation of Language Production: Rehabilitation Applications

ROBERT E. HANLON

Neuropsychological rehabilitation is an expanding field that holds great promise in its primary objective of improving the quality of living of individuals who have sustained neurological insults, particularly traumatic brain injury and stroke. In response to this promise, there is an increasing demand for efficacy and outcome studies unequivocally demonstrating the inherent value of the therapeutic interventions and techniques used with brain-damaged patients. Theoretical models of cognitive processing and neuropsychological function have attempted through detailed analysis and experimentation to explain brain–behavior relationships, cognitive formation, and dissolution of function. However, use of these models for the development of therapeutic interventions with the brain injured, with notable exceptions (Ben-Yishay, 1980; Luria, 1963), has been slow in coming or limited in applicability.

The microgenetic perspective has been the focus of increasing attention of late, which in part is due to the applicability of this approach to neurorehabilitation (see Chapter 2). The microgenetic model of cognition, based on the principles of hierarchical organization and formative processes, progressing through qualitatively different stages, represents a dynamic unitary model of neuropsychological function. A fundamental premise of microgenesis is that the symptoms of brain damage do not necessarily represent deficits or aberrations, but rather, a given symptom reflects the subsurface stage at which the normal process of cognitive formation is disrupted as a result of a lesion. Despite the increased interest in this approach, theoretically, and in terms of clinical application within the realm of rehabilitation, this model remains an alternative view to the more widely accepted connectionistic and modular perspectives on neuropsychological function.

This chapter will proceed with a brief review of the conventional models of cognitive rehabilitation, with a particular emphasis on therapeutic interventions in aphasia. This review will be followed by a detailed description of studies involving the development and application of therapeutic techniques that have been based on microgenetic principles.

## Models of Neuropsychological Rehabilitation

Wilson (1989) recently reviewed the state of the art in cognitive rehabilitation in outlining the models of intervention commonly employed in an attempt to remediate, ameliorate, and alleviate neuropsychological impairments resulting from brain damage. Treatment models in cognitive rehabilitation have emerged from theory and research generated within the disciplines of clinical neuropsychology, experimental cognition, behavioral psychology, and rehabilitation, particularly speech and occupational therapy. The therapeutic application of the theoretical perspective and contributions of each of these disciplines is rarely pure and is generally characterized by considerable overlap and the incorporation of principles and techniques from one or more of these disciplines.

The predominant models of cognitive remediation include the general stimulation model, the functional compensation model, the substitution-transfer model, and behavioral approaches, based on operant conditioning and behavior modification. The general stimulation approach (Sohlberg & Mateer, 1989), an attempt at direct remediation of cognitive deficiency through routine engagement in repetitive drills and exercises (i.e., list learning, vocabulary expansion, computer programs aimed at retraining attention), is probably the most widely used model in cognitive rehabilitation. Despite the practical and straightforward nature of such techniques, there is minimal evidence that practice alone, regardless of the intensity in which such exercises are engaged, leads to meaningful advances in functional performance outside of clinic (Schacter & Glisky, 1986).

Aside from the general stimulation approach, other models employed in cognitive rehabilitation have demonstrated utility, at least with certain patient groups manifesting specific cognitive impairments. The functional adaptation model (Wilson, 1989) probably represents the most useful and effective approach in cognitive rehabilitation. Based on the principles of functional compensation, patients are trained in the use of both external devices (e.g., memory notebooks, checklists) and alternative strategies (e.g., requesting clarification, adopting routine systematic approaches to problem solving) to compensate for deficits in the acquisition, retention, and use of information.

Other models that may be effective in certain situations and with specific patients, but that lack the global applicability of the functional adaptation approach, include approaches based on the substitution of an intact or comparatively intact cognitive function for an impaired cognitive function. Often referred to as *indirect remediation* (Tankle, 1988), techniques such as the use of visual imagery, employed to alleviate the effects of a verbal memory impairment, are attractive but cognitively demanding techniques that often exceed the learning potential of brain-damaged patients.

Luria (1963) presented the most elaborate and indepth model of strategic intervention based on the substitution concept, which is explicitly founded on a unified theory of neuropsychological function. Founded on the theory of dynamic localization of psychological functions (Luria, 1966), a model of neuropsychological restoration based on the reorganization of functional systems was proposed. Following the original work of Anokhin (1947) on the concept of functional systems and the dependence of a functional system on the integrity of its afferent field, combined with the idea of mobile psychological systems, as originated by Vygotsky (1934/1962), Luria delineated three main types of reorganization of functional systems.

According to this model (Luria, 1963), basic intrasystematic reorganization occurs automatically and is exemplified by cases in which, following the onset of hemiplegia, the comparatively preserved proximal motor system begins to be used to compensate for distal functions. Conceptual intrasystematic reorganization may be possible following damage to secondary cortical integration areas but requires intensive and protracted therapeutic training. Interventions of this type may be exemplified by the case of simultaneous agnosia, in which the perceptual field essentially may be widened by restructuring the visual elements into semantically based groups, such as words. Finally, the third type involves intersystematic reorganization. The classic example of this type is that of the Parkinson's patient with a severely dysfunctional gait, who may demonstrate markedly improved walking ability following the incorporation of the visual system by being required to step over lines drawn on the floor. However, aside from the use of Lurian principles of neurologic rehabilitation, which include taking advantage of intact cognitive processes, extended programming of remedial activity, and constant signalization of the defect (Ben-Yishay & Prigatano, 1990), little work has been done on this model outside of the Soviet Union (Luria, Naydin, Tsvetkova, & Vinarskaya, 1969).

In contrast to the models described, which have originated from neuropsychological theory, data derived from experimental cognition, and the application of the fundamental techniques and strategies used in physical rehabilitation, the fourth predominant model of cognitive rehabilitation has emerged from behavioral psychology. Founded on the principles of learning theory and behavior modification, a wide range of interventions have been employed with varying degrees of success, particularly with patients manifesting severe intellectual and behavioral disorders, secondary to brain injury. Approaches include environmental restructuring, various reinforcement schedules, and shaping. Gross and Schutz (1986) elaborated the environmental control approach, based on the strategy of restructuring the patient's enviroment, which includes the prominent display of orientation information, activities of daily living (ADL) reminders in the form of signs and labels, and the consistent provision of information by others, thereby reducing the cognitive demands on the patient. The employment of individualized reinforcement schedules to increase adaptive behaviors and decrease the frequency of maladaptive responses has been advocated by Wood (1987), among others.

## Rehabilitation of Language Disorders

Attempts to increase the functional communicative capacity of aphasic patients through the implementation of various language intervention strategies have proliferated within the fields of speech therapy and neuropsychology. Yet, the efficacy of many of these interventions for improving functional communication remains undemonstrated. Sarno (1981) differentiated two primary models of aphasia therapy, based on the two predominant theoretical perspectives of language dysfunction following stroke. The stimulation–facilitation approach is based on the principle of impaired access to language, whereas the direct-pedagogic approach is founded on the idea that aphasia represents loss of language.

More recently, Basso (1987) reviewed the major approaches in aphasia rehabilitation. The direct stimulation approach in the rehabilitation of language disorders, as in the remediation of other cognitive deficits, is one of the most widely used intervention strategies. Despite the popularity of this approach, however, very little evidence demonstrates that attempts to stimulate language through repetitive verbal exercises results in functional gains in communicative capacity beyond those expected from spontaneous recovery (Miller, 1984).

The psycholinguistic approach has proven to be more fruitful for the development of specific techniques and programs designed to enhance the communication skills of patients with language impairments, particularly global aphasics. Glass, Gazzaniga, and Premack (1973) demonstrated that global aphasics could learn an artificial language system, in which paper symbols represented words, and that these patients were capable of varying degrees of symbolization for communicative purposes. Gardner, Zurif, Berry, and Baker (1976) carried this line of research a step further through the development of a visual communication system. They found that following intensive training, global aphasics could use this system to act on command, respond to questions, and describe situations in their environment. Melodic Intonation Therapy (Sparks & Holland, 1976) and the deblocking technique introduced by Weigl (1981) are additional examples of techniques developed on the psycholinguistic view, which have met with limited success, particularly with severely aphasic patients.

Based on the theory of dynamic organization of functional systems and the capacity for restoration following neurological insult, Luria (1963) proposed elaborate and detailed strategies for aphasia therapy, founded on the concepts of transfer and substitution of function. Through interventions directed toward the systematic reorganization of functions, as described, Luria (1970) presented a comprehensive approach to aphasia rehabilitation. Goodglass (1987) has provided a concise analysis of the Lurian approach to aphasia rehabilitation.

The therapeutic vehicle of behaviorism, behavior modification, which is based on the principles of operant conditioning, particularly the systematic reinforcement of target responses, represents the fourth major approach in language therapy. Examples include use of the shaping technique (Holland, 1967), work on programmed instruction (Holland, 1970; Naeser, 1975), and the functional conditioning of pragmatics (Davis & Wilcox, 1981). These behavioral techniques, among others, have been demonstrated to be effective in advancing communicative capacity with selected aphasic patients. Behavioral techniques in aphasia rehabilitation, however, remain somewhat controversial, as a result of the constraints of the theoretical model, which essentially disregards formative processes and exclusively focuses on units of behavior.

## Applications of the Microgenetic Model to Language Rehabilitation

The application of microgenetic principles to therapeutic interventions in aphasia and other neuropsychological impairments is a relatively recent development in research on this model. The techniques that have been developed represent a marked departure from the conventional approaches to intervention in speech therapy and cognitive remediation. Additionally, unlike the general stimulation approach, which is by far the most common and widely used technique in cognitive rehabilitation (Wilson, 1989), these techniques are based on a unified theoretical model of cognitive formation from which effects may be predicted and further hypotheses formulated.

Microgenesis represents a process model of cognitive formation in which the structural development of mental phenomena evolve through a series of qualitatively different stages following the presentation of a stimulus, to a behavioral response. On this view, all mental representations, including ideas, perceptions, words, and actions are considered to evolve through a process of progressive elaboration that forms the major part of their structure. This microtemporal approach incorporates the Jacksonian principle of hierarchical organization within the stage model of developmental progression (see Brown, 1988; Hanlon & Brown, 1989).

The original microgenetic concepts evolved from the introspectional and gestalt movements around the turn of the century. Influenced by the Würzburger proposals on the dynamic nature of imageless thought and the transitional stages of thought formation, Pick (1913) proposed a multistage theoretical model of language production based on a temporal hierarchy. Heniz Werner (1956) is credited with coining the term *microgenesis* in translation of the German word *Aktualgenese* in a paper on the microgenetic analysis of aphasia (see Flavell & Draguns, 1957).

Brown (1977, 1988) has expanded on the psychological principles of microgenetic theory by providing a neurological framework through which this process unfolds. This structural model of neurocognition holds that the symptoms of brain damage represent the premature exposure of preliminary levels that are normally exceeded and transformed in the process of cognitive formation. On this view, the neurocognitive process unfolds in a unidirectional (bottom-up) progression, traversing neuroanatomical levels and cognitive stages in a manner that recapitulates the course of forebrain evolution.

## *Hemiplegic Writing*

Global aphasia is the largest single diagnostic subtype of aphasia and represents the most severely impaired subgroup of aphasics (Goodglass, 1987). Global aphasics with right hemiplegia, who are agraphic and apraxic on the motorically intact left side, are among the most severely impaired aphasic patients, with regard to communicative capacity. Left-sided agraphia is relatively common in individuals with aphasia of various degrees of severity. The comparatively uncommon nonhemiplegic aphasics with left-sided agraphia and relative preservation of writing on the right side have generally been interpreted as manifesting a disconnection syndrome, caused by a lesion of the corpus callosum (Geschwind & Kaplan, 1962).

Brown, Leader, and Blum (1983) demonstrated that it was possible to train functional hemiplegic writing skills in global aphasics with right hemiplegia and marked left-sided agraphia and apraxia. Based on a technique originally reported by Leischner (1970), Brown et al. (1983) designed a writing prosthesis, which could be moved in all directions, using the residual proximal musculature of the hemiplegic limb. A program was developed for training severe aphasics in the use of the prosthesis. The program systematically progressed from copying letters, shapes, and words, to writing high-frequency and then low-frequency words to dictation, and finally to writing the names of objects presented visually and objects held in the left hand.

In this study (Brown et al., 1983), three patients with global aphasia and right hemiplegia were systematically assessed with respect to their capacity to write with the right limb and prosthesis. All three subjects demonstrated a strikingly well-preserved capacity for copying, writing to dictation, and written naming in response to left-sided palpation. In contrast, all three subjects manifested marked left-sided agraphia, which was pervasive throughout the writing trials.

Left-sided agraphia in nonhemiplegic aphasics with preserved right-handed writing ability is generally interpreted as a disconnection syndrome, caused by the destruction of callosal fibers projecting from left-hemisphere language centers to regions controlling left-hand writing in the right hemisphere. Neuroradiological examination, however, provided no evidence of callosal damage in these three aphasic subjects, and the fact that these patients could write with the hemiplegic right limb argues against a disconnection hypothesis. Additionally, all three cases demonstrated cross-manual transfer when tested with the right limb and prosthesis on the written naming of objects held in the left-hand with their eyes closed. In fact, performance on left-tactile and right-sided written naming was comparable to right-sided written naming of objects on visual confrontation.

Brown et al. (1983) proposed that this finding, which is seemingly incompatible with an interpretation based on a disconnection, could be explained on a microgenetic model. On this view, the finding that global aphasics with left-sided agraphia were able to write with the hemiplegic right limb represented the capacity to access submerged levels in language formation via the functional engagement of proximal limb musculature. The hierarchic organization of motor function composed of a phylogenetically older motor system mediating axial and proximal movement and a comparatively recent motor system responsible for fine distal movements (Kuypers, 1973) may be considered to represent stages in the action microgeny.

If, as the microgenetic view of neurocognitive processing holds, language formation unfolds in a similar manner across neural levels and through cognitive stages, then activation of a preliminary stage in motility (i.e., proximal motor system), following disruption of the end stage (i.e., fine distal motility), may permit access to preliminary stages in linguistic processing, following disruption of the microgenetic end point (i.e., fluent, articulate speech and writing). This phenomenon, however, presumably depends on the destruction of the surface level or end point in the coextensive processes of language formation and motor control.

A follow-up study by Brown and Chobar (1989) confirmed the earlier findings. Ten chronic, predominantly nonfluent aphasic patients underwent a 3-month structured therapy program involving training in the functional use of the prosthesis with the hemiparetic limb. The treatment program consisted of four stages: (1) geometric forms, (2) single letters, (3) high- and low-frequency words, and (4) short phrases. Within each stage, patients systematically progressed through three training phases, including tracing, copying, and writing to dictation. Post-treatment assessment revealed a considerable increase in right-sided writing with the prosthesis, relative to left-handed writing, in all 10 subjects, and generation of spontaneous written expression in 80% of these patients. Additionally, post-testing on the Western Aphasia Battery revealed improvement in other language functions, including oral–verbal expression and auditory comprehension, which was suggestive of a generalization effect. The hemiplegic writing effect was also recently replicated by Friedland (1989).

Beyond the theoretical importance of the phenomenon of hemiplegic writing lie the functional implications that this finding holds for severe aphasic patients. Global aphasics, with left-sided agraphia and apraxia, who are essentially incapable of effectively and reliably communicating through speech, left-handed writing, or left-handed gestures, may be able to write with the right hemiplegic limb with the aid of a prosthesis.

## *Gestural Facilitation of Naming in Aphasia*

The use of gesture and other speech-related body movements in an attempt to improve the communicative capacity of individuals with aphasia following cerebral vascular accidents has received increasing support. Several studies that have examined the efficacy of training in the functional use of gesture and other speech-related movement patterns with aphasic patients have reported increases in oral–verbal expression during the execution of such movements.

Skelly has advocated the therapeutic use of American Indian Sign (Amerind) with aphasics (Skelly, 1979; Skelly, Schinsky, Smith, Donaldson, & Griffin, 1975) and in patients with severe oral apraxia (Skelly, Schinsky, Smith, & Fust, 1974). In addition to the advanced communicative ability provided by acquisition of this signal system, she has consistently reported the concurrent facilitation of verbalization during gestural expression with Amerind.

In studies of pantomime therapy with severely aphasic patients (Schlanger, DiCarrado, & Geffner, 1974; Schlanger & Freimann, 1979), not only could aphasics learn a specific repertoire of pantomimes on which they had been trained, but they could also generalize their gestural expressions to new situations. It was noted that in both of these pantomime therapy studies "aphasics could learn to use pantomime as a substitute for or adjunct to verbal speech, and that pantomime, moreover, facilitated spontaneous verbalization" (Schlanger & Freimann, 1979, p. 35).

Building on the Gardner et al. (1976) work on the visual communication system, Helm-Estabrooks, Fitzpatrick, and Barresi (1982) developed a gestural communication system referred to as "visual action therapy" specifically for global aphasics, in attempt to facilitate gestural expression. With a pre–post-test design using scores on Porch Index of Communicative Ability, (PICA) subtests, they found a strong generalization effect from the training program on the gestural-pantomime subtests scores, as well as improvement on the auditory comprehension scores.

Hadar, Steiner, and Rose (1984) proposed that modulation of suprasegmental control through systematic activation of speech-related movement would enhance oral–verbal expression in nonfluent aphasics. Based on the theoretical view that holds that linguistic and motor processes are interdependent (Fowler, Rubin, Remez, & Turvey, 1980; Turvey, 1980), these researchers found that head movement and postural shifts directly influenced speech production, particularly initiation and fluency (Hadar, Davies, Steiner, & Rose, 1984).

More recently, Johannsen-Horbach, Cegla, Mager, Schempp, and Wallesch (1985) have reported some success in the treatment of global aphasics with Blissymbols, a system of visual–graphic symbols composed of ideograms and pictograms. Interestingly, Johannsen-Horbach et al. (1985) noted that aphasic subjects intermittently emitted correct words while pointing to their corresponding visual symbols. This "simultaneous articulation" of accurate verbal referents during pointing movements was an unexpected and intriguing finding.

Anomia, or word-finding difficulty, characterizes virtually all aphasics in varying degrees of severity and is probably the most common residual deficit following recovery of other language functions. An extensive body of literature exists on the nature of anomia in aphasia. Particular emphasis has been placed on the various forms of disordered naming and paraphasias, the differentiation among aphasia subtypes with respect to naming difficulty, and the stimulus variables and cues that affect naming performance. Goodglass and Geschwind (1976) have suggested that some degree of reduction of available lexical items is a general and essentially invariable symptom of all aphasia subtypes. As such, defective naming ability represents a ubiquitous, functionally limiting symptom that characterizes all types of aphasia.

Among the factors implicated in naming are word frequency and length, context, semantic category, sensory modality of presentation, the inherent sensorimotor characteristics of stimuli, and other behavioral manifestations characteristic of defective naming performance. Aside from variations in and analyses of the effects of the stimuli on naming performance, another branch of research in the area of naming ability has focused on the naming process. Contributions within this vein include studies of tacit knowledge, consistency, naming errors, and responsiveness to various forms of cueing. Approaches to the facilitation of naming in aphasia that have concentrated on cueing have included procedures involving semantic, phonemic, contextual, visual as well as other sensory modalities, and gestural cues.

Hanlon, Brown, and Gerstman (1990) demonstrated that neuromotor activation in the form of gestural production could facilitate linguistic processing, specifically naming performance, in some cases of severe aphasia. Based on the reports of a variable degree of facilitation of verbalization during gestural activity and speech-related movement, and the hemiplegic writing phenomenon discussed previously, Hanlon et al. proposed that engagement of the residual proximal musculature of the hemiplegic limb in the production of a communicative gesture might facilitate naming in aphasic patients. Specifically, they hypothesized that activation of the phylogenetically older proximal motor system of the hemiplegic right limb in the execution of a pointing gesture, which is communicative but nonrepresentational, would have a facilitatory effect on naming ability. This hypothesis was based on the microgenetic model elaborated by Brown (1977, 1988) and described previously. The study is summarized in the following paragraphs.

Twenty-four right-handed aphasic patients with marked naming impairment secondary to a left cerebrovascular accident were selected for inclusion. Subjects consisted of eight Broca's aphasics, six Wernicke's aphasics, four global aphasics, four transcortical motor aphasics, and two anomics. Classification of aphasia subtype was established on the Western Aphasia Battery (Kertesz, 1982). Additionally, a score of 35 or less on the Boston Naming Test (Kaplan, Goodglass, & Weintraub, 1983) was established as criterion for inclusion. The experimental naming stimuli consisted of 138 black-and-white photographs of common objects, representing medium- to high-frequency nouns, which were divided into three sets of 46 items. The stimulus items consisted of words from eight semantic categories, which were matched across the sets for frequency and number of items per category.

The aphasic subjects were assessed on three independent gesture/naming conditions. They were instructed to produce the following movements immediately on visual confrontation with a stimulus item, while attempting to name the pictured object: "point to the pictured object with your right arm" (Condition 1); "make a fist with your right hand" (Condition 2); "point to the pictured objects with your left arm" (Condition 3). The stimulus pictures, which were presented at approximately eye level to the subject, were systematically varied across conditions, with respect to spatial positioning in relation to the subject.

In Condition 1, which required a pointing response with the hemiparetic right limb, primarily generated through activation of the proximal (shoulder) musculature, the pictures were positioned at a 60° to 70° angle to the right of the subject. Such positioning was instituted because lateral rotation of the head to the right, which was necessary to see the stimulus, typically elicited the asymmetrical tonic neck reflex (ATNR). Elicitation of the ATNR resulted in temporary reduction of the flexor synergy and increase in extensor tone in the paralytic limb, which enabled the hemiplegic patients to approximate a pointing gesture. In Condition 3, pointing with the left arm, stimuli were presented at a 60° to 70° angle to the left of the subject. Condition 2, which entailed making a fist or attempting to flex the fingers of the right hand, was included as a control measure, to rule out the effect of generalized activation of the left hemisphere. Stimuli were presented directly in front of the subject in Condition 2.

The results indicated that pointing gestures produced through activation of the proximal musculature of the right hemiplegic limb, in combination with activation of axial musculature and brain-stem reflexes, differentially facilitated naming performance in nonfluent aphasics. This differential effect on naming performance was specific to the anterior aphasics, characterized by nonfluent speech and hemiparesis, and was not demonstrated by the Wernicke's aphasics. The differential effect of right proximal versus left proximal gesturing on naming was significantly greater for the nonfluent subjects ($M = 5.39$) than the fluent aphasics ($M = 1.33$), Mann-Whitney $U = 18$, $p < .02$ (two-tailed) (Hanlon et al., 1990). Figure 9.1 illustrates the difference in mean performance between the nonfluent and fluent aphasic subgroups across the gesture–naming conditions.

Like the differential finding of the right proximal condition relative to the left proximal condition, the differential effect of right proximal gestures versus right distal activation on naming accuracy was significantly greater for the nonfluents ($M = 4.22$) than the fluents ($M = -0.33$), Mann-Whitney $U = 22$, $p < .05$ (two-tailed). Incidentally, no significant difference was observed between the nonfluent and fluent subjects on the left proximal versus right distal differential performance measure.

The difference on the gesture–naming differential measures among the five aphasic subgroups was assessed on a Kruskal-Wallis one-way analysis of variance. Although the subgroups did not differ significantly among themselves, as a result of the consistency of the nonfluent subtypes in generating the proximal right–left differential effect, pairwise comparisons using the Mann-Whitney U test revealed that the Broca's and Wernicke's subgroups differed significantly on both the right proximal versus left proximal differential effect, $U = 8.0$, $p < .05$ (two-tailed) and the right proximal versus right distal differential effect, $U = 6.0$, $p < .05$ (two-

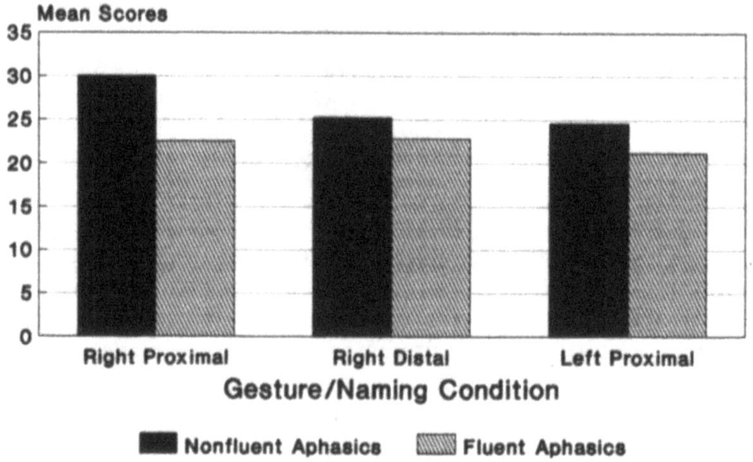


FIGURE 9.1. Performance of nonfluent and fluent aphasic subjects on three gesture–naming conditions. *Note.* Data from "Enhancement of Naming in Nonfluent Aphasia Through Gesture" by R.E. Hanlon, J.W. Brown, and L. Gerstman, 1990, *Brain and Language, 38*. p. 298–314. Copyright 1990 by Academic Press. Adapted by permission.

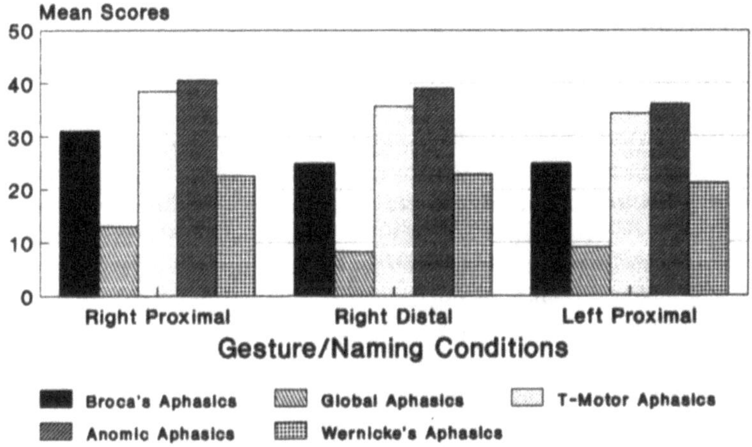


FIGURE 9.2. Performance of five aphasic subtypes on three gesture–naming conditions. *Note.* Data from "Enhancement of Naming in Nonfluent Aphasia Through Gesture" by R.E. Hanlon, J.W. Brown, and L. Gerstman, 1990, *Brain and Language, 38.* p. 298–314. Copyright 1990 by Academic Press. Adapted by permission.

tailed). Figure 9.2 illustrates the relative mean performance of the five aphasic subgroups across the gesture–naming conditions.

A qualitative error analysis revealed expected differences between the nonfluent and fluent aphasics, with regard to the relative proportion of error types. Among the nonfluents, the error distribution across the three gesture–naming conditions was roughly equivalent for most error types, with two notable exceptions. Important differences were revealed with respect to the relative proportion of word production error types (Benson, 1979), specifically initiation and articulation. The number of initiation (i.e., failure-to-respond) errors was comparable under the left proximal gesture (36%) and the right distal activation (34%) conditions. The nonfluents, however, generated comparatively fewer response initiation errors under the right proximal gesture condition (30%). A comparable difference was also demonstrated by the nonfluent subjects in the relative proportion of articulatory errors. No such differences were demonstrated by the fluent aphasics.

These findings support the contention that functional activation of the proximal motor system of the hemiparetic limb in the production of pointing gestures has a facilitatory effect on the naming performance of nonfluent aphasics. This effect was essentially limited to patients with clinical evidence of anterior pathology and was not revealed by fluent (presumably posterior) aphasics. The difference in error patterns revealed by a qualitative error analysis was particularly revealing. Among the nonfluents, the relative proportion of error types across the gesture–naming conditions, with respect to word production errors (i.e., initiation and articulation), strongly supports the idea that engagement of the proximal and axial motor systems in the execution of a communicative gesture with the hemiparetic limb facilitates the execution of articulation.

The facilitatory effect of proximally driven gestural activity on oral naming may be explained through a microgenetic model of neurocognitive processing. The nature of this effect, specifically the influence on naming performance of right-sided pointing gestures, suggests that functional activation of the right proximal limb musculature in the execution of communicative gestures may permit access to submerged levels of language processing in the left hemisphere. Specifically, engagement of the right proximal and axial motor systems in the production of a communicative gesture allows access to preliminary levels in the process of execution of articulation (Hanlon et al., 1990).

The finding of the enhancement of naming through neuromotor activation of the proximal musculature of the paralytic side in the production of communicative gestures suggests that the involvement of the hemiparetic limb in simple gestures has some functional utility during effortful attempts at language production. The effect was demonstrated to varying degrees among the various subtypes of nonfluent aphasia. Conversely, Wernicke's aphasics, in general, were linguistically unaffected by such self-generated communicative gestures. In light of such an apparent dissociation, this gestural intervention technique should be encouraged as an adjunct to conventional speech therapy procedures with nonfluent aphasics, particularly Broca's aphasics, during attempts at word finding.

## Discussion

The concept of interdependence of language processes and motor systems has been proposed and elaborated by others. Kimura (1976, 1979) is a major proponent of this view. Turvey (1977, 1980) has also argued extensively that the organizational properties and formational aspects of language and movement are "qualitatively indistinguishable." This perspective is based on the theoretical principles of dynamic motor control originally proposed by Bernstein (1967). The ideas put forth by Bernstein, including hierarchical organization, dynamic regulation based on the degrees of freedom at a given moment in time, and the cognitive motor act realized through wave-form processes, have strongly influenced microgenetic views on action formation (see Brown, 1988; Goldberg, 1987).

According to the microgenetic perspective, the anterior language–speech formation process sequentially progresses through the stages of intention, initiation, serialization, and articulation (Brown, 1972). Similarly, the process of limb motility unfolds hierarchically through axial movement, involving postural adjustment, trunk rotation, and head orientation, to proximal movements, particularly limb extension and flexion, to distal movements, involving fine adroit, dextrous manipulation. When the individual is engaged in functional communication, the coextensive processes of language formation and motor control unfold in a collaborative progression of gesture, vocalization, and speech (Yakovlev, 1948). Furthermore, if these processes are truncated as a result of a cortical lesion (i.e., nonfluent aphasia and hemiparesis), given the collaborative nature of these processes when the fundamental intent is communication, it is reasonable to assume that functional engagement of archaic proximal and axial motor systems may facilitate language production.

The application of this hierarchically organized process approach to the therapeutic domain, specifically aphasia rehabilitation, represents a marked departure from the conventional linguistic interventions. Based on the findings of the studies discussed, however, the therapeutic implications of the use of the microgenetic model as a model of cognitive rehabilitation represent an intriguing and refreshing alternative to the conventional approaches to intervention with the neuropsychologically impaired.

Like the substitution-transfer approach (Luria, 1963), which is directed toward the reorganization of functions, the microgenetic approach is based on a comprehensive and unitary model of neuropsychology. The focus of intervention is on the facilitation of the transition between processing stages within the progression of cognitive formation. The microgenetic approach stresses activation of specific processing levels based on the determination of the stage at which the formative sequence is derailed, as reflected by error type or symptoms. Unlike the conventional approaches and interventions based on compensatory models, this approach allows the prediction of facilitatory effects based on a structural model of neurocognition.

## References

Anokhin, P.K. (1947). The theory of functional systems as the basis of understanding of compensatory processes in the body. In *Transactions of a Conference on the Restoration of Function after War Injuries*. Moscow: Moscow State University.

Basso, A. (1987). Approaches to neuropsychological rehabilitation: Language disorders. In M. Meier, A. Benton, & L. Diller (Eds.), *Neuropsychological rehabilitation* (pp. 294–314). New York: Guilford Press.

Benson, D. (1979). Neurologic correlates of anomia. In H. Whitaker & H. Whitaker (Eds.), *Studies in neurolinguistics* (Vol. 4, pp. 292–328). New York: Academic Press.

Ben-Yishay, Y. (Ed.). (1980). *Working approaches to remediation of cognitive deficits in brain damaged persons* (Rehabilitation Monograph No. 61). New York: New York University Medical Center, Institute of Rehabilitation Medicine.

Ben-Yishay, Y., & Prigatano, G. (1990). Cognitive remediation. In M. Rosenthal,

E. Griffith, M. Bond, & J.D. Miller (Eds.), *Rehabilitation of the adult and child with traumatic brain injury* (2nd ed.) Philadelphia: F.A. Davis.

Bernstein, N. (1967). *The coordination and regulation of movements.* Oxford: Pergamon.

Brown, J.W. (1972). *Aphasia, apraxia, and agnosia.* Springfield, IL: Charles C. Thomas.

Brown, J.W. (1977). *Mind, brain, and consciousness.* New York: Academic Press.

Brown, J.W. (1988). *The life of the mind.* Hillsdale, NJ: Lawrence Erlbaum.

Brown, J.W., & Chobar K. (1989). Therapy with a prosthesis for writing in aphasia. *Aphasiology, 3,* 709–715.

Brown, J.W., Leader, B., & Blum, C. (1983). Hemiplegic writing in severe aphasia. *Brain and Language, 19,* 204–215.

Davis, G., & Wilcox, M. (1981). Incorporating parameters of natural conversation in aphasia treatment. In R. Chapey (Ed.), *Language intervention strategies in adult aphasia* (pp. 169–193). Baltimore: Williams & Wilkins.

Flavell, J.H., & Draguns, J. (1957). A microgenetic approach to perception and thought. *Psychological Bulletin, 54,* 197–217.

Fowler, C.A., Rubin, P., Remez, R.E., & Turvey, M.T. (1980). Implications for speech production of a general theory of action. In B. Butterworth (Ed.), *Language production* (Vol. 1 pp. 373–420). London: Academic Press.

Friedland, J.F. (1989). *Hemiplegic writing: An access route to language in agraphia?* Paper presented at the Seventeenth Annual Meeting of the International Neuropsychological Society. Vancouver, B.C.

Geschwind, N., & Kaplan, E. (1962). A human cerebral deconnection syndrome: A preliminary report. *Neurology, 12,* 675–685.

Gardner, H., Zurif, E.B., Berry, T., & Baker, E. (1976). Visual communication in aphasia. *Neuropsychologia, 14,* 275–292.

Glass, A.V., Gazzaniga, M.S., & Premack, D. (1973). Artificial language training in global aphasics. *Neuropsychologia, 11,* 95–103.

Goldberg, G. (1987). From intent to action. Evolution and function of the premotor systems of the frontal lobe. In E. Perecman (Ed.), *The frontal lobes revisited* (pp. 273–306). New York: IRBN Press.

Goodglass, H. (1987). Neurolinguistic principles and aphasia therapy. In M. Meier, A. Benton, & L. Diller (Eds.), *Neuropsychological rehabilitation* (pp. 315–326). New York: Guilford Press.

Goodglass, H., & Geschwind, N. (1976). Language disorders (aphasia). In E.C. Carterette & M. Friedman (Eds.), *Handbook of perception* (Vol. 7, pp. 389–428). New York: Academic Press.

Gross, Y., & Schutz, L.E. (1986). Intervention models in neuropsychology. In B.P. Uzzell & Gross, Y. (Eds.), *Clinical neuropsychology of intervention* (pp. 179–204). Boston: Martinus Nijhoff.

Hadar, U., Davies, R.T., Steiner, T.J., & Rose, F.C. (1984). A psychomotor approach to improving speech by modulating suprasegmental control in motor dysphasia and articulatory apraxia. In F.C. Rose (Ed.), *Advances in neurology: Vol. 42. Progress in aphasiology* (pp. 337–351). New York: Raven Press.

Hadar, U., Steiner, T.J., & Rose, F.C. (1984). Involvement of head movement in speech production and its implications for language pathology. In F.C. Rose (Ed.), *Advances in neurology: Vol. 42. Progress in aphasiology* (pp. 247–261). New York: Raven Press.

Hanlon, R.E., & Brown, J.W. (1989). Microgenesis: Historical review and current studies. In A. Ardila & F. Ostrosky-Solis (Eds.) *Brain organization of language and cognitive processes* (pp. 3–15). New York: Plenum.
Hanlon, R.E., Brown, J.W., & Gerstman, L. (1990). Enhancement of naming in nonfluent aphasia through gesture. *Brain and Language*, *38*, 298–314.
Helm-Estabrooks, N., Fitzpatrick, P.M., & Barresi, B. (1982). Visual action therapy for global aphasia. *Journal of Speech and Hearing Disorders*, *47*, 385–389.
Holland, A.L. (1967). Some applications of behavioral principles to clinical speech problems. *Journal of Speech and Hearing Disorders*, *32*, 11–18.
Holland, A.L. (1970). Case studies in aphasia rehabilitation using programmed instruction. *Journal of Speech and Hearing Disorders*, *35*, 377–390.
Johannsen-Horbach, H., Cegla, B., Mager, U., Schempp, G., & Wallesch, C.W. (1985). Treatment of chronic global aphasia: A nonverbal communication system. *Brain and Language*, *24*, 74–82.
Kaplan, E., Goodglass, H., Weintraub, S. (1983). *Boston Naming Test.* Philadelphia: Lea & Febiger.
Kertesz, A. (1982). *Western Aphasia Battery*. Orlando, FL: Grune & Stratton.
Kimura, D. (1976). The neural basis of language qua gesture. In H. Whitaker & A.H. Whitaker (Eds.), *Studies in neurolinguistics* (Vol. 2, pp. 145–156). New York: Academic Press.
Kimura, D. (1979). Neuromotor mechanisms in the evolution of human communication. In H.D. Steklis & M.J. Raleigh (Eds.), *Neurobiology of social communication in primates: An evolutionary perspective* (pp. 197–220). New York: Academic Press.
Kuypers, H.G.J. (1973). The anatomical organization of the descending pathways and their contributions to motor control especially in primates. In J.E. Desmedt (Ed.), *New developments in electromyography and clinical neurophysiology* (Vol. 3, pp. 38–68). Basel, Switzerland: Karger.
Leischner, A. (1970). Seitendifferente Schreibleistungen bei Agraphien. In *Die Rehabilitation der Aphasie in den romanischen Landern* (pp. 70–83). Stuttgart, Germany: Thieme Verlag.
Luria, A.R. (1963). *Restoration of function after brain injury*. New York: Macmillan.
Luria, A.R. (1966). *Higher cortical functions in man.* New York: Basic Books.
Luria, A.R. (1970). *Traumatic aphasia: Its syndromes, psychology and treatment.* The Hague, The Netherlands: Mouton.
Luria, A.R., Naydin, V., Tsvetkova, L.S., & Vinarskaya, E.N. (1969). Restoration of higher cortical function following local brain damage. In R. Yinken & G. Bruyn (Eds.), *Handbook of clinical neurology* (Vol. 3, pp. 368–433). Amsterdam: North-Holland.
Miller, E. (1984). *Recovery and management of neuropsychological impairments.* Chichester, UK: John Wiley.
Naeser, M.A. (1975). A structured approach to teaching aphasics basic sentence types. *British Journal of Disorders of Communication*, *10*. 70–76.
Pick, A. (1913). *Die agrammatischen Sprachstorungen*. Berlin: Springer-Verlag.
Sarno, M.T. (1981). *Acquired aphasia*. New York: Academic Press.
Schacter, D.L., & Glisky, E.L. (1986). Memory remediation: Restoration, alleviation and the acquisition of domain-specific knowledge. In B.P. Uzzell & Y.

Gross (Eds.), *Clinical neuropsychology of intervention* (pp. 257–282). Boston: Martinus-Nijhoff.

Schlanger, P., DiCarrado, C., & Geffner, D. (1974). *A comparison of gestural communication with aphasics: Pre- and post-therapy*. Paper presented at the American Speech and Hearing Association Convention, Las Vegas, NV.

Schlanger, P., & Freimann, R. (1979). Pantomime therapy with aphasics. *Aphasia-Apraxia-Agnosia*, *1*, 34–39.

Skelly, M. (1979). *Amer-Ind gestural code based on universal American Indian hand talk*. New York: Elsevier.

Skelly, M., Schinsky, L., Smith, R., Donaldson, R., & Griffin, J. (1975). American Indian sign: A gestural communication system for the speechless. *Archives of Physical Medicine and Rehabilitation*, *56*, 156–160.

Skelly, M., Schinsky, L., Smith, R.W., & Fust, R.S. (1974). American Indian sign (Amerind) as a facilitator of verbalization for the oral verbal apraxic. *Journal of Speech and Hearing Disorders*, *39*, 445–456.

Sohlberg, M.M., & Mateer, C.A. (1989). *Introduction to cognitive rehabilitation*. New York: Guilford Press.

Sparks, R., & Holland, A. (1976). Method: Melodic intonation therapy for aphasia. *Journal of Speech and Hearing Disorders*, *41*, 287–297.

Tankle, R.S. (1988). Application of neuropsychological test results to interdisciplinary cognitive rehabilitation with head-injured adults. *Journal of Head Trauma Rehabilitation*, *3*, 24–32.

Turvey, M.T. (1977). Preliminaries to a theory of action with reference to vision. In R. Shaw & J. Bransford (Eds.), *Perceiving, acting and knowing*. Hillsdale, NJ: Lawrence Erlbaum.

Turvey, M.T. (1980). Clues from the organization of motor systems. In U. Bellugi & M. Studdert-Kennedy (Eds.), *Signed and spoken language: Biological constraints on linguistic form* (pp. 41–56). Weinheim, Germay: Verlag Chemie.

Vygotsky, L.S. (1962). *Thought and language* (E. Hanfmann & G. Vakar, Trans.). Cambridge, MA: MIT Press. (Original work published 1934)

Weigl, E. (1981). *Neuropsychology and neurolinguistics: Selected papers*. The Hague, The Netherlands: Mouton.

Werner, H. (1956). Microgenesis and aphasia. *Journal of Abnormal Social Psychology*, *52* 347–353.

Wilson, B. (1989). Models of cognitive rehabilitation. In R.L. Wood & P. Eames (Eds.), *Models of brain injury rehabilitation*. Baltimore: Johns Hopkins University Press.

Wood, R.L. (1987). *Brain Injury rehabilitation: A neurobehavioural approach*. Rockville, MD: Aspen.

Yakovlev, P.I. (1948). Motility, behavior and the brain. *Journal of Nervous and Mental Disease*, *107*, 313–335.

# Part II Experimental Methods and Findings

# 10
# Percept-Genesis: A Frame of Reference for Neuropsychological Research

GUDMUND J.W. SMITH

## A Biological Approach

The percept-genetic (or PG) model discussed in the present chapter can be defined as being basically biological. Even if a biological approach has often been associated with a reductionistic, antipsychological one, good reasons support this choice of designation. Biological science need not necessarily be reductionistic. Biology is fundamentally a life science concerned with growth and survival, defense, and adaptation—or, in short, with functional problems in relation to structural differences.

Psychology is also one of the life sciences when it deals not only with traits, dispositions, or skills—that is, consummate mental formations—but with how these formations have come about; not only with the invariant world of perception but with how this world was once built up and is continually being remodeled; and not only with abstract entities such as points on an IQ or anxiety scale but with how intellectual and emotional problems are handled. Unfortunately, too much of today's psychology falls outside this commendable labeling (see Kline, 1988).

The PG model to be outlined here should be considered biological mainly because its central focus is on processes, the very processes of construction supporting our experience of reality. This approach fits hand in glove with neurological analysis, particularly when that science conceives of perceptual acts as being initiated not in the visual cortex but in more ancient parts of the brain, proceeding from the brain stem, via the limbic system and the parietal cortex to the occipital region (Brown, 1988). Similarly, in the PG model, perceptual processes start in the world of subjective representations and end up in the objective world around us.

## What is a Process?

The term *process* has been used in diverse ways, some of them very far from its apposite meaning. In this context, I apply the term primarily in relation to mental events, within or beyond awareness, either directly accessible through the individual's own reporting and behavior, or indirectly, such as by way of experimentation. As just pointed out, processes occupy the center stage in the PG model.

Only an event over time can be designated as a process. Time may represent macro- as well as micro-perspectives, such as years, months, days, hours or—in many instances when the term percept-genesis is used—fractions of a second. The mere passage of time, however, does not constitute a process. Process entails change. And change can be conceptualized in qualitative as well as quantitative terms, the latter often being an abstraction of the former. This is a crucial issue that will be made more explicit when the features of the PG model are brought into focus.

No laudable meaning is inevitably attached to the term *process*. Often, processes are thought of as tools of adaptation, furthering development, and survival. But a process can also be pathogenic, destructive, and turned against the individual.

The most pertinent characteristic of processes is the *successive determination* from one stage to the next, or *cumulation*, as defined in the specific PG context. Thus, one section or phase of a process cannot be conceptualized without reference to the preceding phases. This does not exclude the possibility that a process may superficially appear to be discontinuous (see Hinde & Bateson, 1984). Even if change from one phase to the next looks like a complete metamorphosis, the latter phase cannot be correctly comprehended in isolation. Rather, it must be perceived in the light of previous phases, just as the chrysalid stage in the development of a butterfly must be explained with reference to the seemingly unrelated larval stage.

Thus, relations between stages in a process must be understood in terms of general laws explaining, for instance, the necessity of a chrysalid stage for the production of a butterfly or, to take an example from our studies (Smith & Carlsson, 1990), the role of noncreative periods for the full development of creativity. All too often, psychological researchers have let themselves be confounded by surface contradictions.

## A Brief Historical Perspective

The PG model is concerned with what is happening here and now in a variable present. Perceptual microprocesses had already been described in the 1920s by Gemelli (1928) and Sander (1928/1961), independently of each other. Sander's term for a microprocess was *Aktualgenese*. The explanatory frame of reference of the German school was general psychology. Remnants of this approach can still be found in the USSR.

The term *Aktualgenese* was translated into microgenesis by Heinz Werner (e.g., 1956, 1957). As developmental psychologists, Werner and his associates also tried to relate the formal characteristics of different stages in a microgenesis to stages of development in ontogenesis. For instance, when describing a Rorschach card, a person's tendency to choose childish interpretations would be greater for shorter exposure times than for longer ones (see Friedman, 1953; Phillips & Framo, 1954; Stein, 1949).

These challenging findings did not, however, convince Werner (1956) to use a differential approach. The laws of development were general, as was the parallelism between ontogenesis and microgenesis. On the whole, Werner was not particularly interested in the issue of personality and probably never dreamt of using microgenetic techniques as a gateway to differential diagnosis.

These early investigators employed various methods to reconstruct microprocesses of which the viewer himself was not, or only partly, aware. Fröhlich (1984) describes two main groups. For the *hologenetic* group of methods, the energy level of stimulation is increased from trial to trial "as in tachistoscopic threshold experiments or as when using a polarization device to control the level of luminance—or if the amount of clarity and distinctiveness increases as a result of a refocusing procedure" (p. 25). The *merogenetic* methods seem more questionable as a means of reconstructing a real microgenesis. Here, the stimulus presentation starts with figural fragments and continues in a way that offers increasing detail until a meaningful gestalt can be recognized.

## *Percept-Genesis, a First Look*

The term *percept-genesis* was coined in Lund, Sweden, by Kragh and Smith (1970) to emphasize the specific aim to study the microdevelopment of percepts. The introduction of a new term also marked the difference between the Lund approach and the *Aktualgenese*–microgenesis one.

The frame of reference used in PG analysis is not general psychology. Instead *primary* interest is directed toward the relation between perception and personality. Influence of the so-called New Look school of perception can be detected here (see Blake & Ramsey, 1951). Like the New Look proponents, particularly Klein (1970), the Lund group exploited basic psychoanalytic ideas without feeling bound by psychoanalytic orthodoxy.

Kragh (1955) was the first to describe the relation between perception and personality as developmental. Thus, we do not conceive of two independent entities, the percept and the personality, mutually influencing each other. Instead, the objective (conscious), externalized world is visualized as growing out of a subjective (subconscious) personal core during the course of a PG.

If a subject is presented with a series of exposures such that the first is just below the threshold of recognition but those following are systematically prolonged or intensified, the reports of what he has seen will eventually change, not only quantitatively, that is, with respect to brightness and distinctness, but also qualitatively, with respect to meaning. A process of construction is thus reconstructed.

The early phases in the reconstructed process, the Preliminary-phases, are not just weak transcriptions of stimulus but are stamped by subjective themes, often organized without regard to time and space, having a condensed, synchretic character, reminiscent of dream contents. The late stimulus-proximal phase is called the Concluding-phase. During the PG, the stimulus-distant, subjective formations are gradually *eliminated* and the stimulus-proximal meaning becomes more focal, dominant, and externalized.

The following example is taken from Kragh and Smith (1970, p. 27). The stimulus consisted of a photograph of three braided baskets placed on top of each other, together with a boy and a rather diffuse background of buildings. For the sake of simplicity, only one section of the total picture, the baskets, will be considered here. Four phases of the PG will be presented, including both the subject's description of what he saw and, within parentheses, his associations with what he had seen.

1. A fountain—a monster—a mouth
   (Dragon, vulva, calla-lily, foetus)
2. Three sandbags and a column or niche
   (Tombstone, stamp)
3. Three baskets and a dark wall
   (Same)
4. Three baskets—stimulus-proximal organization
   (Same)
   (Kragh & Smith, 1970, p. 27)

In this way, the real world around us is continually being shaped and reshaped. The process could also be described as successively increasing fovealization, as demonstrated in an experiment by Westerlundh (1983). With progressive retinal centralization of perception—the way percepts are often processed in everyday life—the viewer's impressions of the surrounding world become gradually more intersubjective. But the elimination of the P-phase or marginal meaning is seldom complete. Remnants of the margin may remain as an aura around the central focus. Without these person-proximal, emotionally colored echoes, the real world would be bare and lifeless.

In this context, it is relevant to ask whether a correct focus is present from the very beginning of a PG. We can only surmize that this is true. The focus is, naturally, often deeply embedded in subjective formations, elusive and difficult to descry. But it has a directing influence, setting the limits within which the PG can unfold, limits becoming gradually more constricted the closer the PG approaches the C-phase. This is how the role of stimulus can be described (see Brown, 1988).

It should not be overlooked at this point that the reconstruction of process material always must be brought about within the frame of reference of the present level of experience. An inflexible and narrow frame of reference—too adult and established, perhaps—will obviously bar the admittance of "foreign" and "deviating" material to the reconstructed PG.

## Do Percept-Geneses Really Exist?

One is not generally aware of the existence of PGs. It seems pardonable, therefore, that naively extraverted psychologists often appear to doubt their existence.

Two additional factors are likely to contribute to this doubt. First, PGs are abbreviated when repeated (see Kragh & Smith, 1970). Second, certain fundamentals of perception, necessary for survival, probably do not develop but are instead instantly present to assist the individual. Gibson (1979; see also Reed, 1988) described acts of perception to which the perceiver has little to contribute. What one has in mind is the perception of movement, the detection of certain invariant forms or textures, the adaptive use of important stimulus gradients, and so on.

PGs basically concern the construction of meaningful external objects and are particularly obvious in settings novel to the viewer. In attempts to protract PGs, one should thus avoid geometrical figures devoid of meaning, or stereotyped drawings, and prefer pictures with expressive content, mostly human or clearly physiognomic in character.

Proofs of the existence of PGs have been presented and discussed elsewhere (Kragh & Smith, 1970; Smith & Westerlundh, 1980; Westerlundh & Smith, 1983). Some of the proofs refer to experiments with a stabilized retina (Pritchard, Heron, & Hebb, 1960), demonstrating that without eye movements, that is, repeated fixations of the objects, no stable perception of that object is possible.

The very fact that processes can be reconstructed by means of special methods may be counted as another proof of their existence. To criticism that these processes are likely to be artifacts of little interest, I can offer four possible rejoinders:

1. It has been shown (e.g., Smith, Johnson & Almgren, 1989) that characteristic features of the reconstructed process, such as those interpreted as signs of anxiety or defensive strategies, can be used as efficient predictors in many different settings.

2. Reconstruction is impossible when the situation is well known or empty of meaning. Such would not be the case if the PG was just an artifact generated by nothing but the very technique of protraction.

3. Reconstruction is also difficult in children aged 3 to 4 years, with the result that they do not reach a stable C-phase. This demonstrates the

importance of real PGs for the construction of a stable external world (Smith & Carlsson, 1990).

4. The most functional and simple explanation of the emotional tone surrounding a percept and the associations following its establishment would be that they are remnants of a PG, mostly occurring beyond awareness.

## The Issue of Subliminal Perception

Following Dixon's (1971) theory about subliminal perception, Beloff (1974) has postulated two different perceptual systems, one associated with a relatively low state of arousal and mainly mediated by the limbic and midbrain structures. Subliminal perception is assumed to be associated with this system. This kind of perception allows access to a wide range of information, which otherwise is often excluded by the inhibitory mechanisms of the other perceptual system, associated with a relatively high state of arousal.

Subliminality is not necessarily associated with early PG stages. Subliminal perception may be essentially correct and allow prediction of its effects on simultaneous supraliminal perception, associations, and the like (see Dixon, 1981). This is particularly obvious in experiments with geometric figures (Smith & Henriksson, 1955) for which PGs are brief or nonexistant, that is, subliminal percepts are likely to be close to the C-phase. Recent evidence, however (Westerlundh, 1986) suggests that when meaningful stimulation is presented beyond awareness, the emotional meaning usually has primacy, that is, this meaning is registered and other possible meanings ignored, a conclusion obviously in line with Dixon's postulate. The preceding evidence suggests that subliminal perception can be associated with early as well as late stages of a PG.

## Percept-Genesis, a Closer Look

All PGs build structure. This is not exactly the same as saying that people learn as they go along. Structure is a theoretical construct, sometimes defined as process with a low rate of change. In the present theoretical context, structure building means that one process limits the degree of freedom of subsequent processes by forcing them to follow certain twists and turns, particularly in the beginning of their course.

I subscribe to the psychoanalytic presumption that structure is hierarchically organized. Early structure building corresponds to low levels in the hierarchy, late structure building to higher, more differentiated levels. Thus, primitive structures are superseded by more developed ones as the individual grows older. PGs are supposed, by and large, to reflect this structural hierarchy, from low levels to higher ones, from less adapted to more adapted, from subjective to objective, and so on.

From the preceding discussion, it should be evident that low-level structures are more difficult to obtain by means of reconstruction because of the obstacles erected against these efforts. The degree of reconstruction possible depends on the present situation and the mental condition of the individual. States of reverie are mostly favorable, defensive attitudes unfavorable. As Silverman, Lachman, and Milich (1982) have pointed out, subjects in experiments with verbal activation should be in an optimal receptive mood. Subjects in a PG experiment conducted by a person hostile to basic PG assumptions may be overly apprehensive, leading to a minimum of reconstruction.

Structures are not necessarily inflexible and everlasting. One must presume that even deep-seated structures may change. Because a PG is assumed to reflect the hierarchical arrangement of structures, it cannot, therefore, be an accurate repetition of the life development of the individual, only an approximate one. Another obstructing factor should also be mentioned: Because of the necessarily circumscribed content of any stimulus picture, a single PG can hardly mirror more than a segment of a person's history. Nevertheless, there can still be very striking correspondences between micro- and macro-development, as shown in studies of therapy patients (e.g., Kragh, 1986) and, more convincingly, in studies of groups with important differences in life experience (Kragh, 1955; Westerlundh & Terjestam, 1990). (Westerlundh & Terjestam also offer a more penetrating analysis of this controversial issue than is possible to offer here.)

Freedom of action from structural tyranny exists above all at the spearhead of constructive change, that is during the late phases of a PG. At the same time, a full-fledged PG always reaches back to include previously established structures; while the wind may be bending the branches of a PG tree, it is still rooted in the individual's personal history. How deeply depends on the demands of the present situation. When, however, an individual is challenged to seek radically new solutions to old problems, a deep retreat might be an attempt to take a new run to bypass obstructing structures. This may happen as a result of successful therapy.

As already mentioned, structure is a theoretical construct. At the empirical level, one can discern the visual form reported by the subject, which I call *organization*, and the *meaning* attributed to this form. Meaning may be revealed by the way a subject describes the form or by his associations to it (see the example cited previously). On the basis of organization and meaning, structure can be defined: the richer the pattern of empirical observations, the greater the reliability of the definition.

Organization and meaning are transformed during the course of a PG in three different ways: through *elimination*, *cumulation*, and *emergence*.

Elimination denotes the disappearance of and cumulation, the successive determination of, organization and meaning. In some instances, there seems to be little continuity from one phase to the next. This is defined by the term *emergence*, often corresponding to sudden breaks in the course of a subject's life. The more I deal with meaning instead of organization, the more I move from material typical of the psychology of perception to material typical of the psychology of personality.

When trying to relate the C-phase in a PG to the P-phases, one should not think of the relation of a sum to its parts but rather of the relation of "a differentiated and specified part-component to the complex component pattern from which it has gradually evolved" (Kragh & Smith, 1970, p. 25). (The Kragh & Smith volume also contains more specific analyses not iterated here.)

The abbreviation of PGs through repetition, briefly mentioned before, will hereafter be called *automatization*. To better understand this phenomenon, one also must consider the concept of *stabilization*. The two can easily be confounded. A PG normally leads to more stable perceptions or conceptions of reality. This stabilization occurs not only in the microperspective of a PG but also in the macroperspective of ontogenesis. Concomitant with stabilization in the latter perspective is a growing automatization in the microperspective resulting from repetition of identical or similar PGs. Automatization implies that a process is abbreviated and that originally separate P-phases are shoved into each other and eventually disappear. As a result of automatization, the reflection of ontogenesis in PGs becomes increasingly fragmentary.

Stabilization as well as automatization must be viewed as biological necessities. Through stabilization one not only creates a world recognizable to oneself but a world where one can communicate with others of one's kind with a reasonable degree of mutual understanding. The successive automatization of PGs is the key to an effective energy economy. Energy invested in present enterprises must be released as soon as possible to meet future demands. Automatization facilitates the redistribution of attention and intentional effort (Smith, 1984).

It must also be made clear that a PG cannot lead to a fully stabilized C-phase until ontogenesis has allowed the person the reach a definite conception of reality. And vice versa, as observed, not until the child can anchor his constructive efforts in P-phases can there be a stable C-phase (Smith & Carlsson, 1990).

In this context it might also be necessary to again consider the dominance of C-phase meaning over P-phase meaning. To paraphrase the Finnish philosopher Eino Kaila, one could attribute it to the need for invariance. The C-phase meaning influences the reconstruction of PGs, rendering this process particularly difficult in the face of inhibitions and defenses. This is naturally part of the creativity problem, in as much as creativity presupposes a break with an all-dominant C-phase meaning.

(The topic has been treated at considerable length in Smith & Carlsson, 1990.)

Much PG research has been devoted to the blocking and distorting role of defenses (The Defense Mechanism Test, DMT, Kragh, 1985; The Meta-Contrast Technique, MCT, Smith, Johnson & Almgren, 1989). Less often pointed out is the fact that defenses are not necessarily obstructive. By only partially blocking threatening material actualized in the course of a PG, defenses may increase the individual's possibilities to reconstruct other more useful sides of his PGs. In everyday life, one needs to screen off certain aspects of experience to deal more efficiently with others.

# Techniques of Reconstruction

This discussion has concerned mainly the reconstruction of ultrashort processes, hidden from introspection under ordinary circumstances. The tachistoscope has been the main instrument for presenting stimuli in serials favoring subjective factors at the beginning and objective ones at the end. An alternative so-called amauroscopic technique was successfully applied by Westerlundh and Sjöbäck (1986), who systematically varied the luminance instead of the time duration. A third method was introduced by Westerlundh (1983), who initially presented stimuli in the retinal margin and then gradually moved the stimuli toward the fovea. He proved that this presumably had the same effects as variation in time and luminance. More variation can be found in traditional microgenetic research (Kragh, 1985; Kragh & Smith, 1970; Smith et al., 1989).

I have also tried to study processes of longer duration by observing how subjects gradually, and in different ways, adapt to a mirror-drawing situation, to the well-known conflicts in the (Stroop) color-word test, and to perceptual phenomena like visual afterimages, little known to the average subject. These processes do not differ, in principle, from microprocesses. They are, however, bound to emphasize formal categories more than content, such as continuity versus discontinuity or flexibility versus inflexibility.

One potential advantage of studying these more tangible processes is that they can be more easy to manipulate. One appropriate example is a study of afterimage serials by Smith, Sjöholm, and Andersson (1971). Subjects were instructed to project a visual afterimage of a red face on a screen, the projection distance being longer than the fixation distance. The fixations of the face were repeated 15 times, and the size, brightness, and hue of the ensuing afterimage were recorded each time. The resulting afterimage serials were individually typical, that is, each subject handled the problem of how to fit a subjective phenomenon into a world of physical objects in his own characteristic way.

About half-way through the process, a disturbing auditory signal was given through earphones. The subject immediately responded by starting the afterimage adaptation anew, each subject in his own way. While one could see how the afterimage process repeated the characteristics observed in its original course, one could also see that it was generally abbreviated. If the disruptive signal was applied close to the C-phase, process repetition ceased, except in schizophrenic subjects, who never seemed to become really habituated. This and similar experiments (Andersson, Nilsson, Ruuth & Smith, 1972) clearly demonstrate that it is possible to produce processes for study and that these processes are normally of finite length, gradually become shorter with increasing repetition, and are individually characteristic. These trends provide an additional argument against those who claim that PGs are artifacts of the experimental manipulation.

It might be added that afterimage experiments have also demonstrated the importance of the C-phase for process reconstruction. The subject's conception of the nature of the phenomenon under observation could be regarded as defining his C-phase. By varying the instructions about the "true" nature of afterimages—said to be mainly anchored in outside reality or alternatively, in the subject himself, said to be depending primarily on retinal structures or, alternatively, on the central nervous systems and so on—the experimenter was able to decisively influence the size and color of the images produced, not only in children but in sophisticated adults as well (Smith & Sjöholm, 1974).

## Empirical Support and Neuropsychological Connections

A sizable amount of material has been published in support of the claim that the PG model and the methods operationally defining it are profitable. Some material stems from work with prediction of success and failure in stressful situations—above all, material stemming from the use of the DMT. Other material is more clinical. The MCT (Smith, Johnson & Almgren, 1989) to be presented in detail in Chapter 11 has been employed for decades as a diagnostic instrument. In both these tests, disturbing or threatening stimulation has been exploited to facilitate defensive reactions in the viewer.

Alternative investigations primarily aim at testing theoretical assumptions, mainly psychoanalytic ones. The previously mentioned study using an amauroscopic technique (Westerlundh & Sjöbäck, 1986) is one such example. Andersson's studies employing an alternative DMT method may be cited as another example of how theoretical assumptions can be supported by the application of PG methodology (Andersson, 1984; Andersson & Bengtsson, 1986).

The PG model has not remained untouched by these various empirical efforts. Nilsson (1983) made a thorough attempt at reformulating some of its basic tenets. The developmental perspective with regard to anxiety and defense was influenced by a series of studies of children and youngsters, using both the MCT and an afterimage test (Smith & Danielsson, 1982). By and large, however, the main features have remained the same. The present outline is perhaps more biologically oriented than previous ones (Kragh & Smith, 1970; Smith & Westerlundh, 1980), emphasizing a process perspective. (In line with this partial reorientation, Chapter 11 presents applications in neuropsychology pertaining to laterality, anxiety, and various types of brain dysfunction.)

Why should PG techniques be particularly suited to the field of neuropsychology? The best answer can be given by the just-mentioned empirical studies. Formulated more generally, at least three reasons are evident:

1. The process perspective is consonant in a general way with current approaches to the workings of the brain; that is, it is functional rather than structural.
2. The PG material emphasizes the personality aspect of neuropsychology, often neglected for the benefit of a purely cognitive approach.
3. The PG methods penetrate to the very core of human experience, actualizing hidden material in the context of more adapted conscious material, not abstracting one side from the other but viewing the C-phase and the P-phases as a developmental unit.

The application of PG methodology to neuropsychological problems should not, however, confuse psychology with physiology. What is gained by directly observing the workings of the brain, on the one hand, and what subjects report about their experiences, on the other, are facts belonging to different levels of description. One level cannot be used to explain the other. But a cross-fertilization of theoretical ideas and practical decisions (e.g., regarding rehabilitation) is feasible and desirable. Brown's (1988) microgenetic neurological theory may be cited as an example. Much knowledge about the workings of the brain is produced via psychological experiments (Gazzaniga, 1985). I believe that experiments devised within a process frame of reference, like the one outlined here, may serve this end better than traditional tests. In a similar way, our biological approach to psychology may be particularly suited for using neurophysiological advancements.

## References

Andersson, A.L. (1984). Cognitive growth, psychoanalytic conceptions of the mind, aftereffect experience and disavowal as a defense against threat. In G.J.W. Smith, W.D. Fröhlich, & U. Hentschel (Eds.), *From private to public reality* (pp. 103–114). Bonn: Bouvier.

Andersson, A.L., & Bengtsson, M. (1986). Percept-genetic defenses against anxiety and a threatened sense of self as seen in terms of the spiral aftereffect technique. In U. Hentschel, G.J.W. Smith, & J.G. Draguns (Eds.), *The roots of perception* (pp. 217–246). Amsterdam: North-Holland.

Andersson, A.L., Nilsson, A., Ruuth, E., & Smith, G.J.W. (1972). *Visual after-effects and the individual as an adaptive system*, Lund, Sweden: Gleerup.

Beloff, N. (1974). The subliminal and the extrasensory. In A. Angoff & B. Shapin (Eds.), *Parapsychology and the sciences* (pp. 103–122). New York: Parapsychology Foundation.

Blake, R.R., & Ramsey, G.U. (Eds.). (1951). *Perception: An approach to personality*. New York: Ronald.

Brown, J.W. (1988). *Life of the mind. Selected papers*. Englewood Cliffs, NJ: Prentices-Hall.

Dixon, N.F. (1971). *Subliminal perception: The nature of a controversy*. London: McGraw-Hill.

Dixon, N.F. (1981). *Preconscious processing*. Chichester, UK: Wiley.

Friedman, H. (1953). Perceptual regression in schizophrenia. A hypothesis suggested by the use of the Rorschach test. *Journal of Projective Techniques*, *17*, 171–185.

Fröhlich, W.D. (1984). Microgenesis as a functional approach to information processing through search. In W.D. Fröhlich, G.J.W. Smith, J.G. Draguns, & U. Hentschel (Eds.), *Psychological processes in cognition and personality* (pp. 19–52). New York: Hemisphere.

Gazzaniga, M.S. (1985). *The social brain: Discovering the networks of the mind*. New York: Basic Books.

Gemelli, A. (1928). Il comparire e il scomparire della forme. *Contributi di Laboratorio della Psicologia e Biologia, Università del Sacro Core*, *3*, 385–436.

Gibson, J.J. (1979). *The ecological approach to visual perception*. Boston: Houghton Mifflin.

Hinde, R.A., & Bateson, P. (1984). Discontinuities versus continuities in behavioral development and the neglect of process. *International Journal of Behavioral Development*, *7*, 129–143.

Klein, G.S. (1970). *Perception, motives and personality*. New York: Knopf.

Kline, P. (1988). *Psychology exposed*. London: Routledge.

Kragh, U. (1955). *The actual-genetic model of perception—personality*. Lund, Sweden: Gleerup.

Kragh, U. (1985). *The defense mechanism test*. Stockholm: Persona.

Kragh, U. (1986). Life panorama under the microscope: A paradigmatic case study. In U. Hentschel, G.J.W. Smith, & J.G. Draguns (Eds.), *The roots of perception* (pp. 145–159). Amsterdam: North-Holland.

Kragh, U., & Smith, G.J.W. (1970). *Percept-genetic analysis*. Lund, Sweden: Gleerup.

Nilsson, A. (1983). The mechanisms of defense within a developmental frame of reference. In *Studia Psychologica et Paedagogica, Monograph 64*. Lund, Sweden: Gleerup.

Phillips, L., & Framo, J. (1954). Developmental theory applied to normal and psychopathological perception. *Journal of Personality*, *22*, 464–474.

Pritchard, R.M., Heron, W., & Hebb, D.O. (1960). Visual perception approached by the method of stabilized images. *Canadian Journal of Psychology*, *14*, 67–77.

Reed, E.S. (1988). *James J. Gibson and the psychology of perception*. New Haven, CT: Yale University Press.

Sander, C.F. (1928/1961). Experimentella Ergebnisse der Gestaltpsychologie. *Bericht über den 10 Kongress für experimentelle Psychologie*. (In C.F. Sander & H. Volkelt (Eds.), *Ganzheitspsychologie* (pp. 23–28). Munich: Beck. (Original work published 1928).

Silverman, L.H., Lachman, F., & Milich, R. (1982). *The search for oneness*. New York: International Universities Press.

Smith, G.J.W. (1984). Stabilization and automatization of perceptual activity over time. In W.D. Fröhlich, G.J.W. Smith, J.G. Draguns, & U. Hentschel (Eds.), *Psychological processes in cognition and personality* (pp. 135–142). New York: Hemisphere.

Smith, G.J.W., & Carlsson, I. (1990). *The creative process. A functional model based on empirical studies from early childhood to middle age. Psychological issues, Monograph 57*. New York: International Universities Press.

Smith, G.J.W., & Danielsson, A. (1982). *Anxiety and defensive strategies in childhood and adolescence. Psychological issues, Monograph 52*. New York: International Universities Press.

Smith, G.J.W., & Henriksson, M. (1955). The effect on an established percept of a perceptual process beyond awareness. *Acta Psychologica, 11*, 346–355.

Smith, G.J.W., Johnson, G., & Almgren, P.-E. (1989). *MCT—the meta-contrast technique*. Stockholm: Psykologiförlaget.

Smith, G.J.W., & Sjöholm, L. (1974). Can our theory of reality influence our perception of it? *Psychological Research Bulletin, Lund University, Monograph Series 1*, 1–27.

Smith, G.J.W., Sjöholm, L., & Andersson, A.L. (1971). Effects of extraneous stimulation on afterimage adaptation. *Acta Psychologica, 35*, 138–150.

Smith, G.J.W. & Westerlundh, B. (1980). Perceptgenesis: A process perspective on perception-personality. In L. Wheeler (Ed.), *Review of personality and social psychology* (Vol. 1, pp. 94–124). Beverly Hills: Sage.

Stein, M.J. (1949). Personality factors involved in the temporal development of Rorschach responses. *Journal of Projective Techniques, 13*, 355–414.

Werner, H. (1956). Micro-genesis in aphasia. *Journal of Abnormal and Social Psychology, 52*, 347–353.

Werner, H. (1957). The concept of development from a comparative and organismic point of view. In D.B. Harris (Ed.), *The concept of development: An issue in the study of human behavior* (pp. 125–148). Minneapolis: University of Minnesota Press.

Westerlundh, B. (1983). Personal organization of the visual field: A study of ambient and focal reports of threatening stimuli. *Archives of Psychology, 135*, 17–35.

Westerlundh, B. (1986). On reading subliminal sentences: A psychodynamic activation study. *Psychological Research Bulletin, Lund University, 26*, 10.

Westerlundh, B., & Sjöbäck, H. (1986). Activation of intrapsychic conflict and defense: The amauroscopic technique. In U. Hentschel, G.J.W. Smith, & J.G. Draguns (Eds.), *The roots of perception* (pp. 161–215). Amsterdam: North-Holland.

Westerlundh, B., & Smith, G.J.W. (1983). Percept-genesis and the psychodynamics of perception. *Psychoanalysis and Contemporary Thought, 6*, 597–640.

Westerlundh, B., & Terjestam, Y. (1990). Memory activation and perceptual processing: On the idea of microgeny-ontogeny correspondence. *Psychological Research Bulletin, Lund University, 30*, 6.

# 11
# Application of a Percept-Genetic Methodology to Neuropsychology

INGEGERD CARLSSON, ÅSA LILJA, GUDMUND J.W. SMITH, and AKI M. JOHANSON

This chapter is meant to illustrate, at the level of empirical neuropsychology, the model outlined in Chapter 10. Two studies are reported (Carlsson, 1990; Lilja, Hagstadius, Risberg, Salford, & Smith, 1991a). At first glance, they may appear rather dissimilar, one using normal subjects to study hemisphericity, the other concerning cases of brain tumor. They share at least three common features, however, as follows:

1. Both take account of what has long been known among students of the central nervous system: One learns more from studying systems in dysfunction or under stress than from systems working in perfect balance. This experience is exploited in the first study by forcing normal subjects to engage, "unnaturally," one hemisphere at a time when attending to a complicated perceptual task. In the other study, the manipulation is brought about by pathological processes in the brain.
2. Although much interest in the field of neuropsychology has been devoted to cognitive functioning in isolation, the studies in this chapter are more concerned with a broader personality perspective. That does not mean that cognition has been ignored in these studies. In the first, cognition is associated with creative coping; the second takes account of the fact that serious disturbances in the ability to process disturbing stimulation are not necessarily associated with general intellectual reduction.
3. Both studies exploit a percept-genetic personality test, implying that processes of reality construction are artificially protracted and analyzed. By entertaining threatening stimulation in the test, anxiety and defensive strategies are specifically attended to.

This personality test, the Meta-Contrast Technique (MCT), will be presented in outline form. More specific scoring categories will, however, be reserved for the particular investigation. The second study has also made use of a method allowing the investigator to follow brain activity by measuring the regional cerebral blood flow (rCBF). The rCBF will be presented in the second study. A method for visual half-field stimulation will be described in the first.

## The Meta-Contrast Technique

The MCT was developed based on experiments with subliminal perception (e.g., Smith & Henriksson, 1955). (The percept-genetic model forming the theoretical background of the test is presented in Chapter 10.)

In the present context, the following outline of the model is most relevant. If an individual is confronted with a new situation, he is apt to react with a general state of readiness or arousal, implying mobilization of his accumulated adaptive resources. When, after reiterated fixations, he has received more information, the mobilization is gradually, often rapidly, relaxed, and more specialized functions are delegated to take care of the adaptive task. Or, to view the process from the inside: The initial stages (P-stages) of a percept-genesis are characterized by a varied spectrum of contents, often dominated by primitive levels in the experiential hierarchy and only to a small extent restricted by the actual stimulation. During the ultra-short percept-genesis, however, irrelevant and person-proximal contents are "peeled off," leaving a gradually more prominent nucleus of stimulus-proximal contents. In other words, as the percept-genesis proceeds, it becomes less marked by "subcortical" functions and more by "cortical" ones.

As just mentioned, the MCT was originally based on experiments with subliminal perception. These experiments proved that a supraliminal percept can be affected by a temporally proximal subliminal process. Hence, this technique offered a way to indirectly gain access to early stages in a perceptual process. By combining a subliminal methodology with the percept-genetic one, it might be possible to find out how a new perceptual process might influence the individual's established perceptual frame of reference. If, as in Kragh's (1985) Defense Mechanism Test, the "new" stimulation implied a threat to the established percept, particularly interesting information might be gained about the viewer.

### *Design*

MCT implies repeated tachistoscopic presentations of pairs of stimuli, one exposed immediately after the other. The second stimulus (B) in a pair is intended to represent the established perceptual frame to which the viewer has been adapted in advance. Within this frame, the development of the first stimulus (A) will be followed step by step. Originally, we employed A-stimuli that were incongruent with the content of A (e.g., a car introduced into a living room). In the present experiments, the A-stimuli represent a threat to a person depicted in B. To begin with, A is exposed very rapidly and does not manifest itself as a perceptual structure in its own right but sometimes as changes in the B-percept. With subsequently prolonged exposure times, however, A gradually penetrates B, often in "disguise" to begin with. The test session is concluded when A + B have been correctly reported or when the test must be discontinued for technical reasons (no prolonged exposure times remaining on the scale).

It is unnecessary to dwell on technical details here. The three basic phases of the test session follow: (1) Starting with .01 s, B is presented at gradually prolonged exposure times until the image has been correctly reported. (2) The time for further presentations of B is set at a standardized level where B is presented alone five times in a control series. (3) A is then introduced before B at .01 s. The pairwise A + B presentations are continued, with the exposure time of B held constant and that of A prolonged every second time (according to a geometric scale with a constant of $\sqrt{2}$).

Stimuli are projected on a 35- × 35-cm screen in front of the subject, who describes what he has seen after each presentation. The experimenter not only records what the subject says but also how he behaves (shutting his eyes, sighing, looking panic-stricken, being restless, etc.). These behavior manifestations are of particular interest in the study of patients with cerebral dysfunctions.

There are two MCT series. In the first study, only one of the series was used, in the second study, both series. The A-stimuli in both series depict a threatening face; the B-stimulus, a lonely young person with whom the viewer is supposed to identify (the "hero").

The subject was instructed as follows:

> Pictures will be shown on the screen in front of you. They will be presented at very short exposure times. I'll say "now" before each exposure. Be prepared to look at the screen and then tell me what you saw. Please, make special note of any changes from one exposure to the next.

## *Scoring*

The scoring refers to changes in reports of B and interpretations of A. The sequential aspect is always important. What is scored late in a series is supposed to represent more manifest tendencies than what is reported early, the reason being that late phases are closer to the individual's habitual level of experiencing.

There are two main groups of signs: signs of anxiety and signs of defense against anxiety. The former signs are ordered in a scale from reports of darkness to open manifestations of panic. Disintegrations of the B-picture represent grave anxiety as well as psychotic regressions. The defensive signs range from primitive, behavioral forms to more advanced meaning transformations of A. They are grouped in the following categories: repressive strategies, isolation and negation strategies, projective strategies, depression, regressions, and self-referential sign variants. In some instances, the differentiation between various defense strategies or between defense, on the one hand, and cognitive style, on the other, can be difficult to ascertain, the latter case being exemplified by depressive stereotypies.

### *Standardization Data*

Standardization data have been offered in detail in the most recent MCT manual (Smith, Johnson, & Almgren, 1989). Both interrater and test–retest correlations have been generally high, often close to the statistical ceiling. Validation data have been presented in more than 30 mutually independent studies, typical test-criterion correlations coefficients ranging from .50 to .85. The first validation studies showed, for instance, that people with histrionic characters had more signs of what was called repression than other clinical groups, compulsive–obsessive subjects more signs of isolation-negation, psychotics more signs of regression, and so on. The criterion groups were carefully selected. Later validations also refer to correlations with other tests, to change as a result of therapy, to differences between young children and older ones, and the like.

## Lateralization and Defense Mechanisms in Relation to Creative Functioning

In this study, degree of hemispheric lateralization is tested in a visual half-field design and related to results in a test of creative functioning. The presentation is based on a more comprehensive report by Carlsson (1990).

Various theoretical models have been proposed with regard to the association between hemispheric functions and creativity. Kinsbourne (1982) argues that "Creation may advance while drawing on the specialized processing of one hemisphere only" (p. 418). Others, for instance Arieti (1976), believe that both hemispheres are necessary for creativity.

Bogen and Bogen (1969) discuss the advantage of two independent problem-solving organs—that is, the left, propositional, and the right, appositional, hemisphere—to the solution of a novel situation. They claim that a major obstacle to creative functioning is the inhibitory effect of the left hemisphere's propositionsal thinking on the functions of the right hemisphere.

An experiment giving some support to this model was performed by Martindale and Hasenfus (1978). They found that highly creative subjects, when instructed to be creative, had high levels of electroencephalogram (EEG) alpha-waves in both hemispheres during the inspirational part of a creative task, compared to the elaborational part. Alpha-levels for less-creative subjects did not differ between the inspirational and elaborational parts. This might imply that in highly creative subjects the activity in the left hemisphere was not suppressing activity in the right hemisphere during the inspirational part of the creative process.

Torrance (1982) also emphasizes the right hemisphere. He "reviewed the results of students who were administered a self-report measure of information processing style based on recent hemispheric research" (p. 36) and found "a rather consistent tendency for the measures of creative style to be positively and significantly related to the right hemisphere style" (p. 36).

Thus, it seems likely that the right hemisphere's mode of functioning is important for creative activity, and that mode of interaction between the hemispheres is of interest.

Definitions of creativity vary depending on whether the product, process, or the creative person is emphasized. In this study, priority was given to the creative personality. It is assumed that the creative individual pays attention not only to the objective (intersubjective) reality, but that she or he can make conscious use of subjective ideas and alternative notions of "reality" (Smith, 1981). These aspects of the creative personality are operationalized in the Creative Functioning Test (CFT) (Smith & Carlsson, 1990), described in the following discussion.

The measure of laterality is shown in results on the MCT (described previously), presented in a visual half-field design.

In a previous visual half-field study (Carlsson, 1989), significant laterality effects were found with the MCT. Subjects tested in their right visual half-field (left hemisphere) had more signs of isolation and repression. This was assumed to be due to the left hemisphere being the main center for complex language functions necessary for the operation of developmentally late defense mechanisms.

Subjects who were instead tested in their left visual half-field (right hemisphere) responded with more signs of a developmentally early strategy, namely regression. This was interpreted to be caused by a relative lack of left-hemisphere involvement, allowing latent strategies in the mental apparatus to emerge.

Many subjects in this study, however, responded with a less lateralized pattern. Thus, no matter which visual half-field was stimulated, they responded with defenses typical of both visual half-field groups. These individual differences might have some connection with creativity. In a study of 171 youngsters who were tested with the MCT under regular testing conditions, the highly creative people significantly more often had several different defenses, whereas the uncreative subjects showed a "one-sided" defensive pattern (Carlsson & Smith, 1987).

Because creativity thus implies a flexible shifting between different defensive functions, presumably localized in both hemispheres of the brain, it is assumed that subjects with high scores on the CFT will have analogous responses on the MCT in both visual half-field groups. Subjects low in creativity are instead assumed to have a more lateralized pattern.

## Method

### Subjects

Eighty-four undergraduate students were randomly divided into two groups. The right visual half-field (RVF) group contained 23 women and 19 men. The left visual half-field (LVF) group consisted of 24 women and 18 men. The median age of both groups was 23 years, and age ranged from 18 to 36 years. All subjects were right-handed according to the Edinburgh Handedness Questionnaire (Oldfield, 1971).

### Design

Carlsson (1990) tested half of the subjects with the MCT in the RVF and the other half in the LVF and she tested 60 subjects with the CFT before the MCT or on a follow-up session. The rest (24 subjects) took both the MCT and the CFT in a visual half-field design. For these subjects, Carlsson gave the CFT on two different occasions; the second time with a parallel version of the test. Of the two CFT tests, we will consider the one with the highest score for each subject in the results, because Carlsson discerned no consistent differences between the visual half-field conditions.

#### *The Visual Half-Field Testing With the MCT*

As mentioned, the purpose of the MCT is to evoke anxiety reactions and to study the defense strategies against anxiety.

During testing, the subject rested his head on a support that was placed straight in front of a point of fixation. This point was marked only on the left (or right) edge of the picture screen showing a threatening face. The picture was thus exposed in only one or the other visual half-field, and stimulation entered the opposite hemisphere first. For the subjects tested in their RVF, the examiner turned the pictures around. The angle from the point of fixation to the edge of the threatening face was 3.1°, and to the far end of the face, 6.4°.

The examiner instructed the subject to look at the point of fixation each time a picture was shown. During the testing, the experimenter reminded the subjects once or twice not to move their eyes. Only very few subjects reported occasional difficulties with the fixation.

#### *Scoring Dimensions in the MCT*

The following categories taken from the MCT manual were most common in the subjects in this study: regression, projection, isolation, repression, and anxiety.

*Regressive strategies* imply that the subject regresses to infantile modes of perceiving (e.g., reporting colored objects in the black-and-white picture) or that the continuous reporting of the stabilized hero-picture is broken. The subject either cannot see at all what it depicts or believes that it is an entirely new picture. Vague answers are scored as tendencies toward regression.

*Sensitivity and projection*: A sensitive person reacts to the threat very early but instead interprets it as changes occurring in the hero-picture. This strategy can be seen as a means to locate worrying stimulation in the outside world. When these changes get stronger they are interpreted as more clearly projective defensive maneuvers. Uncertain answers are scored as tendencies toward projection.

*Isolation* varies from infantile strategies to more mature efforts to keep threat and hero apart. Tendencies toward isolation are scored when an answer is vague or when the subject tries to give a "rational" explanation of the phenomena on the screen.

*Repression* implies efforts to decathect, or drain the threat of strength and life. It contains a spectrum of reactions from those primarily found in children to more mature symbolic answers. Vague answers are scored as tendencies toward repression.

*Anxiety* varies from mild, moderate, to grave signs. Anxiety often implies partial blackening of the picture.

The experimenter and an independent judge scored all MCT protocols. The agreement was generally good. In a few cases of dissension, a third judge was called in.

*The Creative Functioning Test*

The CFT was also developed within the percept-genetic tradition. In most instances, the percept-genesis has been studied in relation to various threat situations, but in the CFT, another approach is tried. Here, particular attention is paid to the subject's attitude to early, idiosyncratic stages in his percept-genesis. A creative person is defined as having an inclination to loosen himself from reality and to engage in subjective interpretations instead.

The CFT has been validated in a series of investigations (for a thorough review, see Smith & Carlsson, 1990). Different outside judges have evaluated criteria like originality, richness in ideas, expressiveness, or renewal. Correlations have been high, for example, .72 between an outside judge of artists' productions and CFT.

To formulate matters more closely in relation to the CFT: The subject is presented with a picture motif, which is shown at initially very short presentation times, which are successively prolonged. After a series of divergent interpretations, the subject can perceive and describe the picture correctly. Thereafter, the testing continues uninterrupted but with gradually shortened exposure times to withdraw outside support for recognition.

The stimulus motif in the CFT is a black-and-white photograph of a still-life depicting a rounded glass bottle with a wide bowl beside it. The parallel version depicts an armchair with a round table beside it. Both pictures are somewhat vague with clear physiognomic qualities.

The prolonged, or *upward*, part of the test elucidates whether the subject can offer alternative interpretations before the correct report; in other words, it may be considered a test of imagination. The most important measure of creativity, however, is what happens in the successively abbreviated or *downward*, part of the test. The question is: Does the subject regard the interpretations from the upward series as "wrong," and will he therefore hold on to the correct motif? The other possibility is a willingness and interest in returning to early conceptions of the picture or to new inventions. In other words, a creative person can see *both* the reality ("facts") *and* disregard it in favor of his own imagination ("fantasy").

The technical equipment is the same as with the MCT. The testing began with an exposure time of .01 s and was prolonged with a quotient of $\sqrt{2}$. The upward series ended when the subject described the picture correctly three times in a row. The testing continued with the downward series and ended when the subject no longer saw anything on the screen.

The subjects were instructed to report after each exposure what they thought was depicted, even if uncertain.

*Scoring Dimensions in the CFT*

The CFT protocols can be scored in both the upward and downward parts because these correlate with different aspects of the creative personality. The results in the downward series correlate with the most clearly creative features, like originality and richness in ideas (Smith & Danielsson, 1978), and in the present study only the downward series was scored. The degree of abandonment of the correct stimulus meaning is measured in a scale that originally contained six steps: high, medium, and low creativity.

*High Creativity*. The subject interprets the whole picture in a completely different way during one or several exposures. For example, "Now it was the person with the car, like in the beginning."

*Medium Creativity*. The subject interprets only part of the picture differently, or his interpretation is rather vague or only implies plastic changes of the picture's content: "A cross in front of an ellipse, very weak."

*Low Creativity*. The subject reports that the picture gets dimmer, darker, or disappears piece by piece.

The experimenter scored the CFT protocols. For the most part, the scoring was easy, but in a few cases of doubt, an independent judge decided. No names were attached to the protocols, and in most instances, the scoring was done several months after the testing.

## Results

### Creative Functioning in the Visual Half-Field Groups

The visual half-field groups had equal proportions of differently creative subjects. In the RVF group, 13 subjects had high, 17 had medium, and 12 subjects had low creativity. In the LVF group, the corresponding results were 12, 17, and 13 subjects.

The relatively high degree of creative and medium-creative subjects probably depends on the kind of subjects who participated. About half were students of architecture and the rest students of medicine.

### Single Defense Categories Compared With Creativity

The high-, medium-, and low-creative groups were compared concerning laterality in the MCT. Table 11.1 shows the number of subjects with signs in each defensive category.

The low-creative LVF group tended to have more subjects with regression plus tendencies to regression than the low-creative RVF group ($p < .10$, Fisher's exact test, two-sided), whereas medium- or highly creative subjects did not differ between the visual half-field groups.

For sensitivity and projection, Carlsson (1990) found no laterality effects. Instead, the low-creative subjects, irrespective of visual half-field group, had less sensitivity projection than more creative subjects. For both visual half-field groups jointly, a chi-square calculation yielded 6.88, $df = 2$, $p < .05$.

Carlsson (1990) found a marked difference between the low-creative groups for isolation, which was predominant in the RVF group ($p = .02$, Fisher's test, two-sided). In medium-creative subjects, the isolation scores tended to differ ($p < .10$, Fisher's test), whereas no contrast was obserred between highly creative subjects.

Table 11.1. Number of subjects with regression, projection, isolation, and repression compared with degree of creativity in the visual half-field groups.

| | RVF group ($n$) | | | LVF group ($n$) | | |
|---|---|---|---|---|---|---|
| CFT | With defensive category | Tendency | No sign | Defensive attribute | Tendency | No sign |
| | | | **Regression** | | | |
| High | 1 | 5 | 7 | 5 | 1 | 6 |
| Medium | 1 | 8 | 8 | 3 | 3 | 11 |
| Low | 1 | 0 | 11 | 5 | 1 | 7 |
| | | | **Sensitivity and projection** | | | |
| High | 2 | 6 | 5 | 3 | 5 | 4 |
| Medium | 0 | 7 | 10 | 3 | 8 | 6 |
| Low | 1 | 2 | 9 | 1 | 3 | 9 |
| | | | **Isolation** | | | |
| High | 5 | 6 | 2 | 6 | 5 | 1 |
| Medium | 10 | 4 | 3 | 6 | 6 | 5 |
| Low | 8 | 1 | 3 | 2 | 4 | 7 |
| | | | **Repression** | | | |
| High | 11 | 0 | 2 | 7 | 1 | 4 |
| Medium | 12 | 3 | 2 | 6 | 9 | 2 |
| Low | 8 | 1 | 3 | 2 | 6 | 5 |

CFT, Creative Functioning Test; LVF, left visual half-field; RVF, right visual half-field.

Repression was more common in the low-creative RVF group than in its LVF counterpart ($p = .02$, Fisher's test). In the medium-creative groups, we found a tendency ($p < .10$, Fisher's test). The highly creative subjects did not diverge.

### Nonhemisphere-specific Defenses Compared With Creativity

Another way to study differently creative subjects is to see to what extent they use defenses typical of the not-directly stimulated hemisphere. These strategies are regression in the RVF group and isolation plus repression in the LVF group.

For this comparison, isolation and repression were considered jointly, and the subjects were divided at the best median: Subjects with repression plus a tendency toward isolation (or vice versa), or with both isolation and repression, were placed above the median for isolation plus repression.

Table 11.2 shows the number of subjects with scores above or below the median for isolation plus repression and with or without scores for regression plus tendencies toward regression. Only three low-creative subjects responded with nonhemisphere-specific defenses, whereas 13 subjects high in creativity did so. A chi-square calculation yields $p < .01$ ($\chi^2 = 10.43$, $df = 2$). The skewed median cut for isolation plus repression in the LVF group could possibly influence the result. The balance can be improved if those subjects in the LVF group who have at least one defense (but with no additional tendency), are placed above the median. The contrast becomes approximately the same ($\chi^2 = 11.36$, $df = 2$, $p < .01$).

### Results in Anxiety

Carlsson (1990) discerned no significant differences between the subjects, neither between visual half-field groups nor between levels of creativity.

TABLE 11.2. Number of subjects in the creativity groups with or without regression, combined with results in isolation plus repression.

| | RVF group | | LVF group | |
|---|---|---|---|---|
| | Isolation plus repression above median | Below median | Isolation plus repression above median | Below median |
| | **High creative subjects** | | | |
| All signs of regression | 4[a] | 2[a] | 4[a] | 2 |
| No signs of regression | 5 | 2 | 3[a] | 3 |
| | **Medium creative subjects** | | | |
| All signs of regression | 8[a] | 1[a] | 2[a] | 4 |
| No sign of regression | 4 | 4 | 5[a] | 6 |
| | **Low creative subjects** | | | |
| All signs of regression | 0[a] | 1[a] | 1[a] | 5 |
| No sign of regression | 6 | 5 | 1[a] | 6 |

[a] These subjects have nonhemisphere-specific defenses.
LVF, left visual half-field; RVF, right visual half-field.

## Discussion

This study supported the assumption that highly creative subjects would have less asymmetry between LVF and RVF than low-creative subjects. Carlsson (1990) found no differences when comparing the visual half-field groups at the high end of the creativity scale. Moderately creative subjects tended to differ, whereas Carlsson found significant differences between the visual half-field groups in low-creative subjects. Also, highly creative persons more often responded with nonhemisphere-specific defenses than low-creative ones.

The visual half-field groups did not differ in sensitivity and projection. Instead, these signs diminished with diminishing creativity. This result could reflect a lower stimulus threshold in creative people, not necessarily differing between the hemispheres. A related finding was made by Sackeim, Packer, and Gur (1977). These authors describe their results as follows:

> Left movers, or right hemisphericity people, showed the subliminal effect when encouraged to think in a holistic and intuitive fashion. This effect was predicted. Surprisingly, right-movers (left-hemisphericity people) tended to show the subliminal effect when encouraged to think in an organized and logical manner, indicating that hemisphericity and cognitive set may be more mutually interdependent in affecting susceptibility to subliminal stimulation than was originally expected. (p. 628–629)

A sensitive disposition has previously been assumed to characterize creative people (e.g., Greenacre, 1957). Analogous results were obtained in studies of professional artists and youngsters (Smith & Carlsson, 1990). In both groups, repression and sensitivity in the MCT correlated positively with creativity.

A possible neuropsychological explanation of the results in the present study concerns mode of information transfer between the hemispheres; the main connection being the corpus callosum. It is well-established that speech is a left-hemisphere function in almost all right-handed people. When the subjects in the present study are, for instance, stimulated in their right hemisphere, the transmission of information to the left hemisphere becomes crucial, because the subjects are requested to report verbally what they see on the screen. It may be proposed that in low-creative subjects transmission of information is of insufficient detail or intensity to enable certain functions in the other hemisphere to become fully activated.

Martindale and Hines (1975) described their highly creative subjects as having a higher rate of disinhibition and "a slight deficit in cortical self-control" (p. 98) when trying to suppress alpha-waves in an EEG feedback task.

The results in Carlsson (1990) study could perhaps be worded in the following way: Whereas the low-creative people adhered strictly to the directly stimulated function, highly creative people more often shifted between different styles, that is, they responded more flexibly.

## Anxiety and Coping Strategies in Brain Tumor Patients

Lilja et al. (1991a; cf. also 1991b) used the MCT to penetrate emotional disturbances and personality changes in 25 patients suffering from various forms of brain tumor, in a pre- and post-operative design. This section is based on their reports.

They intended to describe the brain tumor patient's subconscious and conscious world of experience and the process in which it is constructed and reflected and to study how surgery might influence this process and how the patients were able to cope before and after the operation.

The patients also were administered a standardized battery of cognitive assessment.

The measures of emotion and perception, unexpectedly, enabled the differentiation of specific dimensions of anxiety, regressive personality disturbances, and immature defensive strategies in patients with highly malignant astrocytomas as compared to patients with less-malignant or benign brain tumors. These results were partially substantiated by neurophysiological findings.

The study was initiated by the clinical observations that patients with supratentorial, highly malignant cerebral tumors display specific affective changes, including "inappropriate" cheerfulness and euphoria and diminished insight in sickness. Distractibility, loss of initiative, and inertia, perhaps resulting from a decrease in cortical tonus, were also noted. Similar clinical features have been described in association with frontal lobe disturbances (Christensen, 1979; Goldberg & Costa, 1987; Luria, 1981), sometimes also in association with right hemisphere lesions (Gainotti, 1972).

In addition, several patients spontaneously reported sudden, unpredictable, and unmotivated panic attacks, often as long as 2 years before admission. Various anxiety states have been shown to involve frontal lobe functioning, as measured by both psychological and neurophysiological methods (Hagstadius, 1989; Johanson, Gustafson, & Risberg, 1986; Nauta, 1971; Reivich, Gur, & Alavi, 1983).

This prompted Lilja et al. (1991a) to ask how the tumor, irrespective of localization, affects the vulnerable frontal lobe system (Goldberg & Bilder, 1987) in terms of functional, neurophysiological disturbances coupled to anxiety and other behavioral manifestations indicating frontal lobe (or right-hemisphere) disturbances.

## Aims

The primary aim of the investigation was to elucidate the brain tumor patient's preconscious and conscious processing in terms of possible emotional disturbances such as anxiety as reflected by the MCT and associated with changes of (frontal) rCBF. A second aim was to study the effects of surgery as measured by these methods. Finally, Lilja et al. (1991a) wanted to compare patients with highly malignant gliomas with those with other forms of brain tumor, regarding the psychological and neurophysiological measures.

## Materials and Methods

As mentioned, Lilja et al. (1991a) analyzed the MCT without knowledge of tumor malignancy and the following two groups could be distinguished:

*Group HM* consisted of patients with highly malignant astrocytomas (Kernohan, grade III to IV); ($n = 17$). The group comprised 6 women and 11 men, with a mean age of 55 years (range 32 to 74). In five patients, the tumor involved diencephalic brain structures. Fourteen patients had nonfrontal tumors: three had tumors located in or involving the frontal lobes. Ten patients had a tumor in the right hemisphere and seven, in the left.

*Group LM* consisted of patients with less-malignant or benign brain tumors and also included two cases of metastases ($n = 8$). The group comprised four women and four men, with a mean age of 43 years (range 26 to 61). Four patients had nonfrontal and four, frontal tumors. Seven had a left-hemisphere tumor localization and one patient had a right-hemisphere tumor.

All operated tumors had a diameter exceeding 4 cm. Increased intracranial pressure was controlled by steroid medication, and no patients had remaining symptoms of increased intracranial pressure at the time of preoperative testing.

In all, 25 patients with brain tumor, 16 men and 9 women, aged 26 to 74 years, were studied with the MCT, preoperatively (17 HM and 8 LM patients). Postoperatively, eight HM patients and seven LM patients were followed up. Lilja et al. (1991a) investigated rCBF in 22 patients, preoperatively (15 HM patients and 7 LM patients). Postoperative rCBF values were determined in 16 patients (10 HM and 6 LM patients).

### Personality Assessment: The Meta-Contrast Technique

The general description of the MCT can be found in the introduction of this chapter. Scoring classes relevant for this study were: 1, anxiety; 2, regression; 3, repression; 4, isolation; 5, projection. A scoring class may be hierarchically organized, that is, arranged from anxiety manifestations and defensive strategies typical of preschool children, stepwise to those typical of adults (up to old age). This way of arranging permits us to retrace a pattern of maturation growth of anxiety and defenses, beginning at the behavioral and ending at an internalized level. Anxiety manifestations begin at the external (behavioral) level (open fear or primary anxiety). The patient shows marked signs of fear (sometimes panic) obviously connected with the appearance of stimulus A (the threatening face). At the internalized level, we score *a*, pathological signs (e.g., "zero-phases" that imply a complete breakdown of the perceptual input, holes or cracks in the wall in B, fusion of the threat and hero, etc.) and *b*, moderate signs (e.g., hero is reported absent, dark structures in the last third of the series, etc.). We scored other signs of anxiety as well.

Regressive strategies involve regression from a habitual level to a more immature one and usually are manifested in the test as breaks of the continuity in the series, discontinuity. The most pathological form of regression has been noted in psychotic subjects; that the B-stimulus is not recognized from one exposure to the next (e.g., the patient might report that "this is a totally different picture") is common in cases of nonparanoid schizophrenia (Cesarec, Nyman, & Nyman, 1988; Smith, 1968). The previously mentioned "zero-phases" are also scored in this category.

Repression retraces a scale of manifestations. The external level, called "direct denial," implies, for instance, eye-shutting behavior. The internalized (or symbolic) levels follow: *a*, low level (e.g., hero shuts his eyes as the threat becomes liminal); *b*, middle level (e.g., A is reported as a statue, etc.); and *c*, high level (e.g., A is reported as a tree or an object). Genuine repression implies in general that A becomes "stiff" or "lifeless." This strategy is ontogenetically developed before the isolation and negation strategies: On the external (behavioral) level, the patient (or the normal preschool child) isolates literally, for example, with his hands on the screen at the place of the threat. At the internalized level we scored as follows: *a*, low level (e.g., when the distance between hero and threat is reported increased); *b*, middle level (e.g., when A is reported as a "white object" etc.); and *c*, high level, genuine signs (e.g., stimulus A becomes a bright surface or an empty face or is hidden by protecting curtains). The isolation strategies are not fully developed until late latency or prepuberty. Typically, picture A and picture B are kept separated by the viewer.

Projective strategies are common at the age of 5 and peak again at puberty. When the 5-year-old's signs are scored in adulthood, they might be considered more or less pathological, sometimes regressive. We divide this scoring class as follows: *a*, sensitivity when the A stimulus influences the frame percept subliminally (e.g., the subject reports changes of perspective, light, posture of the hero); *b*, moderate signs, implying unconscious identification with the threatening stimulus, which is interpreted as "cheerful," "friendly," or "my doctor," and so on; *c*, marked signs (e.g., reports of pronounced movement, additional persons, etc.).

### Regional Cerebral Blood Flow

As mentioned, Lilja et al. (1991a) used rCBF as the neurophysiological measurement of functional changes in the cortex. They employed the $^{133}$xenon-inhalation technique. This is a well-established method for the study of brain circulation in normal people and in patients with and without brain damage (Risberg, 1980). The technique was outlined by Mallet and Veall (1965) and further developed by Obrist, Thompson, Wang, and Wilkinson (1975) and Risberg, Ali, Wilson, Wills, and Halsay (1975).

The subject inhales a mixture of $^{133}$xenon and air for 1 minute via a face mask and a rebreathing spirometer system, followed by 10 min of normal air breathing. The inert, emitting tracer diffuses into brain tissue from arterial blood and is cleared by venous blood. The gamma-radiation emitted by the tracer is continuously monitored either by 32 or, with a new high-resolution system, by 254 extracranial scintillation detectors (Risberg, 1987).

Lilja et al. (1991a) measured rCBF while the patient was in a resting state, lying supine on a comfortable bed, with eyes closed and a minimum of external stimulation. The measurement was preceded by some time of adjustment to the measurement situation.

Patients with highly malignant, nonfrontal tumors were analyzed separately (preoperatively, $n = 12$; postoperatively, $n = 7$).

## Design and Statistics

All measurements were made 1 to 2 days before surgery and 7 to 8 days after. In the MCT material, comparisons between the groups were made using Fisher's exact probability test for 2 × 2 contingency tables. Threshold comparisons were made, using a binomial test. Paired and unpaired *t* tests were used in the statistical analyses of the rCBF data. Neither the patients nor the examiner were verbally informed of the final diagnosis regarding tumor malignancy at the testing occasions.

## Results

### MCT Findings

Lilja et al. (1991a) made three different types of group comparisons: (1) Presurgery comparisons between the HM and LM groups, (2) Postsurgery comparisons between the groups, (3) Pre- to post-surgery comparisons in the HM group.

An overview of the studied variables is provided in Figures 11.1A and B, which show pre- and post-surgery comparisons between the HM and the LM groups. In Figure 11.1b, behavioral, low-, and middle-level repression form one variable, called "*immature repression*"; behavioral, low-, and middle-level isolation form another, called "*immature isolation.*"

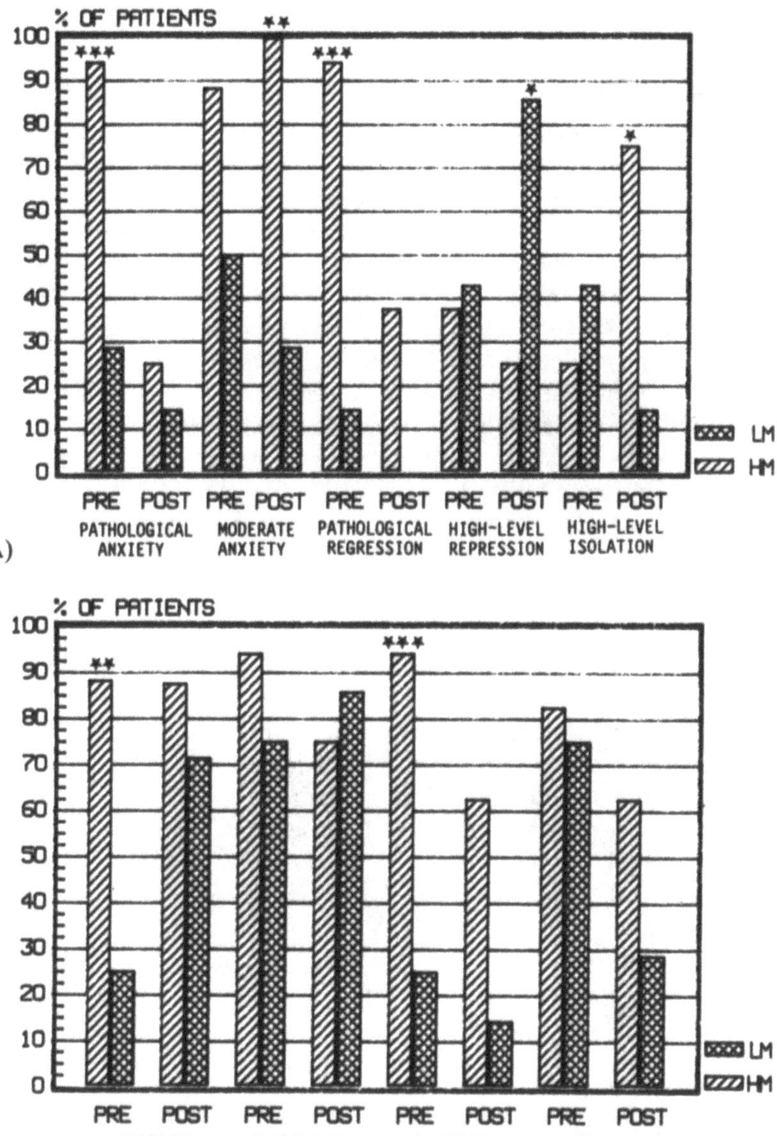


FIGURE 11.1. Results are shown for the Meta-Contrast Technique, pre- and post-surgery comparisons between the groups. (A) Before surgery, the HM group (patients with highly malignant astrocytomas) showed more pathological anxiety as compared to the LM group (patients with less-malignant or benign brain tumors) $p = .001$. Pathological regression was mostly observed in the HM group, $p < .001$. After surgery, the HM group showed more moderate anxiety, $p = .007$, and more genuine signs of isolation were found in this group, $p = .032$. The LM group used more symbolic (high-level) repression, $p = .032$. (B) Before surgery, the HM group showed more signs of moderate projection, $p = .035$, and immature repression was also more common in this group, $p = .001$ (***, $p \leqslant .001$; **, $p \leqslant .01$; *, $p \leqslant .05$).

*Presurgery Comparisons Between the Groups*

Sixteen out of 17 patients in the HM group displayed pathological anxiety and two out of eight in the LM group. This contrast is significant at the .001 level. Zero-phases as well as open fright or panic reactions were typical. Sixteen out of 17 patients in the HM group and four out of eight in the LM group showed moderate anxiety (not significant). All patients except one in the HM group, but only one in the LM group, had pathological regression ($p < .001$). The specific regressive strategy was abrupt changes in the meaning of the B-stimulus. As mentioned, this strategy has previously been scored in cases of schizophrenia (Cesapec et al., 1988; Smith, 1968). High-level (mature) repression and isolation were uncommon in both groups. Moderate projection was a strategy used by 15 patients in the HM group and by two patients in the other group ($p < .0035$). Immature forms of repression were more frequent in the HM group (16 patients) versus two patients in the LM group ($p < .001$).

*Postsurgery Comparisons Between the HM and LM Groups*

Lilja et al. (1991a) found pathological anxiety in two patients in the HM group and in one in the LM group. Moderate anxiety was present in all patients in the HM group and in two patients in the LM group ($p < .007$). Two patients in the HM group had pathological regression compared to none in the other group. High-level (genuine) repression was a defensive strategy used by the LM group (six out of seven patients) and two of eight patients in the HM group ($p < .05$). High-level isolation was more common in the HM group ($p < .05$). Seven out of eight patients in the HM group and five out of seven in the LM group showed moderate signs of projection after surgery. Sensitivity was common in both groups, as before surgery. Immature repression was found in five patients in the HM and in one patient in the LM group.

*Pre- to Post-surgery Differences in the HM Group*

Pathological anxiety, pathological regression, immature isolation, and repression were less accentuated postoperatively ($p < .001$) (weighed comparison).

In spite of the fact that the *threshold* for the correct identification of the B-stimulus was slightly higher in the HM group than in the LM group, the threshold for the identification of the A-stimulus was lower. Postsurgery, the threshold for the identification of B was significantly lowered in the total group of patients ($p < .003$).

### rCBF in HM Patients With Nonfrontal Tumors

Before surgery, the 12 HM patients with nonfrontal tumors showed significantly lower rCBF distribution values than controls in superior frontal

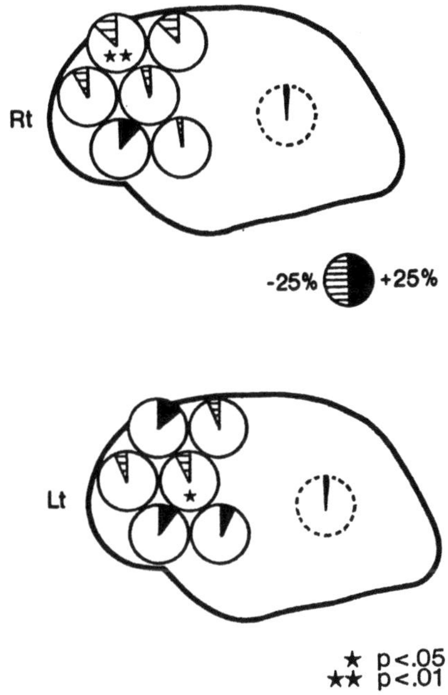


FIGURE 11.2. Differences in preoperative regional cerebral blood flow (rCBF) among 12 patients with highly malignant tumors with nonfrontal tumor localization and age-matched controls are shown. Differences are shown as clock symbols; black angles denote higher rCBF in the patients and striped angles lower rCBF (180° = 25% difference). The posteriorly located dotted circles denote the mean difference of the 10 nonfrontal detectors (*, $p < .05$; **, $p < .01$).

areas of the right hemisphere ($p < .01$) and in the left midfrontal area ($p < .05$). Distribution values in inferior-frontal areas were higher than in controls both in the right and in the left hemisphere. We saw no differences in the remaining areas (10 detectors combined) (Figure 11.2).

The seven patients with postoperative assessments showed significant pre- to post-operative decreases of rCBF in inferior-frontal ($p < .01$) and midfrontal areas of the right hemisphere. rCBF in the left frontal lobe as well as in the other areas (remaining detectors combined) showed no postoperative changes. In the superior frontal parts of the right hemisphere, the preoperatively low flow persisted (Figure 11.3).

Three HM patients with frontal tumors showed more marked superior-frontal and prefrontal flow reduction in both hemispheres compared to controls and patients with nonfrontal tumors, a pattern that was essentially unchanged after surgery.

A comparison between the HM and LM patients revealed that for the group with nonfrontal tumor localization, there were no significant differences in frontal rCBF preoperatively. There was, however, a tendency to

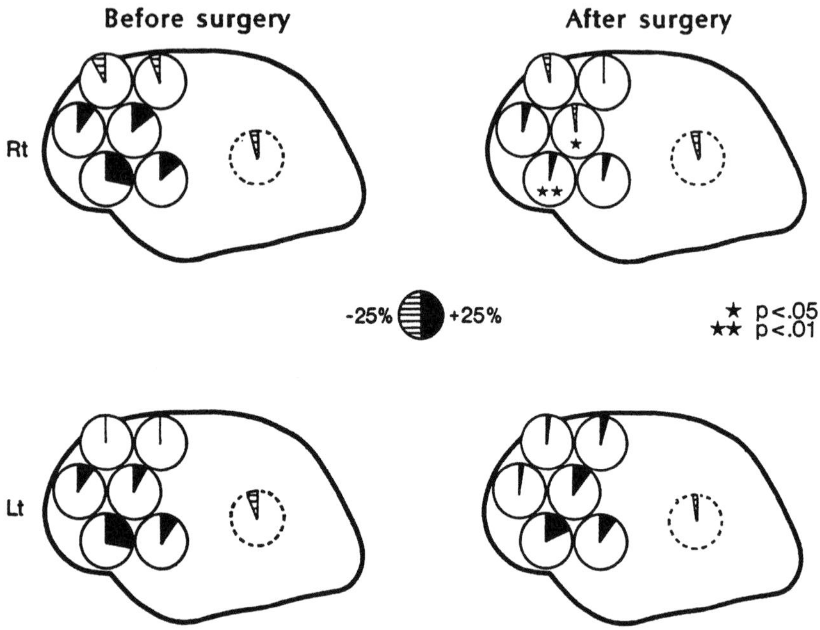


FIGURE 11.3. Pre- and post-operative regional cerebral blood flow (rCBF) levels, in seven patients with highly malignant tumors with nonfrontal tumor localization. Striped angles denote rCBF, lower than the hemispheric mean; and black angles denote rCBF higher than the mean. The postriorly located dotted circles denote the mean of the 10 nonfrontal detectors (*, $p < .05$; **, $p < .01$).

higher rCBF in inferior-frontal areas and lower in superior-frontal areas in the HM group, which was more marked in the right hemisphere. Postoperatively, rCBF was significantly lower in midfrontal and inferior-frontal areas of the right hemisphere in the HM group ($p < .05$).

## Discussion

Preoperatively, all cognitive assessments in both groups of patients were within normal range, except for verbal short-term memory, which was grossly impaired in both the HM and LM groups. Postoperatively, these results were essentially unchanged.

For the MCT, however, Lilja et al. (1991b) observed a clear difference between these two groups, with the HM group showing a higher incidence of schizoid-like regression as well as panic-related anxiety preoperatively. The rCBF recordings support the MCT as far as this difference is concerned, both pre- and post-operatively, indicating deviations in ventral and dorsal frontal areas in patients with highly malignant gliomas, not located in or involving the frontal lobes.

The nature of the regression found in the HM group appears consistent with the regression concept in the microgenetic theory of cognition (Brown, 1988). Brown holds that the regression seen in cases of brain damage is microstructural and not ontogenetic. One interpretation of this concept, applied to the present results, is that patients with highly malignant gliomas lose control of reality occasionally, revealed in the perceptual process as discontinuity, perceptual breakdowns, and so on.

The regression, however, is also in a wider meaning "ontogenetic" in the sense that both the HM and the LM groups (before surgery) showed lack of mature defenses, that is, the kind of repression and isolation expected in the well-adapted adult. This does not imply that these patients have generally "regressed" to a more "archaic" or primitive way of handling reality in general but that they may employ primitive defense strategies in an unknown, stressful, or anxiety-provoking situation.

Another interpretation of this specific kind of regression, implying that the patient loses control of the content in the B picture occasionally, is that the disturbances merely reflect fluctuations in attentional control of perceptual input. Such an explanation, however, seems insufficient in view of the fact that the picture is not even recognized from one exposure to the next. Such a disturbance must be considered as a regressive, psychotic-like reaction, the subjective world taking over reality control. As mentioned, this kind of regression has previously almost exclusively been found in cases of psychoses, above all, schizophrenia (Cesarec et al., 1988; Smith, 1968). The rCBF findings of low-flow activity, in dorsal frontal areas of the right hemisphere and in left-midfrontal areas both pre- and post-operatively are, at least partially, in line with previous rCBF findings of a hypofrontal flow pattern in cases of chronic schizophrenia (Ingvar & Franzén, 1974).

According to the evolutionary cytoarchitectonic dual-frontal lobe hypothesis (Pandaya & Barnes, 1987), the dorsal trend is involved in, among other things, attention and initiation of behavior (Pandaya, 1988). Following this hypothesis, the more organic-related interpretation that disturbances in attentional control could be a factor in the regression seen in the HM group seems possible. This, in turn, is supported by other rCBF results. The dorsal frontal areas of the right hemisphere become activated in high-anxiety–prone normal subjects during activation with a highly attention-demanding task (Hagstadius, 1989). The patients also, as mentioned, showed loss of initiative, clinically.

The presurgery elevated blood flow in inferior frontal areas could be associated with the preoperatively high incidence of panic-related anxiety in the HM group. The fronto-orbital and midfrontal areas, described as the neocortical representation of the limbic system, have been shown to be involved in anxiety states (Nauta, 1971).

Frontal rCBF changes have been reported earlier in different states of anxiety. Normal subjects who are highly anxiety prone have been reported to have higher mean flow and higher relative flow in superior frontal- and fronto-temporal areas of the right hemisphere, compared to a group that was low-anxiety prone. The magnitude of the frontotemporal asymmetry was related to degree of anxiety (Hagstadius, 1989). These results confirm those of Reivich et al. (1983), who, using position emission tomography (PET), found a similar association between degree of frontal asymmetry (right over left) and anxiety level in normals.

In cerebral-intact patients with anxiety neurosis, Johanson, Risberg, Silfverskiöld, and Smith (1986) found a left-sided, orbitofrontal flow increase during elevated anxiety. Level of anxiety was assessed by means of the MCT. The anxiety signs from the MCT were cross validated in situ during the rCBF recording.

The rCBF was recorded before and after stereotactic psychosurgery in patients with pathological anxiety. Postsurgery flow reductions were seen in frontal areas, bilaterally, with a parallel reduction in anxiety (Kullberg & Risberg, 1978). Thus, evidence exists for both left, right, and bilateral frontal lobe involvement in attentional, motivational, and emotional processes.

Following the dual-frontal lobe hypothesis, the ventral frontal lobe trend is closely tied to a synthesis of object–emotion relationships, sequential processes, drive, motivation, and will (Pandaya, 1988). There could be a disturbance in the habituation process, leading to the patient's experiencing the stimuli in the MCT as new at each exposure step. This fact alone might imply a higher degree of anxiety proneness that would interfere with the synthesis of object–emotion relations in the MCT. The results of Lilja et al. (1991b) indicate that brain tumor patients, perhaps more than normal subjects, are inclined to react faster to subliminal stimulation and hence to have a higher degree of access to deeper or preliminary stages in cognition.

The backward pattern-masking paradigm, used in the MCT, does not only require a high amount of attention. The object identity of the stimuli presented at the screen is also meaningful in character, that is, affectively laden. The microgenetic approach holds that the experiential or affective level in cognition would be the first (or deepest) level to be activated in any cognitive act. These subcortical or preprocessing stages would thus be elicited by means of emotionally meaningful subliminal stimulation.

The present HM patients showed a postoperative inferior-frontal decrease of flow in the right hemisphere, parallelled by normalized (moderate) anxiety. This fact supports the assumption that the frontal flow characteristics, pre- and post-operatively, are related to the patient's emotional functioning in general and particularly to pathological anxiety.

If panic-anxiety is one of the initial symptoms of malignant tumor growth, it might well be a primary (organic) symptom and not a reaction, which has been suggested by Brown:

> The anxiety in brain disorder is a symptom and not a reaction. . . . It is an "in-between" stage . . . and the form taken by the affect when an object [image] is positioned between external and mental space, i.e., when the image is just exteriorizing as an object, or the object recedes to the underlying image." (Brown, 1985, p. 125)

This is in perfect accordance with the MCT way of provoking anxiety. The present results also show that the method is suitable for eliciting anxiety manifestations in patients with this kind of central nervous system (CNS) disorder. It could be mentioned that the number of peripheral benzodiazepine receptors (not situated in the CNS) increase in number as the tumor grows more malignant (Black et al., 1989). This might have a relation to panic anxiety in patients with highly malignant gliomas (Black, personal communication, May 1990), although the precise function of these receptors are unknown at present.

The so-called "catastrophic reaction" (Goldstein, 1952/1973) in the testing situation and in the rehabilitation process is a well-known phenomenon. This "reaction" might be due to the inability of the brain-damaged patient (in general) to cope with external and internal stress (indicated by present results), and a panic will occur.

Preoperatively, both groups of patients showed lack of mature defenses. The HM group showed significantly more immature repression as compared to the LM group. This is not surprising. Mature repression implies a high level of symbolic transformation of the threatening stimulus. It is known that patients with frontal lobe dysfunction often lose the ability of abstract thinking such as required in, for example, logic, the construction of logic-grammatical sentences (Christensen, 1979; Luria, 1981), and the interpretation of proverbs. The HM patients might also have lost the ability to interpret and express emotionality in language, an impairment associated not only with frontal lobe dysfunction but also with right-hemisphere disturbances.

Both groups of patients showed sensitivity and an increased susceptibility to the subliminal stimulus both before and after surgery. Several explanations may apply: According to the dual-frontal lobe hypothesis, the dorsal frontal lobe trend is related to peripheral vision. The stimuli in the MCT are not presented parafoveally, but other studies have shown that centrally microgenetically presented stimuli engage the peripheral visual system, at least in the early phases (Westerlundh, 1983). Increased sensitivity to subliminal stimulation might also be due to hypermetamorphosis, that is, a tendency to take notice of and attend to every visual stimulus, part of the Klüver-Bucy syndrome.

In the MCT, sensitivity is, however, interpreted as a projective-defensive strategy. In the study of Lilja et al. (1991a), before surgery, the HM group showed significantly more signs of moderate projection compared to the LM group. Postoperatively, the sensitivity in both groups persisted, and in the LM group, the signs of moderate projection increased. Because both groups of patients showed sensitivity and moderate projection we cannot, based on the present material, conclude anything about possible relations between frontal lobe dysfunction and sensitivity-projection. *Projection* in general implies that the distinction between the internal and external world could disappear and be manifested in a state of confusion. Stroke patients tested with the MCT show more marked signs of projection (movement, additional persons in the picture, etc.). These patients also differ from the brain tumor patients with respect to other defenses as well as pathological anxiety.

## General Discussion

Interest in personality as a reflection of brain functioning is not new. Personality, however, usually has been studied in a very general way as an echo of experienced clinicians' observations of patients with brain injuries or dementia. It has been demonstrated here that more precise personality descriptions are indeed possible.

Personality can be depicted in many different ways. It is still common to exploit self-reports as a basis for enumeration of traits, present or absent, in analogy with the static way in which the landscape of cognitive skills has usually been conceptualized. Projective or other psychodynamically oriented methods have been avoided. The empirical investigations included in this chapter are unique in their use of a percept-genetic methodology, which (as discussed in Chapter 10) cannot be fully taken advantage of except in combination with a psychodynamic (but not necessarily psychoanalytic, in the orthodox meaning of the term) approach to personality functioning. Contrary to common belief, the combination of brain research and percept-genesis seems self-evident, as has also been pointed out by the neurologist Jason Brown (e.g., 1988). As stated in Chapter 10, the percept-genetic perspective is basically biological because its main object of interest is live processes of reality construction not hypostatized abstract entities.

Previous neurological research has often concerned cognitive aptitudes in isolation from personality. Our attention to personality functioning does not imply that, in a similar manner, we want to exclude cognitive functioning from our field of attention. In the study of brain tumor patients (Lilja et al., 1991b), it was of particular interest that the personality disturbances were accompanied by cognitive disturbances only to a small extent. The results of the laterality study also reflected "cognitive" differences between the hemisphere groups. As we see it, cognitive and personality functioning must be considered as complementary aspects of the same parcel. An emotional disturbance, for instance, acquires a different meaning, depending on the quality of cognitive functioning in the affected individual, and vice versa.

It is remarkable that the MCT has proved to be a useful test not only in patients with an intact intellect but, as shown in a recently published study (Johanson, Smith, et al., 1990), in demented patients as well. In these patients, the usual types of psychometric testing were mostly difficult to carry out. Many of them found it very arduous to talk about themselves, about their anticipations and anxieties, and to describe how they tried to cope with these frustrations. The MCT is easy to administrate, because it only requires of the test person that he describe a picture appearing on a screen. Furthermore, the MCT offers an indirect access to the demented patients' inner worlds when other channels become increasingly blocked up and unreliable.

The aim of the first study (Carlsson, 1990) was not to formulate the problem of hemisphericity in general terms. Instead, degree of cooperation between the two hemispheres was analyzed in relation to creativity. The more creative the individual, the more open the communication between the two hemispheres appeared to be, at least with respect to the use of defenses. As far as hemisphericity is concerned, there can obviously be distinctive group differences. Thus, conclusions about functional localization might be very misleading if such possible differences are not taken into account, one group of subjects generating results very different from another group.

Applied to dysfunctional cerebral states, the MCT can disclose anxiety reactions and defensive strategies, varying with both the etiology and localization of the damage. In the study of dementia just referred to, localization determined the personality changes no matter if the damage was degenerative, that is, influencing the very structure of the brain, or caused by the blood vessels as infarcts or hemmorhages. In contrast, the second study in this chapter (Lilja et al., 1991a) revealed a marked difference in, for example, anxiety reactions, depending on the degree of malignancy of brain tumors with approximately the same localization. A possible explanation of this could be that the toxic influence emanating from the tumor changes the brain chemistry (the transmittor substances) in such a way as to transform the anxiety reactions reported and the types of defenses used to control them.

The second study demonstrated that the mental dysfunction was clearly associated with the severity of the brain pathology. Although important aspects of cognitive functioning, such as reasoning, appeared to be little affected by the tumor growth, the constructive processes of the most deeply disturbed patients showed near-psychotic discontinuities in MCT. In previous investigations, summarized in Smith et al. (1989), these discontinuities were associated with psychotic, particularly schizophrenic regressions. This association has been borne out by a recent clinical study (Cesarec et al., 1988). The fact that many of the patients with highly malignant tumors performed poorly on a verbal memory task seems to indicate that subcortical areas, secondarily connected with the frontal lobe, are affected by the tumor growth.

The brain tumor patients were more inclined than normal subjects to use primitiye defensive strategies. One typical primitive defense is projection, localized by psychoanalysts at an early stage of ontogenesis; a typical representative of the more advanced defenses is isolation. The latter type of defense was often registered in the left-hemisphere group in the lateralization study. Even in these normal subjects, however, the engagement of the right hemisphere elicited the use of more primitive defenses, although within a normal repertoire.

A differentiation between hemispheres is not enough to explain the difference between conscious and preconscious processing. The right hemisphere is assumed to have better access to deeper layers of the CNS than the left one (Brown, 1988). More ancient parts of the brain are thus involved. As mentioned, the threatening stimulus in the MCT not only engages the visual cortex in early phases of the process but also, and probably to a higher degree, the brain stem. Brown has described the successive engagement of the brain stem, the limbic system, the parietal part of the cortex and, last, the occipital part in terms of space perception: a two-dimensional map of body and body space, an ego-centered volumetric space, a three-dimensional object-centered space, and a final analysis and exterioration of the object. Obviously, in a percept-genetic experiment, the visual cortex does not respond adequately to an outside stimulus until after phylogenetically older stages have reacted to the message and initiated defensive measures, if necessary. These measures may be reshaped as the process continues, becoming more and more mature. When the cortex is affected by pathological processes, the individual still tries to defend himself, but in a more primitive manner and not always successfully.

It should be obvious by now that we recommend a combination of psychodynamic and cognitive perspectives for future neuropsychological research. It is not enough, however, to employ any personality and cognitive methodology. The studies included in this chapter seem to us to have convincingly demonstrated the intrinsic possibilities of percept-genetic tools, particularly the MCT. The cognitive data to be produced with the process-oriented PG descriptions should allow a qualitative as well as quantitative differentiation. One recent example of such an exploitation of traditional cognitive tests is the study by Johanson, Brun, Gustafson, Risberg, and Tideman (1990). In their handling of a cognitive test battery, they were also aided by a flexible frame of reference for the observation of behavior in the test situation. In addition, process-oriented methods might provide valuable tools for our understanding of the nature of, for instance, language, memory, and learning disorders.

Finally, we wish to emphasize the need to include more normal subjects in neuropsychological research to allow for sensible conclusions about what is really pathological.

## *References*


Arieti, S. (1976). *Creativity, the magic synthesis*. New York: Basic Books.

Black, K.L., Ikezaki, K, Toga, A.W., Santori, E.M., Becker, D.P., & Smith, M.L. (1989). In vitro binding characteristics of peripheral benzodiazepine receptor ligands to brain tumors [Abstract]. *Journal of Cerebral Blood Flow and Metabolism*, *9*(Suppl. 1), 222.

Bogen, J.E., & Bogen, G.M. (1969). The other side of the brain: 3. The corpus callosum and creativity. *Bulletin of the Los Angeles Neurological Societies*, *34*(4), 191–203.

Brown, J.W. (1985). Imagery and microstructure of perception. *Journal of Neurolinguistics*, *1*, 89–141.

Brown, J.W. (1987). The microstructure of action. In E. Perecman (Ed.), *The frontal lobes revisited* (pp. 251–272). New York: IRBN Press.

Brown, J.W. (1988). *The life of the mind. Selected papers*. Englewood Cliffs: Prentice-Hall.

Carlsson, I. (1989). Lateralization of defence mechanisms in a visual half-field paradigm. *Scandinavian Journal of Psychology*, *30*, 296–303.

Carlsson, I. (1990). Lateralization of defence mechanisms related to creativity. *Scandinavian Journal of Psychology*, *31*, 241–247.

Carlsson, I., & Smith, G.J.W. (1987). Gender differences in defence mechanisms compared with creativity in a group of youngsters. *Psychological Research Bulletin, Lund University*, *27*, 1.

Cesarec, Z., Nyman, R.A., & Nyman, G.E. (1988). Differentiation and prediction of schizophrenia by means of the Meta-Contrast Technique. In Z. Cesarec (Ed.), *Varieties of schizophrenic disease* (pp. 253–268). Lund, Sweden: Department of Psychiatry and Neurochemistry.

Christensen, A.-L. (1979). *Luria's neuropsychological investigation. Text*. Vojens, Denmark: P.J. Schmidt.

Gainotti, G. (1972). Emotional behavior and hemispheric side of the lesion. *Cortex*, *8*, 41–55.

Goldberg, E., & Bilder, R.M. (1987). The frontal lobes and hierarchical organization of cognitive control. In E. Perecman (Ed.), *The frontal lobes revisited* (pp. 159–187). New York: IRBN Press.

Goldberg, E., & Costa, L. (1987). Qualitative indices in neuropsychological assessment. Executive deficits following prefrontal lesions. In K. Adams & J. Grant (Eds.), *Neuropsychological assessment in neuropsychiatric disorders* (pp. 48–64). New York: Oxford University Press.

Goldstein, K. (1973). Effect of brain damage on personality. In T. Millon (Ed.), *Theories of psychopathology and personality*. Philadelphia: W.B. Saunders. (Original work published 1952)

Greenacre, P. (1957). The childhood of the artist, libidinal phase development and giftedness. *The Psychoanalytic Study of the Child*, *12*, 47–72.

Hagstadius, S. (1989). *Brain function and dysfunction*. Doctoral dissertation, Lund University, Lund, Sweden.

Ingvar, D.H., & Franzén, G. (1974). Abnormalities of cerebral blood flow distribution in patients with chronic schizophrenia. *Acta Psychiatrica Scandinavica, 50*, 425–462.

Johanson, A., Brun, A., Gustafson, L., Risberg, J., & Tideman, E. (1990). *A longitudinal study of Alzheimer dementia in Down's syndrome.* Unpublished manuscript.

Johanson, A.M., Custafson, L., & Risberg, J. (1986). Behavioural observations during performance of the WAIS Block Design Test related to abnormalities of regional cerebral blood flow in organic dementia. *Journal of Clinical and Experimental Neuropsychology, 8*, 201–209.

Johanson, A.M., Risberg, J., Silfverskiöld, P., & Smith, G. (1986). Regional changes in cerebral blood flow during increased anxiety in patients with anxiety neurosis. In U. Hentschel, G.J.W. Smith, & J.G. Draguns (Eds.), *The Roots of Perception* pp. 353–360. Amsterdam: North-Holland.

Johanson, A., Smith, G.J.W., Gustafson, L., Hagberg, B., Nilsson, B., & Risberg, J. (1990). Adaptation in different type of dementia and normal elderly subjects. *Dementia, 1*, 90–101.

Kinsbourne, M. (1982). Hemispheric specialization and the growth of human understanding. *American Psychologist, 37*(4), 411–420.

Kragh, U. (1985). *The defense mechanism test.* Stockholm: Persona.

Kullberg, G., & Risberg, J. (1978). Changes in regional cerebral blood flow following stereotactic psychosurgery. *Applied Neurophysiology, 41*, 79–85.

Lilja, Å., Hagstadius, S., Risberg, J., Salford, L., & Smith, G.J.W. (1991a). Frontal lobe dynamics in brain tumor patients: A study of regional cerebral blood flow and affective changes in brain tumor patients before and after surgery. *Neuropsychiatry, Neuropsychology and Behavioral Neurology*, in press.

Lilja, Å, Smith, G.J.W., & Salford, L.G. (1991b). Microprocesses in perception and personality. *Journal of Nervous and Mental Disease*, in press.

Luria, A.R. (1981). *The working brain: An introduction to neuropsychology.* London: Penguin Books.

Mallet, B.L. & Veall, N. (1965). Measurement of regional cerebral clearance rates in man using 133-Xenon inhalation and extracranial recording. *Clinical Science, 29*, 179–188.

Martindale, C., & Hasenfus, N. (1978). EEG differences as a function of creativity, stage of the creative process, and effort to be original. *Biological Psychology, 6*, 157–167.

Martindale, C., & Hines, D. (1975). Creativity and cortical activation during creative, intellectual and EEG feedback tasks. *Biological Psychology, 3*, 91–100.

Nauta, W.J.H. (1971). The problem of the frontal lobe: A reinterpretation. *Psychiatric Research, 8*, 167–187.

Obrist, W.D., Thompson, H.K., Wang, H.S., & Wilkinson, W.E. (1975). Regional cerebral blood flow estimated by 133-Xenon inhalation. *Stroke, 6*, 245–256.

Oldfield, R.C. (1971). The assessment and analysis of handedness: The Edinburgh inventory. *Neuropsychologia, 9*, 97–113.

Pandaya, D.N. (1988). *Frontal lobe architecture and connections.* Paper presented at the 16th Annual INS meeting. New Orleans, LA.

Pandaya, D.N., & Barnes, C.L. (1987). Architecture and connections of the frontal lobe. In E. Perecman (Ed.), *The frontal lobes revisited* (pp. 41–72). New York: IRBN Press.

Reivich, M., Gur, R., & Alavi, A. (1983). Positron emission. Tomographic studies of sensory stimuli, cognitive processes and anxiety. *Human Neurobiology*, *2*, 25–33.

Risberg, J. (1980). Regional cerebral blood flow measurements by 133-Xe inhalation. Methodology and applications in psychology and psychiatry. *Brain and Language*, *9*, 9–34.

Risberg, J. (1987). Development of high resolution two-dimensional measurement of regional cerebral blood flow. In J. Wade et al. (Eds.), *Impact on functional imaging in neurology and psychiatry* (pp. 35–41). London: John Libbey.

Risberg, J., Ali, Z., Wilson, E.M., Wills, E.L., & Halsay, J.H. (1975). Measurement of regional cerebral blood flow by 133-xenon inhalation: Preliminary evaluation of an initial slope index in patients with unstable flow compartments. *Stroke*, *6*, 142–148.

Sackeim, H.A., Packer, J.K., & Gur, R.C. (1977). Hemisphericity, cognitive set, and susceptibility to subliminal perception. *Journal of Abnormal Psychology*, *86*, 624–630.

Smith, G.J.W. (1968). Differentiation of psychotic subjects by means of the Meta-Contrast Technique. *Scandinavian Journal of Psychology*, *9*, 39–44.

Smith, G.J.W. (1981). Creation and reconstruction. *Psychoanalysis and Contemporary Thought*, *4*, 275–286.

Smith, G.J.W., & Carlsson, I. (1990). *The creative process. A functional model based on empirical studies from early childhood up to middle age. Psychological Issues, Monograph 57.* New York: International Universities Press.

Smith, G.J.W., & Danielsson, A. (1978). Richness in ideas, ego-involvement and efficiency in a group of scientists and humanists: A study of creativity using a process-oriented technique. *Psychological Research Bulletin*, *Lund University*, *18*, 4–5.

Smith, G.J.W., & Danielsson, A. (1982). *Anxiety and defensive strategies in childhood and adolescence. Psychological Issues, Monograph 52.* New York: International Universities Press.

Smith, G.J.W., & Henriksson, M. (1955). The effect on an established percept of a perceptual process beyond awareness. *Acta Psychologica*, *11*, 346–355.

Smith, G.J.W., Johnson, G., & Almgren, P.E. (1989). *MCT—the Meta-Contrast Technique*. Stockholm: Psykologiförlaget.

Torrance, E.P. (1982). Hemisphericity and creative functioning. *Journal of Research and Development in Education*, *15*(3), 29–37.

Westerlundh, B. (1983). Personal organization of the visual field: A study of ambient and focal reports of threatening stimuli. *Archives of Psychology*, *135*, 17–35.

# 12
# Microgenesis in Visual Information Processing: Some Experimental Results

TALIS BACHMANN

Hardly anyone in contemporary psychology would be willing to reject the notion of cognitive processes (including perception) as representing events in time, having their beginning, duration, and end. Many of us still believe that these cognitively specified segments of time are filled with processes that are qualitatively different and follow one another either by the strict rules according to the "complete-previous-stage-then-go-to-the-next" law, or by the indiscrete process of transition and change between the stages. All this can be termed the *formal* acceptance of the microgenetic imperative, either implicit, or explicit. (In information-processing psychology, e.g., this idea has been touched or briefly mentioned by Chastain, 1977; Eriksen & Schultz, 1979; Forgus & Melamed, 1976; Haber & Hershenson, 1980; Hoving, Spencer, Robb, & Schulte, 1978; Uhlarik & Johnson, 1978; Murch, 1973; Shekhter, 1981; Uttal, 1988; Watt, 1988; Zusne, 1970). But relatively few scholars take, as one would call it, the *radical* standpoint regarding these cognitive processes in time and regard microgenesis (MG) as the basic characteristic or central theoretical idea behind the process(es) under consideration. Interestingly enough, these researchers do not represent so much the mainstream cognitive psychology as they represent—or their academic origins are within—neuropsychology, clinical psychology, or developmental psychology (cf. Arieti, 1962; Brown, 1977, 1983; Conrad, 1947; Froehlich, Smith, Draguns, & Hentschel, 1984; Hentschel, Smith, & Draguns, 1986; Kragh & Smith, 1970; Sergent, 1986; Werner, 1948, 1956, 1957).[1] The discussion of the reasons for this situation remains beyond the scope of this chapter, however.

What are the conceptions we meet most often in the works of the followers of the radical idea of MG? This chapter concerns primarily the

[1] The German tradition of studying cognitive processes, where the microgenetic (the *Aktualgenese*) problems have always been of high importance, represents an exception to this rule (cf. Froehlich & Laux, 1969; Graumann, 1959; Linschoten, 1959; Sander, 1928; Undeutsch, 1942; Werner, 1948).

process of visual perception; the reader may wish to consult other works concerning more general aspects of MG (see Bachmann, 1980, 1988a, 1990; Flavell & Draguns, 1957; Froehlich et al., 1984; Hentschel et al., 1986; Kragh & Smith, 1970; Smith, 1957). As for the process of perception, the radical stance includes the following: (1) The perceptual process consists of rapid alternation of several moments and stages where each preceding stage represents a mental state of a less concrete, more general character and *each succeeding one—more concrete and differentiated* (articulated) (Brown, 1977; Lange, 1893; Werner, 1957). (2) The perceptual act includes alternation of stages, which represents not so much a succession of completely different cognitive structures as activated (e.g., A, B, C) but a succession of stages whereby each successive stage unfolds from the previous one, thus carrying on some of its contents and repeating its functions at the next, higher level (e.g., A, BA, CBA; or - A, A', A"). This idea, the idea of *recapitulation* or cognitive cycling has its roots in several classic studies (Lange, 1893; Werner, 1948), is discussed or developed further in contemporary research (Brown, 1977, 1983; Froehlich et al., 1984), bears strong psychobiological foundations (MacLean, 1990), and has some formal affinities with the models of perceptual activity offered by contemporary cognitively oriented ecological psychology (cf. Neisser, 1976; Shaw & Turvey, 1981). (3) The active process of specific use of cognitive representations in terms of neural coding does not go hand-in-hand with the dynamics of *conscious experience*. The systems for the former and the expression of the latter are (a) partially independent, relatively *autonomous*, (b) represent a *continuum*, and (c) can be (re)combined, (re)coupled and (re)activated in *multiple flexible* ways, including simultaneous activity at different levels and interlevel facilitation or interlevel interference (Allport, 1987; Brown, 1983; Dixon, 1981; Kalmus & Bachmann, 1980).

As the next step of this presentation, these basic characteristics of MG are discussed in the light of experimental evidence from perceptual information-processing psychology.

## Microgenetic Regularities as Revealed by the Experiments on Visual Information Processing

### *Paradigms of Visual Masking and Rapid Serial Presentation*

Suppose you face the task of measuring the average duration of the microgenetic process of perceiving an image of some more or less common visual object (the test). In perceptual sciences, the most common method for reaching this aim used to be the method of retroactive (backward) masking. A stimulus image of the test object is shown for a brief time (e.g., for

10 ms) as the first stimulus ($S_1$), and within a short interval, it is followed by another, masking, image as the second stimulus ($S_2$), which interferes with the perception of the test. If the test were presented without a succeeding mask, it would have been perceived with 100% accuracy, but in the condition of backward masking, the percentage of correct responses with regard to $S_1$ is considerably lowered or can even reach the level of random guessing. If we now gradually increase the stimulus onset asynchronies (SOAs) between $S_1$ and $S_2$, then we finally reach the value of SOA that is sufficient for $S_1$ to escape from masking. I have analyzed 138 functions of backward masking from the studies that have been published in the highest ranking experimental psychology journals beginning with 1960 and have calculated the generalized average functions of masking (see Bachmann, 1989b). Based on this, I conclude that in most cases the masking functions become asymptotic with the SOA values of about 200 to 250 ms. Thus, indeed, perception requires time to be completed and, operationally, the average duration of a microgenetic cycle can be equalled to this interval.

Perhaps, however, this is just a *latency,* needed for reaching a decision with regard to an *invariant* image of the perceptual object or merely a time for preparing a response to this image, without any relation to the hypothetical evolution through the *variable* states of the subjective image itself? Let us look at some experiments more closely.

In the study by Kirkham (1977), the subjects were presented with different regular black-and-white patterns ($S_1$; e.g., checkerboard), which were backward-masked by a bright flash ($S_2$). The SOA between the $S_1$ and $S_2$ was varied, and confusion matrices of the subjects' responses were developed for each SOA condition. The procedures of multidimensional scaling enabled Kirkham to show that at the different epochs of MG different aspects of $S_1$ dominated the perceptual image. At first, randomness versus *regularity* of image elements' arrangement was represented, followed by visual representation of *orientation* and number of spatial directions, which in turn was followed by the next stage—representation of *local details*.

In the study by Kissin (1976), the transient, backward-masked exposures of short lines were employed. The lines may have been tilted away from the vertical at various degrees (up to 30°). If the subjects were unsure about their responses, they had to indicate the smallest range of the stimuli to which they would ascribe their response (e.g., "0° to 12°, but no more"). Kissin found that, with increasing the SOA, this range (the "zone of presence") systematically narrowed down within the 50 ms of MG, ending up in adequate percepts. (See also Andrews, 1967a, b.)

In the work presented by Krol and Tanenholtz (1979), subjects had to respond also by producing drawings of the $S_1$ as perceived, in addition to their verbal responses. The stimuli were texture-like patterns, composed of different texture patches, which were arranged spatially in alternative ways. Four stages of MG were pointed out by the authors: (1) segregation of the areas with different brightness (39 ms); (2) fragmentary characterization of the texture samples (55 ms); vague segregation of the "poles" of different textured areas (63 ms); (4) precise specification of the borderlines between the areas (179 ms).

Pairs of successive, spatially overlapping human faces as $S_1$ and $S_2$ were exposed for identification in our study (Bachmann, 1989a). The SOAs ranged from 20 to 160 ms, thus falling within the interval of unitary MG duration. The luminance of the $S_1$ was considerably higher than that of the $S_2$. If presented with the stimuli, subjects effectively perceived one face, which at short SOAs mostly resembled the first stimulus (the one with higher intensity, naturally, dominated perception if images were integrated at very short SOAs) but with increasing SOA systematically shifted toward the appearance of the second stimulus. The overall level of efficiency remained the same, however. In Figure 12.1, one can see the basic results in the form of the identification functions, which could be considered as a quantitative demonstration of the microgenetic focus transition in real

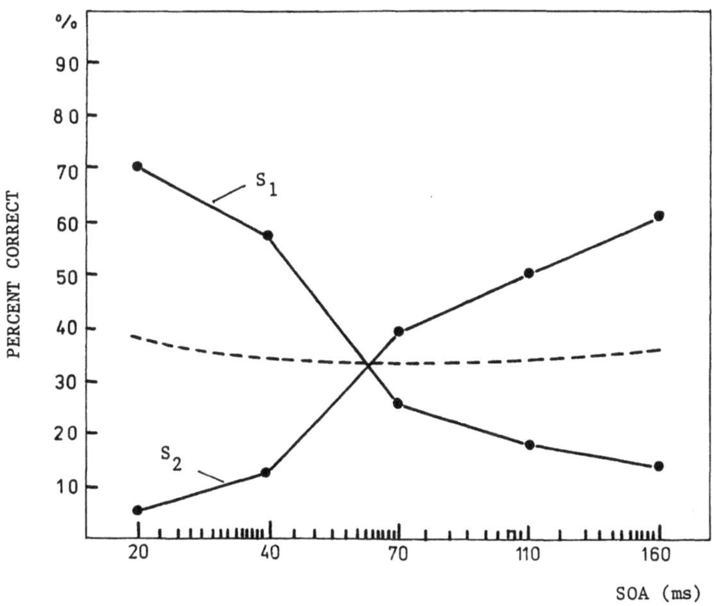


FIGURE 12.1. Percentage of correct identification of human faces, presented transiently as successive, spatially overlapping stimuli ($S_1$ and $S_2$), as a function of stimulus-onset asynchrony (SOA). The dashed line refers to the percentage correct, averaged for both $S_1$ and $S_2$. Note that $S_1$ had higher luminance than $S_2$. *Note.* From "Microgenesis as Traced by the Transient Paired-Forms Paradigm" by T. Bachmann, 1989, *Acta Psychologica*, *70*, pp. 3–17. Copyright 1989 by Elsevier Science Publishers B.V. (North-Holland). Adapted by permission.

time. The temporal value of the cross-over point of the first- and second-stimulus identification functions can be taken as the index of the half-cycle of perceptual MG within the constraints set by present experimental variables. MG, being started by $S_1$, gradually gets over to $S_2$.

Several other studies demonstrate that during MG qualitative changes in the percept occur: Perceptual representation of location precedes that of the class of visual form, which in turn precedes the identity stage of the form (Dolan & Mayzner, 1978; Solman, 1977). The perceived quality of the surface of a form and of the form itself depends on MG of the contour, which defines this form (Cheatham, 1952; Imada & Yodogawa, 1984; Werner, 1935). The degree of expression of the visual illusions and perceptual constancies develops through the MG stages (Epstein & Hatfield, 1978; Epstein, Hatfield, & Muise, 1977; Reynolds, 1978, 1981). The apparent size of a stimulus increases throughout the stages of MG and approaches gradually the adequate measure (Kostelyanets & Kamenkovich, 1986; Wilding, 1982a; cf. also Holt-Hansen, 1980, on the "expansion" of the form through MG). During MG, the reduction of the degrees of freedom of the elements of the image takes place according to the lawful alternation of stages in the sequence—topological invariant, projective invariant, affine invariant, invariant of similarity, and metric invariant (Vekker, 1974).

A considerable amount of experimental work therefore supports the statement that MG proceeds from the less-differentiated, more general, to the more-differentiated, concrete quality of the perceptually represented objects and features. The $S_2$ in the shape of the masking stimulus, however, may only create artificial perturbations, which have nothing in common with "normal" perception; addition of an extra energetic input a few moments after the test may artificially "create" MG.

Highly important, though often overlooked, studies by Cohene and Bechtoldt (1974, 1975) help to clarify some of these problems. These authors designed an elegant backward-masking experiment whereby, in a physical sense, no additional stimuli were made to succeed the $S_1$. How can this be done? Suppose we create $S_1$ by superimposing (integrating) two quasirandom coveys ($C_1$ plus $C_2$) of dots so that some of the dots of $C_1$ and some of the dots of $C_2$ form a bigram for recognition. We expose this $S_{1(C_1+C_2)}$ for a short time and then *switch out* one of the constituent coveys (e.g., $C_1$). Now we have $S_{2(C_2)}$, which no longer likens to bigram and which also does not constitute new energetic input to the visual system. Nevertheless, pronounced backward masking of the bigram by the remaining dots was observed. Again, the situation is very much like the integrated $S_1$ switches in the time-consuming first stages of the MG process, which will be realized not until the moment when only the remaining portion of the dot structure— the $C_2$—is well represented in the perceptual system and the subject consciously perceives it at the terminating stage(s) of MG.

I have completed a study by combining mutual masking of $S_1$ versus $S_2$ and the registration of the visual-evoked potentials from the occipital and vertex sites of the human scalp (see Bachmann, 1989b). With short and intermediate SOAs, strong backward masking was observed but also the gradual improvement of perceptibility with the increase in SOA from shortest to intermediate. There were practically no qualitative differences, however, between the $N_{150}$ components in the condition of paired $S_1-S_2$ presentation with SOAs less than or equal to 70 ms and the condition of single $S_1$ exposure. It seems as if only the $S_1$ is critical in switching in the MG process, and the main portion of the nonspecific, modulatory thalamocortical ascending impulses (which can be considered as the main source of $N_{150}$ generation) reach the cortical specific representations some time later. In one instance, these modulatory inputs find undisturbed $S_1$-related specific representations (expressed, e.g., as the excitatory postsynaptic potentials?), in another instance they find only the $S_2$-related, "fresh" activity with higher signal/noise ratio in comparison with that of the $S_1$. As a consequence, either $S_1$-related or $S_2$-related processes are enhanced (the latter being more pronounced) and integrated with consciousness-related higher levels of neurophysiological activity. Regardless, however, this difference in psychological contents of the percept with changing SOA or manipulation of $S_1$-alone versus paired $S_1-S_2$ conditions, the evoked potentials (EP) component $N_{150}$ remains invariant.

Thus, the effects of the addition of the $S_2$ to the display in succession to $S_1$ seem not to cause some "acting backward" extra perturbations—as is conceptualized in many of the masking theories—but only seem to constitute a material to be used by the processes that are characteristic to the end-stages of MG. With regard to visual backward masking, this means that masking is not so much a process of inhibition as it is a process of transition of the microgenetic focus from the first segments of visual information to the succeeding ones. This hypothesis presupposes a decisive role to be rendered to the nonspecific, phasic thalamocortical modulatory activities that mediate the dynamics of perceptual conscious experience in real time. (For more detailed discussion of this conceptualization, see Bachmann, 1984, 1989b; Crick, 1984.)

If this is so, then one could find some evidence in neurosurgery, given the nonspecific, consciousness-critical functional units (included in the energetic block, to use Luria's [1973] terms) are implied. I studied volunteers among a group of patients who were undergoing stereotactic surgery to treat Parkinson's symptoms (Bachmann, 1989b). The eight volunteers with multiple chronically implanted electrodes (the targets being in *globus pallidus, nucleus centrum medianum, nucleus reticularis thalami, nucleus ventralis lateralis thalami*) participated in the masking experiment just after they had been subjected to the treatment of Parkinson's symptoms by the activating electrostimulation (for the details of the method see Smirnov & Resnikova, 1985). In this situation, when the subjects' nonspecific system had been just activated, I found that the psychophysical masking functions had changed considerably. Backward masking almost disappeared, and already at short SOAs, the $S_1$ was clearly perceived. Given that this treatment indeed enhances nonspecific thalamocortical input, then the results are in accordance with my hypothesis. Nonspecific modulatory mechanism, if heavily preactivated, could cause speed-up of the MG for $S_1$, and it will be perceived at the first place, without the need to evoke the secondary activation, which otherwise, if evoked by $S_1$ itself, would lead to better perception of the $S_2$ instead of the $S_1$, which, paradoxically enough, should be the instigator of the activating cycle in ordinary circumstances.

Additional support for this conceptualization came from another experiment of caffeine and chlorpromazine treatment (cf. Bachmann, 1989b). Chlorpromazine treatment of the subjects did not change the relative effectiveness of the perception of $S_1$ and $S_2$ in the mutual masking situation. (In this procedure, subjects must report both the $S_1$ and the $S_2$, which are the stimuli of the same general class, e.g., a square and a triangle, or a ring and a rhombus, exposed successively at the same location in the visual field.) The caffeine treatment, however, yielded qualitative differences in the masking functions: As compared to the placebo control condition, I found relative release from masking (facilitation of MG). The more interesting aspect of this study, however, was that for the $S_2$, the facilitation was found to begin with shorter SOA values (80 ms) than for the $S_1$ (facilitation for $S_1$ began with SOA equal to 120 ms). These regularities again point to the possibilities that (1) only the thalamocortical phasic nonspecific activation (cf. caffeine vs. chlorpromazine difference) can be considered as one of the crucial mechanisms of MG and that (2) MG indeed takes some time, which means that the indicators of certain experimental effects on MG could be found only after some temporal interval has elapsed between the beginning of the presentation of the first, MG–evoking stimulus and the second, MG "probe," stimulus. In case of mutual masking with intermediate SOAs, the $S_2$ could take the advantage of the enhanced activation. Only with longer SOAs, the $S_1$ itself can be enhanced, because the nonspecific processes, which are necessary for conscious MG, have had enough time to "find" intact $S_1$-specific representations without any "surrogate activities" from the succeeding signals, which carry information about $S_2$. All this applies to the exogeneously evoked MG cycle. In case of strong endogeneous activation (cf. as fostered by the stereotactic procedure), the MG duration could appear to be minimized as much as possible.

Several predictions may be derived from the proposed hypothesis. The first presupposes that, in case of rapid successive exposure of spatially overlapping $S_1$ and $S_2$ with $S_1$ being more intense a stimulus than $S_2$, the subjective contrast of the $S_2$ at intermediate SOAs—characteristic of uncompleted MG temporal value—should be higher than it would be in the control condition, where $S_2$ is exposed singly. This prediction contradicts any masking theory but is consistent with the interactive MG model, because the MG process, if it is evoked by a more intense $S_1$, realizes itself more conspicuously, which should be evident at later stages when dealing with signals from $S_2$. The other prediction states that the subjective moment of "conscious arrival" (actualization) of $S_2$ could be faster if it is presented after the MG-inducing $S_1$ rather than in isolation (in which case the "surrogate" preliminary MG is absent). These predictions were tested experimentally and received factual support (Bachmann, 1988b, 1989a).

Until now, we have discussed mostly the *energetic* interaction between $S_1$ and $S_2$ as the "probes" of the course of the compound MG process, which elaborates signals from both of the stimuli as if they are the successively arriving input of an invariant processing cycle for some perceptual object. But is there any *informational* interaction? The studies by Lawrence (1971), Intraub (1981, 1985), Calis and Leeuwenberg (1981), Calis, Sterenborg, and Maarse (1984), and Styles and Allport (1986) provide evidence allowing a positive answer. This research supports the continuous informational interaction of rapid successively presented stimuli in a way that preceding items could act as informational units that provide "starting cues" and/or contexts for certain cognitive perceptual operations, which then are carried out and/or realized later on on the basis of succeeding items. Particularly, Calis and Leeuwenberg (1981), in a Wernerian tradition, note that developing a perceptual structure—a process that is initiated by the first stimulus and that proceeds on the following one—could be considered as a specific operation in a more general knowledge-driven process. So the true direction of cognitive activity may quite well be an outer directed, intrinsic process of cuing the arriving input, rather than a stimulus–response type of activity. The seminal paper by Nikitin (1905) on percept-genesis was one of the first to show this possibility. If the subjects in his study already began to grasp the tentative meaning of the tachistoscopic stimulus exposed, then their drawings of the exposed objects became *less* accurate as compared to the drawings made according to the perceptual experience at previous stages. In other words, if higher order cognitive search for meaning initially went in the wrong direction, the physical stage of representation suffered too (in comparison with the stages, where iconic aspects "were on their own," without top-down control.

The data referred to here leave no room for the conceptualization of perceptual processing as a tightly stimulus-bound event *a la* there are as many percepts as there are stimuli. The nature of the genesis of the subjective perceptual image of a stimulus can be understood only as an interactive, multifaceted process depending on other inputs and directed by the (results of) previous microgenetic operations. Especially so, if we present stimuli within the temporal interval, which specifies the duration of an elementary microgenetic cycle. And, as a matter of fact, most of the information-processing studies of perception, attention, and short-term memory do just so. It is rarely accepted that iconic memory could be just incompleted microgenesis, selective spatial attention could be continuation of MG for the signals from the locus, microgenetic analysis of which was started by a selective precue, and that visual masking is just a phenomenon whereby the MG cycle, started on the first stimulus, continues on the following one thus leaving the first without service of consciousness.

## *The Paradigm of Binocular Rivalry*

Suppose you face the task of finding an easy way to present two competing stimuli for two competing MG processes to be observed simultaneously. One of the solutions to this problem is exemplified in the well-known experimental technique termed *binocular rivalry* (for reviews see Levelt, 1968; Uttal, 1981; Walker, 1978). If the two images (patterns) that are presented to alternative retinas have very large disparities or—even better—if the disparities consist in the forms being completely different, then instead of subjective fusion of the two images, as would be in normal visual process with images of minor disparity, there will be rivalry between the patterns: Either subject consciously perceives one stimulus, or another (and they may alternate), but not both at once. Several problems arise out of this paradigm. What happens to information provided by the currently suppressed stimulus? What are the mechanisms of the process of rivalry? Is it an instantaneous and spontaneous phenomenon of alternation based on inhibition of some low-level processes or a result of more higher level analysis signifying the ontological impossibility of having two different objects occupying the same space at once? How does the state of rivalry develop? Because the elementary MG process, as we saw, is characterized by considerable speed (about 150 to 200 ms in usual circumstances), then the simple subjective observation of rivalry does not help very much in answering even a single one of these questions. We need some additional, more sophisticated experimental procedures.

Jeremy Wolfe from the Massachusetts Institute of Technology presented rivalrous stimuli dichoptically for short duration (less than 150 ms, i.e., less than the duration of a MG cycle) and found what he called "abnormal fusion" (Wolfe, 1983). He essentially repeated the results obtained earlier by Goldstein (1970) and Anderson, Bechtoldt and Dunlap (1978). Only if the duration of these stimuli exceeded 150 to 200 ms, the ordinary rivalry appeared. It seems as if the rivalry process itself is an event that undergoes microgenetic development. If the stimuli are exposed for a shorter period than ordinary MG would take, then the simultaneous MG process for both of the alternative stimuli has not yet had the opportunity to reach the final stages (i.e., to give a perceptual evidence of two *incompatible* inputs), and we observe this abnormal fusion. One possible conclusion is that rivalry as a microgenetic phenomenon presupposes some top-down control from higher levels of analysis to the lower level ones. This hypothesis has received strong support from the neurophysiological study by Varela and Singer (1987). These authors showed that before the rivalry state develops, signals from both inputs reach cortex and only after corticosubcortical feedback is provided, the rivalry will be established.

Of course, this should not mean that the information from the suppressed input is totally filtered out from the nervous system. Evidence to the contrary is provided by Dixon (1981), Uttal (1981), Wilding (1982b) and others. For example, visual information presented to the suppressed eye takes part in determining stereoscopic depth; the meaning of a word that was exposed to the suppressed eye can cause increase of reaction time to a word that is presented to the dominant (conscious-experience-related) eye, given that these words are semantic associates. What is interesting in the latter effect (data by Abbot, cited in Wilding, 1982b) is that if subjects were administered caffeine, the effect disappeared. We can interpret this according to our nonspecific model of MG. If the nonspecific activity of the dominant channel is increased by the caffeine intake, it resists better the competing tendencies of the currently suppressed but still information-carrying channel.

Important data regarding the conditions enabling "abnormal fusion" of submicrogenetic competing stimuli was provided by Wolfe (1986). If the submicrogenetic, abnormally fusing stimulus images were exposed within 200 ms after the 2-s pair of another stimuli that yielded normal rivalry, then the phenomenon of "abnormal fusion" disappeared. It seems that if the perceptual system already is in a rivalrous state, then it takes some time—about 200 ms—to restore the capacity for fusion (note again the value of 200 ms, which is equal to my measured ordinary MG cycle).

Thus far it is obvious that information, provided by the input to the suppressed channel, should not be totally inaccessible for the perceptual processing. But how can one demonstrate experimentally the time course of MG for the input signals presented to the suppressed channel, given that there will be a switch of the MG focus to this channel? For this purpose, I have tried to employ the mutual masking procedure described in the preceding discussion in combination with binocular rivalry (Bachmann, 1989b). Subjects were presented with the succession of spatially overlapping $S_1$ and $S_2$ (different geometric forms, 7-ms duration for each) with varying SOAs. The stimuli were exposed either to the dominant eye, or to the suppressed eye. Figure 12.2 shows the results in terms of the function of recognition. The $S_2$ is perceived much better in comparison with $S_1$ at all SOA values except for SOA = 220 ms, where—at the end of the MG cycle—masking disappears. The process of MG, started by $S_1$, goes on to

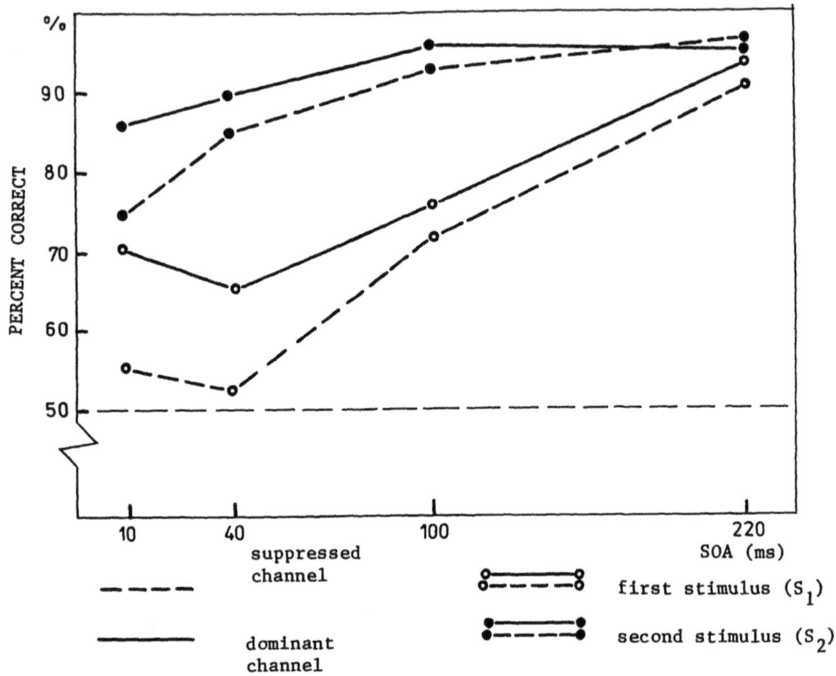


FIGURE 12.2. Percentage of correct identification of geometric forms, presented transiently as successive, spatially overlapping stimuli ($S_1$ and $S_2$), as a function of stimulus-onset asynchrony (SOA) and the condition of binocular rivalry. (Dashed line, the stimuli, presented to the suppressed channel; continuous line, the stimuli, presented to the nonsuppressed, dominant channel.) *Note*. From *Psychophysiology of Visual Masking. The Fine Structure of Conscious Experience* (in Russian) by T. Bachmann, 1989, Tartu: University of Tartu Press. Copyright 1989 by T. Bachmann. Adapted by permission.

realize itself with $S_2$ as the main material for perception, and its efficiency is higher at the intervals inclusive to the MG cycle but not more. Furthermore, the stimuli that were exposed to the dominant channel are perceived better at all SOAs where masking takes place. The MG for dominant-channel stimuli should, of course, be faster and/or more efficient in terms of microgenetic activation. With long SOA, however, the difference in favor of the stimuli presented to the dominant channel disappears. This may indicate that in the conditions where the $S_1$ and $S_2$ no longer interact within the same MG cycle (cf. 220 ms as an interval sufficient for MG to be completed on $S_1$ before the $S_2$ arrives), the interchannel, retroeffective microgenetic activation of the traces of the stimuli that were exposed to the suppressed channel could be as effective as the activation of the stimulus representations in the conditions where the stimuli are exposed to the dominant channel.

The results, as taken together, support the radical idea of MG as to the relatively autonomous nature of conscious processes and preconscious perceptual coding. Additionally, the results support the flexibility of the conscious MG focus in terms of the possibility for it to be applied to either one of the alternative perceptual evidence represented in different cortical subsystems (the combination of information from the alternative retinas takes part not earlier than at the cortical level in case of dichoptic presentations and binocular rivalry), and the possibility to retroeffectively develop an MG process for the perceptual information that is no longer physically present in the subject's visual field but is stored in specific perceptual systems. Indeed, as is persuasively argued by Brown (1983), each new state in MG time develops over the previous states, which are attenuated, either by virtue of belonging to the past ($S_1$ vs. $S_2$) or by virtue of not being the material for the MG focus to be applied on (suppressed channel information vs. the dominant-channel information). But neither the temporal-domain nor the neuroanatomy-domain foci of MG processes could do their job without the alternatives they depend on or grow out from.

## *The Paradigms of Global Versus Local Processing of Visual Information*

One of the few representatives of cognitive psychology who has explicitly acknowledged the MG imperative is David Navon. His now-classic experiments have demonstrated that in visual perception global levels of form are processed before the local levels (the global precedence, or "forest before trees," phenomenon, cf. Navon, 1977, 1981). If a stimulus letter, such as *E*, is formed from the small constituent stimulus letters, then one can ask subjects to respond as quickly as possible to either the globally defined stimulus or to the locally defined one. The local constituent letters can be (1) congruent with the global one, or (2) incongruent (see Fig. 12.3). So in case of incongruity between the global and local levels of form, one could expect interference that should show up in the increase in reaction times to these compound letters as compared to reaction time in congruous or neutral control condition. Navon found evidence supporting this prediction, but the main result of his study consisted in the asymmetric nature of the interference: If subjects had to respond to local level, then there was clear interference from the global level, but the opposite was not found. Thus, the conclusion seems pretty natural: To be able to interfere, the information contained in certain spatial level should be perceptually represented not later than information contained in another level, and whereas the interference was unidirectional—from the global to the local level but not vice versa—then the global information should have been represented earlier than the local one.

```
EEEEEEEEEEE     NNNNNNNNNNN
EEEEEEEEEEE     NNNNNNNNNNN
EEE             NNN
EEEEEEEEE       NNNNNNNNN
EEEEEEEEE       NNNNNNNNN
EEE             NNN
EEEEEEEEEEE     NNNNNNNNNNN
EEEEEEEEEEE     NNNNNNNNNNN

(A)             (B)

EEEEEE     NNNNNN
E          N
EEEEE      NNNNN
E          N
EEEEEE     NNNNNN
```

FIGURE 12.3. Examples of the typical stimuli used in the Navon's *global precedence paradigm*. (A) Local and global levels of form are congruent; (B) local and global levels of form are incongruent.

Despite the lively discussions and further specifications (cf. Boer & Keuss, 1982; Hughes, Layton, Baird, and Lester 1984; Kinchla & Wolfe, 1979; Miller, 1981; Ward, 1983), the general results concerning the global precedence remain valid. Other methods, including multidimensional similarity judgments, reactions to gratings, and other psychophysical procedures have also proved the progression of visuospatial MG from large-scale, global analysis to fine-scale, locally differentiated analysis (Breitmeyer, 1975; Petersik, 1978; Vasilev & Mitov, 1976; Watt, 1988).

Another way to study the relative impact of global or large-scale versus local or fine-scale spatial levels of pattern or form on visual perceptual processes is to use the procedure of quantizing half-tone TV or photographic images into isoluminant, square-shaped pixels (cf. Harmon & Julesz, 1973; Sergent, 1986; see Fig. 12.4). One can vary both the spatial level of quantization (the more pixels the original picture has been divided into, the finer the upper level of spatial articulation, adequately preserved through this procedure) and the temporal variable of exposure duration (the longer the exposure, the fuller the possibilities for a stimulus to go through the sufficient amount of MG stages to reach recognition or some other measure of perceptual adequacy).

I have performed several experiments of pattern recognition or identification by systematically varying the spatial and temporal parameters as described here (Bachmann, 1987, 1991; Bachmann & Kahusk, 1987). The basic results are depicted on Figure 12.5. With fine quantization, if the quality of the quantized image of the test object is practically close to the original, nonquantized version in terms of visual familiarity, the efficiency of recognition or identification increases systematically with increase in exposure duration, which is a fairly common result from the classic visual MG experiments. However, with coarse quantization (e.g., 36 pixels by 36

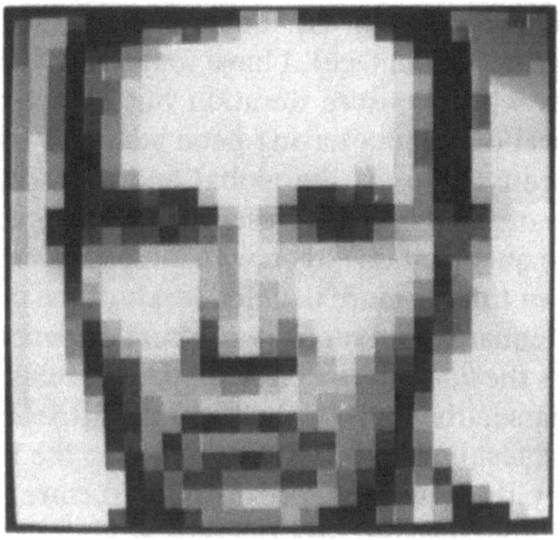

FIGURE 12.4. An example of the spatially quantized visual stimulus image (in this case a human face) with the level of spatial quantization equal to approximately 20 pixels per face along the horizontal dimension.

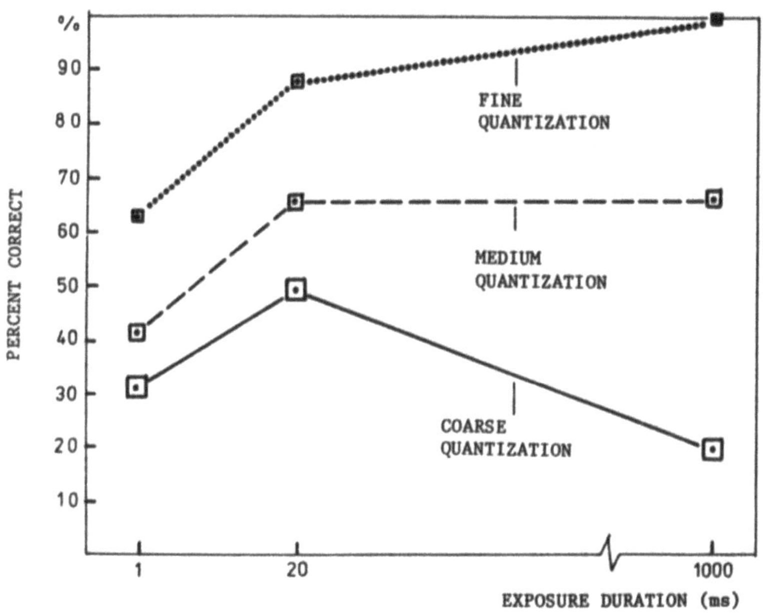


FIGURE 12.5. Percentage of correct identification (recognition) of the spatially quantized images of stimulus objects as a function of exposure duration and level of spatial quantization. (Adapted and generalized from Bachmann, 1987; Bachmann, 1991; Bachmann & Kahusk, 1987.)

pixels for the quantized image of an human eye or $15^2$ pixels per face for the quantized image of human face), I have found that initially recognition efficiency increases with exposure duration but then begins to *decrease* with additional duration quanta having been added to stimulus' on-time. Conclusions are pretty clear. If the global and local levels of form are congruous in terms of signifying the presence of an invariant object (which is the case with fine quantization), then with increasing exposure duration, MG—proceeding on to ever more detailed levels of the stimulus—gathers more and more adequate, congruous perceptual evidence to reach a correct decision as to the identity or class of the stimulus exposed. If the quantization is coarse, then the global spatial distribution of contrast, characteristic to the test image, is less distorted than the local distribution, which is masked by the square-shaped pixels' structure. With increasing exposure duration, initially, the MG buildup of global form leads to the increase in recognition, but later, with MG proceeding on local, fine-grain levels, recognition is impaired, because the spurious masking structure of the pixels' corners and straight edges will now dominate the perceptual image. The process is similar to the MG in case of interaction of $S_1$ and $S_2$ (as described previously here): Global level could be considered as $S_1$ and local level as $S_2$, but now the temporal dispersion is not introduced by the independent experimental variable of SOA, but by the MG itself, working sequentially at different levels of the stimulus that was presented in a single exposure. The most intriguing feature of the results (cf. Fig. 12.5) is that at the intermediate exposure durations, where coarsely quantized images are recognized best, the fine-quantized images are still recognized much more efficiently than the coarsely quantized images. This regularity includes an apparent paradox, because with such short exposure durations, where the decrease for the coarse-quantized recognition function has not started yet, the fine-scale features of stimuli should not be represented in perception and there would not be any advantage for the fine-quantized images. (Otherwise, there should have been already some decrease in the recognition functions for coarse-quantized images!) But one still sees the conspicuous difference in favor of the fine quantization at all exposure durations. The only answer to this paradox originates from the conceptualization of MG as the process that *uses* (and takes time to use) perceptual evidence of different spatial quality at different moments of time, this evidence having been preconsciously already *represented* in the specific modules of the nervous system. So with shorter exposure durations, the fine-scale information "is already there," but will be used (actualized) at later moments as MG proceeds on to ever finer scales of spatial representation. If it were simply for filtering out the high spatial frequencies (i.e., the fine scale of image) at short exposures, then the image with, quantization equal to, for example, 128 by 128 pixels would not have lead to better recognition at short exposures than an image with 36 by 36 quantization. (A remark of certain importance would be to notice that the same results were obtained when using the isobrightness regime of exposures so that increase in exposure duration was counterbalanced by decrease in luminance by suitable neutral density filters; cf. Bloch's law for the brightness of exposures less than 100 ms. This means that the temporally accumulating MG process seems to matter indeed, not only the simple experimental succession of different sensory states with different quality as based on objective energetic differences.)

The similar process whereby cognitive operations proceed from more "global" to differentiated quality can be found also in other areas of research, e.g. psychosemantics and experimental aesthetics. In an elegant experiment psychologists from Moscow, Petrenko and Vasilenko (1977) presented tachistoscopic images of different objects for recognition. In addition to the task of recognition (i.e. finding correct denotative meaning) subjects had to give ratings to the seen stimuli with using the semantic differential scales (i.e. connotative meaning was being measured). The most curious result was that at the intermediate stages of MG where correct denotative meaning was still not grasped yet, the connotative meaning started to show shift towards the "right direction"; e.g. if a picture of the belt was shown tachistoscopically, the subjects still recognized it as the snake, but the SD ratings already shifted more towards inanimate connotative quality in comparison with the earlier stages. The capacity to apprehend the general qualities of an artistic style of the paintings already at the first stages of MG together with the process of differentiation of SD ratings were demonstrated by Bachmann and Vipper (1983).

The results of the experiments from global versus local processing paradigms, as taken together, support the main postulates of the radical MG theory. Perception develops from more general to more differentiated. Each succeeding stage is based on and grows out of the preceding ones. Information at the preceding levels could be considered as the context or the "stratification frame" for the information that is elaborated at the succeeding stages and most probably is guided by the results of the previous analyses. The MG proceeds as a flexible process of rendering conscious quality to alternative perceptual representations (or representations as combined) that already are represented simultaneously in the specific cortical centers but have not yet been serviced (or praised!) by consciousness. Continuity between the processing at different stages and levels, as well as facilitation or interference between the levels—given the evidence of congruity or its absence—constitutes a normal picture of MG.

## Concluding Remarks

Clearly, at the present stage of development, the MG theory still lacks much of the needed specificity and terminological unity that would help to put forward precise hypotheses and test them in the collective efforts to reach unequivocal, precise answers to the exactly raised problems. The noogenesis of microgenesis has not reached the advanced epoch (but neither is at its origins). Moreover, there are several important methodological pitfalls in MG research, as is persuasively pointed out by Prinz

(1986). In the light of this, my listing of experimental results can be considered more as an illustration than firm proof. I showed that the same general laws of microgenetic nature could be found within a diverse variety of cognitive processes, including visual perception. But even with the concept of perception, I have some methodological difficulties. Who has the courage to claim that in visual perception it is easy to separate "pure" vision from semantic aspects of cognition and also from the response generation processes (as researchers, we all rely on the *answers* of the subjects). Because of the fairly integral nature of these aspects, it is often hard to tell what subdivisions of MG we should regard as the source of our results or object of study or what kinds of processes we are dealing with primarily. The theoretical picture will be even messier if one stresses that one must not confuse the two principal perspectives of MG progression (cf. Kalmus & Bachmann, 1980): (1) between-levels, or interlevel, MG; for example, from *features* to *objects* to *meanings* to *knowledge* and/or to *responses* (or from *sensory analysis* to *sensory-objective synthesis* to *concrete image* to *abstract knowledge*); (2) within-level, or intralevel, MG; for example, from global to local features; from general, large-scale object representation to specific and/or fine-scale object representation; from vague, generalized, connotatively sensitive meaning to precise conceptual specification or identity. In the actual perceptogenetic process, one should consider the heterarchic, "vertical" (cf. 1) plus "horizontal" (cf. 2) progression of temporally overlapping activities within the nervous system. In the present chapter, I have dealt mostly with intralevel aspects of MG on features' or concrete image representation levels, occasionally touching on the problems of interlevel heritage. But even the within-level analysis reveals fairly complex, multistage progression of the perception with feedback-type regulatory processes and temporally overlapping activity. Indeed, what, then, should one term *levels* and what the *stages*? And so on. However, one cannot escape feeling that behind the terminological and methodological relative disorder, one still has, first, one's imagination as to how things happen in reality (which is very much the same regardless of how one terms it) and, second, the systematically growing data about the brain structures involved in MG-like processes. These factors should sooner or later lead to some consensus with regard to the basic problems of microgenesis and basic methods of its study, many of them touched on in the present publication. The experimental evidence from visual information processing research at least supports many of the basic principles of the microgenetic approach, if not more.

## References

Allport, A. (1987). Selection for action: Some behavioral and neurophysiological considerations of attention and action. In H. Heuer & A.F. Sanders (Eds.), *Perspectives on perception and action* (pp. 395–419). Hillsdale, NJ: Erlbaum.

Anderson, J.D., Bechtoldt, H.P., & Dunlap, G.L. (1978). Binocular integration in line rivalry. *Bulletin of the Psychonomic Society, 11*, 399–402.

Andrews, D.P. (1967a). Perception of contour orientation in the central fovea: Part 1. Short lines. *Vision Research, 7*, 975–997.

Andrews, D.P. (1967b). Perception of contour orientation in the central fovea: Part 2. Spatial integration. *Vision Research, 7*, 999–1013.

Arieti, S. (1962). The microgeny of thought and perception. *Archives of General Psychiatry, 6*, 454–468.

Bachmann, T. (1980). Genesis of a subjective image. *Acta et Commentationes Universitatis Tartuensis. 522. Problems of Cognitive Psychology*, 102–126.

Bachmann, T. (1984). The process of perceptual retouch: Nonspecific afferent activation dynamics in explaining visual masking. *Perception & Psychophysics, 35*, 69–84.

Bachmann, T. (1987). Different trends in perceptual pattern microgenesis as a function of the spatial range of local brightness averaging. Towards an empirical method for the differentiation between global and local levels of form as related to processing in real time. *Psychological Research, 49*, 107–111.

Bachmann, T. (1988a). The microgenetic approach to studying cognitive processes. II. Current state of the research as based on classical methods. III. Overview of contemporary methods and some generalizations (in Russian). *Acta et Commentationes Universitatis Tartuensis. 796. The Problems of the Development of Cognitive Processes*, 3–55.

Bachmann, T. (1988b). Time course of the subjective contrast enhancement for a second stimulus in successively paired above-threshold transient forms: Perceptual retouch instead of forward masking. *Vision Research, 28*, 1255–1261.

Bachmann, T. (1989a). Microgenesis as traced by the transient paired-forms paradigm. *Acta Psychologica, 70*, 3–17.

Bachmann, T. (1989b). *Psychophysiology of visual masking. The fine structure of conscious experience* (in Russian). Tartu: University of Tartu Press.

Bachmann, T. (1990). The microgenetic approach to studying cognitive processes. I. Historical review. (in Russian). *Acta et Commentationes Universitatis Tartuensis, 894. Cognition and regulation of activity*, 34–60.

Bachmann, T. (1991). Identification of spatially quantized tachistoscopic images of faces: How many pixels does it take to carry identity? *European Journal of Cognitive Psychology*, 3(1), 34–60.

Bachmann, T., & Kahusk, N. (1987). *Nonmonotonic microgenetic function for the perceptual representation of quantized visual images of objects*. Paper presented at the workshop on Knowledge Representation and Information Processing, Berlin, Abstracts, p. 45.

Bachmann, T., & Vipper, K. (1983). Perceptual rating of paintings from different artistic styles as a function of semantic differential scales and exposure time. *Archives of Psychology, 135*, 149–161.

Boer, L.C., & Keuss, P.J.G. (1982). Global precedence as a postperceptual effect: An analysis of speed–accuracy tradeoff functions. *Perception & Psychophysics, 31*, 358–366.

Breitmeyer, B.G. (1975). Simple reaction time as a measure of the temporal response properties of transient and sustained channels. *Vision Research, 15*, 1411–1412.

Brown, J.W. (1977). *Mind, brain, and consciousness*. New York: Academic Press.

Brown, J.W. (1983). Emergence and time in microgenetic theory. *Journal of the American Academy of Psychoanalysis, 11*, 35–54.
Calis, G., & Leeuwenberg, E. (1981). Grounding the figure. *Journal of Experimental Psychology: Human Perception & Performance, 7*, 1386–1397.
Calis, G., Sterenborg, J., & Maarse, F. (1984). Initial microgenetic steps in single-glance face recognition. *Acta Psychologica, 55*, 215–230.
Chastain, G. (1977). Feature analysis and the growth of a percept. *Journal of Experimental Psychology: Human Perception & Performance, 3*, 291–298.
Cheatham, P.G. (1952). Visual perceptual latency as a function of stimulus brightness and contour shape. *Journal of Experimental Psychology, 43*, 369–380.
Cohene, L.S., & Bechtoldt, H.P. (1974). Visual recognition as a function of stimulus offset asynchrony and duration. *Perception & Psychophysics, 15*, 221–226.
Cohene, L.S., & Bechtoldt, H.P. (1975). Visual recognition of dot-pattern bigrams: An extension and replication. *American Journal of Psychology, 88*, 187–199.
Conrad, K. (1947). Über den Begriff der Vorgestalt und seine Bedeutung für die Hirnpathologie. *Nervenarzt, 18*, 189–193.
Crick, F. (1984). Function of the thalamic reticular complex: The searchlight hypothesis. *Proceedings of the National Academy of Sciences, 81*, 4586–4590.
Dixon, N.F. (1981) *Preconscious processing*. Chichester: Wiley.
Dolan, T.R., & Mayzner, M.S. (1978). Detection and recognition of alphabetic characters: Simultaneous and contiguous. *Bulletin of the Psychonomic Society, 12*, 430–432.
Epstein, W., & Hatfield, G. (1978). The locus of masking shape-at-a-slant. *Perception & Psychophysics, 24*, 501–504.
Epstein, W., Hatfield, G., & Muise, G. (1977). Perceived shape at a slant as a function of processing time and processing load. *Journal of Experimental Psychology: Human Perception & Performance, 3*, 473–483.
Eriksen, C.W., & Schultz, D.W. (1979). Information processing in visual search: A continuous flow conception and experimental results. *Perception & Psychophysics, 25*, 249–263.
Flavell, J.H., & Draguns, J.G. (1957). A microgenetic approach to perception and thought. *Psychological Bulletin, 54*, 197–217.
Forgus, R.H., & Melamed, L.E. (1976). *Perception. A cognitive-stage approach*. New York: McGraw-Hill.
Froehlich, W.D., & Laux, L. (1969). Serielles Wahrnehmen, Aktualgenese, Informationsintegration und Orientierungsreaktion: I. Aktualgenetisches Modell und Orientierungsreaktionen. *Zeitschrift für Experimentelle und Angewandte Psychologie, 16*, 250–277.
Froehlich, W.D., Smith, G., Draguns, J.G., & Hentschel, U. (Eds.). (1984). *Psychological Processes in Cognition and Personality*. Washington, DC: Hemisphere.
Goldstein, A.G. (1970). Binocular fusion and contour suppression. *Perception & Psychophysics, 7*, 28–32.
Graumann, C.F. (1959). Aktualgenese: Die descriptiven Grundlagen und theoretischen Wandlungen des aktualgenetischen Forschungsansatzes. *Zeitschrift für Experimentelle und Angewandte Psychologie, 6*, 410–448.
Haber, R.N., & Hershenson, M. (1980). *The psychology of visual perception*. New York: Holt, Rinehart & Winston.
Harmon, L.D., & Julesz, B. (1973). Masking in visual recognition: Effects of two-dimensional filtered noise. *Science, 180*, 1194–1197.

Hentschel, U., Smith, G., & Draguns, J.G. (Eds.). (1986). *The roots of perception. Individual differences in information processing within and beyond awareness.* Amsterdam: North-Holland.

Holt-Hansen, K. (1980). How does a figure appear and disappear in visual perception? *Perceptual & Motor Skills, 32*, 27–55.

Hoving, K.L., Spencer, T., Robb, K.Y., & Schulte, D. (1978). Developmental changes in visual information processing. In P.A. Ornstein (Ed.) *Memory development in children* (pp. 21–67). Hillsdale, NJ: Erlbaum.

Hughes, H.C., Layton, W.M., Baird, J.C., & Lester, L.S. (1984). Global precedence in visual pattern recognition. *Perception & Psychophysics, 35*, 361–371.

Imada, T., & Yodogawa, E. (1984). Critical SOAs in pattern-by-pattern and pattern-by-flash masking: A study on contour formation process. *Psychologia, 27*, 22–29.

Intraub, H. (1981). Rapid conceptual identification of sequentially presented pictures. *Journal of Experimental Psychology: Human Perception & Performance, 7*, 604–610.

Intraub, H. (1985). Visual dissociation: An illusory conjunction of pictures and forms. *Journal of Experimental Psychology: Human Perception & Performance, 11*, 431–442.

Kalmus, M., & Bachmann, T. (1980). Perceptual microgenesis of complex visual pattern: Comparison of methods and possible implications for future studies. *Acta et Commentationes Universitatis Tartuensis. 529. Studies in Psychology IX.* 135–159.

Kinchla, R.A., & Wolfe, J. (1979). The order of visual processing: "Top-down," "bottom-up," or "middle-out"? *Perception & Psychophysics, 25*, 225–231.

Kirkham, R.W. (1977). Perceptual priority in pattern vision. In R.H. Day & G.V. Stanley (Eds.), *Studies in perception* (pp. 80–92). Nedlands: University of Western Australia.

Kissin, M.E. (1976). Tachistoscopic study of identification of simple visual stimuli (in Russian). *Voprosy Psikhologii, 1*, 122–126.

Kostelyanets, N.B., & Kamenkovich, V.M. (1986). Estimation of the size of the contoured test image in the conditions of identifying the masker (in Russian). *Fiziologiya Cheloveka, 12*, 301–304.

Kragh, U., & Smith, G.J.W. (Eds.). (1970). *Percept-genetic analysis*. Lund, Sweden: Gleerup. Krol, V.M., & Tanenholtz, L.I. (1979). The peculiarities of Tachistoscopic perception of textures (in Russian). *Fiziologiya Cheloveka, 5*, 281–285.

Krol, V.M., & Tanenholtz, L.I. (1979). The peculiarities of tachistoscopic perception of textures (in Russian). *Fiziologiya Cheloveka, 5*, 281–285.

Lange, N.N. (1893). *Psychological investigations. The law of perception* (in Russian) Odessa: Tipografiya Odesskogo Voyennogo Okruga.

Lawrence, D.H. (1971). Two studies of visual search for word targets with controlled rates of presentation. *Perception & Psychophysics, 10*, 85–89.

Levelt, W.J.M. (1968). *On binocular rivalry*. The Hague: Mouton.

Linschoten, J. (1959). Aktualgenese und heuristisches Prinzip. *Zeitschrift für Experimentelle und Angewandte Psychologie, 6*, 449–473.

Luria, A. (1973). *The working brain*. New York: Basic Books.

MacLean, P.D. (1990). *The triune brain in evolution: role in paleocerebral functions*. New York: Plenum.

Miller, J. (1981). Global precedence in attention and decision. *Journal of Experimental Psychology: Human Perception & Performance, 7*, 1161–1174.

Murch, G.M. (1973). *Visual and auditory perception*. New York: Bobbs-Merrill.

Navon, D. (1977). Forest before trees: The precedence of global features in visual perception. *Cognitive Psychology, 9*, 353–383.

Navon, D. (1981). The forest revisited: More on global precedence. *Psychological Research, 43*, 1–32.

Neisser, U. (1976). *Cognition and reality*. San Francisco: Freeman.

Nikitin, M.P. (1905). On the problem of formation of visual perceptions. An experimental investigation (in Russian). *Vestnik Psikhologii, Kriminal'noy Antropologii i Gipnotizma, 2*, 112–122.

Petersik, J.T. (1978). Possible role of transient and sustained visual mechanisms in the determination of similarity judgments. *Perceptual & Motor Skills, 47*, 683–698.

Petrenko, V.F., & Vasilenko, S.V. (1977). On perceptual categorization (in Russian). *Vestnik Moskovskogo Universiteta. Seriya—Psikhologiya, 1*, 26–34.

Prinz, W. (1986). Looking at some New Look problems from an information processing point of view. In U. Hentschel, G. Smith, & J.G. Draguns (Eds.), *The Roots of Perception* (pp. 419–426). Amsterdam: North-Holland.

Reynolds, R.I. (1978). The microgenetic development of the Ponzo and Zöllner illusions. *Perception & Psychophysics, 23*, 231–236.

Reynolds, R.I. (1981). Perception of an illusory contour as a function of processing time. *Perception, 10*, 107–115.

Sander, F. (1928). Experimentelle Ergebnisse der Gestaltpsychologie. In *Bericht über den 10. Kongress für experimentelle Psychologie*. (pp. 23–87). Jena Germany: Verlag von Gustav Fischer.

Sergent, J. (1986). Microgenesis of face perception. In H.D. Ellis, M.A. Jeeves, F. Newcombe, & A. Young (Eds.), *Aspects of face processing* (pp. 17–33). Dordrecht, The Netherlands: Martinus Nijhoff.

Shaw, R.E., & Turvey, M.T. (1981). Coalitions as models for ecosystems: A realist perspective on perceptual organization. In M. Kubovy & J.R. Pomerantz (Eds.), *Perceptual organization* (pp. 343–415). Hillsdale, NJ: Erlbaum.

Shekhter, M.S. (1981). *Visual recognition: Regularities and mechanisms* (in Russian). Moscow: Pedagogika.

Smirnov, V.M., & Resnikova, T.N. (1985). Artificial stabile functional links as a method of study and medical treatment in the conditions of a pathological state (in Russian). *Vestnik Akademii Meditsinskikh Nauk SSSR, 9*, 18–23.

Smith, G. (1957). Visual perception: An event over time. *Psychological Review, 64*, 306–313.

Solman, R.T. (1977). Evidence that focal processing involves a build-up of a visual object. *British Journal of Psychology, 68*, 305–310.

Styles, E.A., & Allport, D.A. (1986). Perceptual integration of identity, location and colour. *Psychological Research, 48*, 189–200.

Uhlarik, J., & Johnson, R. (1978). Development of form perception in repeated brief exposures to visual stimuli. In D. Walk & H. Pick (Eds.), *Perception and experience* (Vol. 1, pp. 347–360). New York: Plenum.

Undeutsch, U. (1942). Die Aktualgenese in ihrer Allgemein-Philosophischen und ihrer characterologischen Bedeutung. *Scientia, 72*, 37–42, 95–98.

Uttal, W.R. (1981). *A taxonomy of visual processes*. Hillsdale, NJ: Erlbaum.

Uttal, W.R. (1988). *On seeing forms*. Hillsdale, NJ: Erlbaum.
Vasilev, A., & Mitov, D. (1976). Perception time and spatial frequency. *Vision Research, 16*, 89–92.
Varela, F.J., & Singer, W. (1987). Neuronal dynamics in the visual corticothalamic pathway revealed through binocular rivalry. *Experimental Brain Research, 66*, 10–20.
Vekker, L.M. (1974). *Mental processes* (Vol. 1). (in Russian). Leningrad: University Press.
Walker, P. (1978). Binocular rivalry: Central or peripheral selective processes. *Psychological Bulletin, 85*, 376–389.
Ward, L.M. (1983). On processing dominance: Comment on Pomerantz. *Journal of Experimental Psychology: General, 112*, 541–546.
Watt, R. (1988). *Visual processing: Computational, psychophysical and cognitive research*. London: Erlbaum.
Werner, H. (1935). Studies on contour: 1. Qualitative analyses. *American Journal of Psychology, 47*, 40–64.
Werner, H. (1948). *Comparative psychology of mental development*. New York: International Universities Press.
Werner, H. (1956). Microgenesis and aphasia. *Journal of Abnormal Psychology, 52*, 347–353.
Werner, H. (1957). The concept of development from a comparative and organismic point of view. In D.B. Harris (Ed.), *The concept of development* (pp. 125–148). Minneapolis: University of Minnesota Press.
Wilding, J. (1982a). The effect of forward and backward masking by flash on apparent size. *Perception, 11*, 153–162.
Wilding, J.M. (1982b). *Perception. From sense to object*. London: Hutchinson.
Wolfe, J.M. (1983). Influence of spatial frequency, luminance, and duration on binocular rivalry and abnormal fusion of briefly presented dichoptic stimuli. *Perception, 12*, 447–456.
Wolfe, J.M. (1986). Stereopsis and binocular rivalry. *Psychological Review, 93*, 269–282.
Zusne, L. (1970). *Visual perception of form*. New York: Academic Press.

# 13
# Anxiety, Defense, and Attention Control

UWE HENTSCHEL, MANFRED KIEẞLING, and
ARN HOSEMANN

Having read the title of this chapter, the reader might expect a rather short story, some kind of condensed, shorthand information on the theoretical and empirical interrelatedness of the variables in question. This could be seen as an easy task, but our experience during the time of planning the study, the data recording, and interpretation has convinced us that for the story to be understandable, it will have to be rather complex. The first reason for this concerns the theoretical part of the study and its relation to the experimental design; the second is more a question of adequately describing the necessary technical details.

Variables in an experiment are the direct offspring of the operationalizations chosen, and ideally, it should also be possible to delineate the operationalizations directly from a theory with its specific statements and definitions. In most fields of psychology, however, matters are still not that simple, and the more complex the phenomena to be studied are, the greater the theory–operationalization gap can become. A variety of definitions are available for each construct, and most of these definitions are inherently vague. Unfortunately, this is not immediately apparent from verbal communication. In this regards, we think that the three sets of variables in our study are rather prototypical examples of the difficulties starting empirical research from a well-defined theoretical basis.

Theories can, however, be used as global stimulating ideas, models or guidelines, while precision in an experiment must come from specific operationalizations. In that case, it would be better not to refer to it as *theory testing* in the proper meaning of the term. Nevertheless, these experiments—such as the one presented here—can have a strong impact through their potential applications in reality-related fields.

The aim of our experiment was to test the effect of anxiety and defense mechanisms on a cognitive-performance task. The task was designed to

---

The study was supported by a grant from Daimler-Benz AG, Stuttgart, West-Germany.

simulate the attention-related part of driving a car, with the situations varying from normal to various states of inadequate stimulation.

Although it is not specifically theory testing, some remarks on the theoretical background for the empirical elements of the study seem in order. We will try to do this by starting with the dependent variable (performance scores in an attention task under different conditions of stimulation) and its hypothetical relation to the behavior that should be simulated by it, that is, car driving.

Driving a car is a habitual behavior for most people. It is under normal circumstances not an especially dangerous activity, but it can become very dangerous under certain circumstances. Under which conditions do the circumstances change from safe to dangerous? Regarded from a systems approach, the car, the driver, and the outside conditions (e.g., road and weather) are potentially influential elements with more or less important subelements and differing states. It is self-evident that the activity of driving becomes extremely dangerous if the brakes or the steering fail, or to take a more sophisticated example, if the driver does not notice that the road is slippery. Prevention of the first two kinds of danger seems to be a task for technicians rather than for psychologists, and consequently the analysis of the behavior of the driver is psychologically much more interesting than the analysis of the mere technical elements in the system. Moreover, by official statistics, estimations of the causes of accidents tend to be attributed to the driver in a very high proportion of cases (for West Germany, these estimations are in the range of 85% to 90%, Rompe & Heißing, 1985).

Seen from the systems perspective, the person-related part of the task of driving a car is a complex input–output process with a continuous feedback loop. The input encompasses attention-related information processing, and motor reactions are the output. Because motor reactions that are not too complicated, when trained, become automatized after some time and do not show large individual differences any longer (e.g., Fleishman & Hempel, 1956), we decided to neglect them in our experiment.

An important basic factor for the successful processing of information seems to be the degree of incoming stimulation with possible effects on the driver's attention, his evaluation of the situation and its specific elements, and his decision making. Concentrating on this dimension has the additional advantage that the complexitiy of real driving can be reduced in a meaningful manner and that it is consequently also better suited for an experimental study using a simulation approach. Because attention and information processing make up the central frame of reference for our dependent variable, some theoretical reference seems necessary in regard to these topics.

Everyone obviously seems to know what attention is, to paraphrase a statement of William James (1890), but when it comes to definitions, it is still necessary to make a choice among them. Restricted definitions aim at a momentary conscious state (focus definitions) or the process aspect of this state (process of focusing) (Meldman, 1970). Other definitions take into account the multidimensional features of attention (Fröhlich, 1978); Pribram's (1981) definition of attention, stressing the holding to one rather than another program with the implication of span, competency, effort, and consistency over time belongs to this kind. Also of note are the definitions including phenomena of unconscious selective attention (dual-process theories of attention) (N.F. Dixon, 1981; N.F. Dixon, Hentschel, & Smith, 1986); the definitions extending the concept to an organized set of procedures (Glass, Holyoak, & Santa, 1979); and attempts to regard attention in relation to its contribution to "resources of ability" (Cooper & Regan, 1982; Hunt, 1980).

We agree with Eysenck's (1982) general critique on most theory constructions for human information processing in that they basically neglect the noncognitive links in the interrelation of motivation, emotion, and cognition. Orientation reactions in reality are embedded in a social environment (Chance, 1976), and in that they make up a part of complex human behavior. For our purpose of studying the attention control of rather complex tasks, it seems absolutely necessary to use one of the more complex definitions as a theoretical frame of reference, such as, for example, that of Glass et al. (1979). We also adhere to the dual-process idea. The disadvantage with such a complex definition is that it is not possible at this moment to describe these organized sets of procedures in terms of a physiological process. The use of such a complex definition makes it much more plausible, however, to postulate a hypothetical relation to our independent variables that also are not suited for a complete description in mere physiological terms. Moreover, with regard to the experimental variation of the situation, we will have to refer to other theories in which attentional functions are at best implicit elements.

For one of our independent variables, anxiety, a lot of research has been done on the physiological level, but anxiety is regarded by most psychophysiologists as a complex reaction, the signs of which can be observed on a subjectively verbal level in particular forms of expression and behavior and in central and peripheral psychophysiological measures (Birbaumer, 1977; Fröhlich, 1983). Although some evidence indicates that anxiety may be an inborn characteristic (Gray, 1971), anxiety is regarded in most theories as a learned behavior, a signal to indicate the perception of a dangerous external stimulus, and in S. Freud's (1926/1959) anxiety theory, it is also the potential sign for threat from within. Cattell and Scheier (1961) have first made the distinction between state and trait anxiety for which Spielberger and his co-workers (Spielberger, Gorsuch, & Lushene, 1970) then have constructed two separate inventories (A-state and A-trait). Because we did not plan to include in our study a definite form of ego threat, which is seen as a crucial differential factor for A-state (e.g., Heinrich & Spielberger, 1982) we decided instead to choose a trait inventory covering potentially anxiety-eliciting situations with as many aspects as possible.

Looking for other potential predictors in the personality domain with reference to our psychodynamic orientation, we have decided to choose defense mechanisms as the second construct that also shows some theoretical links to anxiety. Defense mechanisms were defined by S. Freud (1894/1949) on the basis of individual reports of patients. Anna Freud (1946), in her elaboration of the concept, adhered to the same principle. Defense mechanisms registered in that way served as indicators for the dynamic functioning of the patients and were hypothetically related to symptoms of psychopathology (Eriksen & Pierce, 1968). Because they were deducted as intrapsychic constructs, they also can be regarded as classic personality variables.

Traditional psychoanalysts really never were troubled by the problem of whether the persons themselves or the situational variance was more important for people's behavior. The focus of their attention was the person. If you change the viewpoint with the aim of making predictions of behavior in general, the borders of the intrapsychic island are transcended, and the basic question arises of whether defense mechanisms are also valuable constructs to explain some part of the variance in person–situation interactions. To make this a specific hypothesis, an answer to this question requires, of course, some specification of the kind of situation and the situational demands, and last but not least, a reliable operationalization of the mechanisms of defense to be registered. One now may choose between the traditional psychoanalytic approach (A. Freud, 1946), including the extended version of using vignettes (Vaillant, 1974), and the use of tests. The test approach can be divided into paper-and-pencil measures, projective tests and the percept-genetic techniques of the Defense Mechanism Test (DMT) (Kragh, 1969) and the Meta-Contrast Technique (MCT) (Smith, Johnson, & Almgren, 1982).

We decided for our study to use the DMT, which will be described later in more detail, but at this point some remarks on the general approach seem appropriate. Microgenesis can be defined as an approach aiming at the explanation of general psychological phenomena, showing in that respect, some similarity to the information-processing approach (Hentschel, Smith, & Draguns, 1986), while percept-genesis has from its very beginnings stressed individual differences and personality (see Chapter 10). As in the past (Hentschel et al., 1986), microgenesis will be used as the general term for both in this text. The basic idea behind both approaches, microgenesis and percept-genesis, is clearly related to process, which can be regarded as an umbrella concept for different microgenetic and percept-genetic techniques as long as these processes are not expected to be identical. Some of the implicit phenomenological differences between them have been discussed earlier (Hentschel, 1984).

In all microgenetic techniques with meaningful pictorial stimuli, the main interest of the observing experimenter is usually aimed at the evolvement of meaning in the different stages of the perceptual process. This is elicited through a series of tachistoscopically presented stimuli, which are usually threatening in one way or another. The exposure times increase, covering a range from very short to sufficient for clear recognition. It is the effort in search of meaning (Draguns, 1984; Kreitler & Kreitler, 1984; Linschoten, 1959) that keeps the subjects motivated and lets them strive stepwise for a better recognition and at the same time makes it a diagnostically relevant process from the metaperspective of the experimenter.

It has been doubted on good grounds that the subjects' reports about what they have seen in the different expositions reflects "mere perception" (e.g., Prinz, 1986). It is the interdependence of the subject and his milieu that essentially characterizes perceptual adaptation, for the explanation of which Hentschel et al. (1986) have referred to two biological models, the model of the functional circle (*Funktionskreis*, von Uexküll, 1921) and the Gestalt region theory (*Gestaltkreis*, von Weizsäcker, 1947). Another more formal way, but at the same time more restricted, to represent the interdependence between perceiver and stimulus, is provided by Brunswick's (1955) lens model (cf. Hentschel & Schneider, 1986). If the gradually adapted assignment of meaning is to be seen as the most central constituent in the process, then the question of whether or not this reflects mere perception is not so important for its diagnostic relevance. It is the reference to reality that forms the crucial critical element in that case. It is to the merit of Ulf Kragh (1955) to have recognized this and at the same time to have developed a "translation" into mechanisms of defense.

The sequence postulated by Kragh (1970b) is the following: (1) subliminal threat (against the hero, with whom the subject is supposed to identify); (2) submanifest anxiety; (3) defensive processes. The hypothetical linkage between anxiety and defense becomes obvious in this sequence also. It has been repeatedly questioned, however, if this is the only possible explanation of what is happening in the actual situation. On the objective output side, there are only the reports that the experimenter gets from the subject, and thus for the moment, no definite conclusion seems possible in that discussion. There is, however, on rational grounds no good reason not to use the concept of defense to explain the results. There is sufficient proof that defense mechanisms defined in such a way as traits are valid predictors for danger involving normal behavior, like piloting or diving. Ulf Kragh's (1970a) results are still astonishing in that even in a highly selected group of specialists, stress tolerance and accident proneness can be predicted by means of perceptual defense mechanisms. This has been well cross-validated in the meantime by among others, Neuman (1978) and Vaernes (1982). Hentschel and Kießling (1990) could show that defenses also are exerting an influence on less dangerous activities like taking an intelligence test and solving a concept-formation task.

If defense mechanisms must be given a place among the relevant moderator variables in a number of tasks in different areas, then it is probably their reality-distorting effect that gives them their predictive power, and this is also one of the reasons that we have included them in the present study. To repeat the general goal of the study: we planned to design a task that could be regarded as a good simulation of the attention-related part of the task of driving a car, providing different conditions (normal, two forms of understimulation, and two forms of overstimulation), and to predict the performance in that task by means of self-reported anxiety and perceptual defenses.

## Method

### *Experimental Conditions for Measuring the Dependent Variable.*

Because driving a car under the conditions of normal load of information, understimulation, and overstimulation was our analogy for the information-processing task to be simulated, we first had to construct a task that fulfilled the respective requirements. We decided to use a computer-controlled experiment with the specific conditions as given in Table 13.1.

The basic design of the task as presented to the subject is schematically given in Figure 13.1. The subjects saw a rectangle with nine separated fields on the monitor. They were told that three simple geometrical figures (a square, a circle, and a triangle) could appear in changing intervals in any of these nine fields. Whenever the relevant symbol (which was different in four of the five specific conditions) appeared, they had to press the corresponding key on the number part of the keyboard (see Fig. 13.1).

In Table 13.2, the specifications for the different conditions are listed. (The computer program comprising these specifications was developed by B. Kraas.) In the normal condition, the subjects were constantly busy throughout the whole period. The intervals between exposures became

TABLE 13.1. The five specific conditions in the attention-control experiment.

| Demarcation of conditions | Attempt to achieve |
|---|---|
| Monotony | A state of lower activation, unvoluntarily lowered vigilance |
| Satiation | Decrease in task valence with tendency to go out of the field by introducing variations against the rules (connected symptoms: inattention, forgetting, fatigue) |
| Normal | Normal level of activation, manageable task requirements |
| Stress-level 1 | Unmanageable information load with resulting conflictual disregulation (connected symptoms: anxiousness, nervous tension, hyperactivity) |
| Stress-level 2 | Increase in conflictual disregulation as compared to stress-level 1 by heightened strain through larger information load |

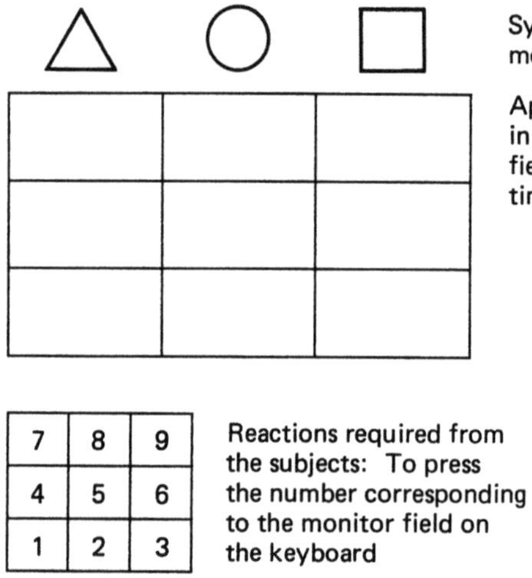


FIGURE 13.1. Schematic presentation of the attention-control task as given to the subjects.

shorter (15% acceleration from the beginning to the end), but the task remained manageable without any difficulties. The monotony situation was experienced through the long intervals between trials as boring, and satiation was introduced by presenting the relevant stimulus in a restricted area in a time pattern with minor variation, which required the subjects to press the keys in serial reactions with the following order: 7, 8, 4, 5, 7, 5.

Stress was introduced on level 1 (stress 1) through different colors and a large gradual decrease (50%) of the intervals between the trials from the beginning to the end, so that the subjects had to work twice as fast at the end in comparison to the beginning of the stress 1 condition.

On the second level of stress (stress 2), the background colors of the field in which the relevant symbol appeared were also changed. The minimum interval between the different exposures had the same large decrease (50%) as in the stress 1 condition.

The effect of the different conditions on the subjects was tested in a pilot study (n = 5), after which the subjects were asked about their impressions and feelings. From that study, it could be concluded that the conditions of understimulation were experienced as boring, the normal condition requiring routine attention was manageable, and the two stress conditions were experienced as hardly manageable with the corresponding feeling of becoming nervous and not being at ease (see Table 13.1).

The experiment was run individually, the computer registered automatically the reaction times and the errors made. An error was also scored when the reaction was not given within the limit of two times the exposure

TABLE 13.2. Characteristics of the different conditions in the attention-control task.

<table>
<tr><td></td><td>Normal</td></tr>
<tr><td>Relevant symbol:</td><td>Green triangle in combination with 0–2 irrelevant symbols, same color</td></tr>
<tr><td>Number of trials:</td><td>200</td></tr>
<tr><td>Exposure time:</td><td>8/10 s</td></tr>
<tr><td>Interval between trials:</td><td>11/10–20/10 s</td></tr>
<tr><td>Acceleration:</td><td>Factor 15</td></tr>
<tr><td>Error feedback:</td><td>Yes</td></tr>
<tr><td></td><td>Monotony</td></tr>
<tr><td>Relevant symbol:</td><td>Green square, no irrelevant symbols</td></tr>
<tr><td>Number of trials:</td><td>25</td></tr>
<tr><td>Exposure time:</td><td>7/10 s</td></tr>
<tr><td>Interval between trials:</td><td>300/10–600/10 s</td></tr>
<tr><td>Acceleration:</td><td>Factor 1</td></tr>
<tr><td>Error feedback:</td><td>No</td></tr>
<tr><td></td><td>Satiation</td></tr>
<tr><td>Relevant symbol:</td><td>Yellow circle appearing in predetermined sequence in a restricted area of the whole field<table><tr><td>7</td><td>8</td><td></td></tr><tr><td>4</td><td>5</td><td></td></tr><tr><td></td><td></td><td></td></tr></table></td></tr>
<tr><td>Number of trials:</td><td>594</td></tr>
<tr><td>Exposure time:</td><td>5/10 s</td></tr>
<tr><td>Interval between trials:</td><td>11/10–20/10 s</td></tr>
<tr><td>Acceleration:</td><td>Factor 1</td></tr>
<tr><td>Error feedback:</td><td>No</td></tr>
<tr><td></td><td>Stress 1</td></tr>
<tr><td>Relevant symbol:</td><td>Circle (green, red, or yellow) in combination with 0–2 irrelevant symbols, changing colors</td></tr>
<tr><td>Number of trials:</td><td>250</td></tr>
<tr><td>Exposure time:</td><td>4/10 s</td></tr>
<tr><td>Interval between trials:</td><td>5/10–10/10 s</td></tr>
<tr><td>Acceleration:</td><td>Factor 50</td></tr>
<tr><td>Error feedback:</td><td>Yes</td></tr>
<tr><td></td><td>Stress 2</td></tr>
<tr><td>Relevant symbol:</td><td>Circle (green, red, or yellow) in combination with 0–2 irrelevant symbols, changing colors and changing background colors</td></tr>
<tr><td>Number of trials:</td><td>300</td></tr>
<tr><td>Exposure time:</td><td>4/10 s</td></tr>
<tr><td>Interval between trials:</td><td>3/10–6/10 s</td></tr>
<tr><td>Acceleration:</td><td>Factor 50</td></tr>
<tr><td>Error feedback:</td><td>Yes</td></tr>
</table>

time, starting with the onset of the stimulus. The order of the different conditions was the following: monotony, stress 1, normal, satiation, and stress 2. The different parts of the computer-controlled experiment were separated by other tests and periods of rest.

## The Independent Variables in the Study

### Anxiety

The anxiety inventory used was the Interaktions-Angst-Fragenbogen [Interaction Anxiety Questionnaire] (IAF) scale (Becker, 1982). It comprises 55 items, which are grouped into six subclasses of anxiety on a habit level. These subclasses are contained in the following scales (the figures in parentheses indicate the internal consistency reliabilities of the respective scales): 1, anxiety of physical injury (.84); 2, stage-fright (.86); 3, anxiety to violate moral norms (.75); 4, anxiety of illness and medical treatment (.75); 5, anxiety to be too self-assertive (.77); 6, anxiety of self-devaluation (.81). In addition, the manual describes two second-order factors: scale 7, summarizing scales 1, 4, and 6, and scale 8, summarizing scales 2 and 5. The scales 1 to 6 may be summed up to provide a trait anxiety score (internal consistency: .74). We have chosen this method because it covers a rather broad range of potentially anxiety-related habits. Separate norms for men and women are available and were also used in this study in order to avoid the problem with higher raw scores of women subjects which are usually observed. According to the different norms, the raw scores were transformed into *T*-scale values.

### The Defense Mechanism Test

The DMT is a percept-genetic test with the aim of exploring the whole perceptual process from the very subjective beginning to "public reality" (Smith, Fröhlich, & Hentschel, 1984). The test consists of a tachistoscopic presentation of a stimulus configuration starting with very short exposure times (10 ms), gradually increasing to 2 s over a total of 20 trials. The stimulus configuration shown in this way consists of a young person with an older person to the left or to the right of the younger, who looks in a threatening manner at the younger one. In the middle part of the picture there is an object (e.g., a car, a ball, a plate), which can be seen as "belonging" to the younger person.

The terminology used to describe the elements of this configuration is in part borrowed from the Thematic Apperception Test (TAT) (Murray, 1938): the younger person defined as hero, the object before the younger person as instrument, and the second person as the peripheral or threatening person. The stimulus configuration is sex specific (i.e., both persons are male or female and the respective instrument is also designed to evoke male or female associations). A complete test series consists of two pictures of the same kind (i.e., the same elements in the stimulus configuration) but with different persons and instruments. The test series is started with a distractor slide (a nonthreatening harmonious "mother–child" scene), followed by the series with test picture 1, the distractor slide, the series with test picture 2, and at the end again the distractor slide. The subjects are seated in a rather dimly lighted room (2.8 lux) with the experimenter at their side. After every exposure they must report what they have seen (or believe to have seen as the instruction underlines the point that they also should tell their subjective impressions and report things on the picture of which they are not certain) and to make a simple drawing after each exposure. The experimenter awaits the subjects' spontaneous response and then is allowed to ask clarifying questions regarding, for example, the sex and the age of the persons in the picture in the case that "two persons" are reported without specifics. The time for taking the test varies, but nonpathologic subjects need roughly 1 hour. Verbal reports and drawings can be scored according to the manual (Kragh, 1985) into 10 main categories of mechanisms of defense: repression, denial, isolation, reaction formation, identification with the aggressor, turning against the self, introjection of the opposite sex, introjection of another object, projection, and regression.

Control of the reliability of the DMT implies at least two problems: the interscorer reliability and the retest or parallel test reliability. Because the basic idea of the test is to reflect a process, repetitions of the test are unlikely to give the same or very similar results. Results with a parallel version, however, showed satisfying reliabilities even for a longer period of time (Neuman, 1967). Interrater-reliability estimates depend on the training of the raters. The DMT is in that respect not comparable to a questionnaire, where the only relevant question is whether one has used the scoring sheets correctly. Very good results (>.90) can be obtained, however, if the raters have received a training with the coding system (cf. Smith, Kragh, & Hentschel, 1980).

### Sample and Testing Procedure

One hundred subjects took part in the experiment. The age and sex distribution is given in Table 13.3. Their mean age was 34 years. They all had to have a driver's license, the acquisition of which dated back from 1 to 20 years with a mean of 13.5 years. Because we did not want to have a mere student sample, the number of students was limited to 25, although when compared to a representative German sample, the educational level nevertheless was higher in our sample. Another 22 subjects had already finished their studies. The testing was done in a quiet room in the University of Mainz. As a result of technical problems, the data were incomplete for five subjects and therefore had to be excluded from the sample (see Table 13.3). All subjects volunteered to take part in the experiment and received financial compensation.

### Study Design and Hypotheses

Concerning the dependent variable, the performances in the computer-simulated attention task can be regarded separately with the conditions of

TABLE 13.3. Age and sex distribution of the subjects in the experiment.

| | Sex | |
|---|---|---|
| Age | Female | Male |
| 20–35 | 24 (0) | 25 (2) |
| 36–55 | 28 (1) | 23 (2) |

Figures in parentheses indicate subjects with missing data.

monotony and satiation on the one hand, and the two stress situations on the other. The normal situation serves as base line in both conditions of understimulation and both conditions of overstimulation.

The number of independent variables is a problem for an analysis of variance design, especially the 10 defense mechanisms of the DMT. Different solutions to this problem are possible. One is to choose some defense mechanisms on theoretical grounds and exclude the others. Another is to reduce the number of necessary analyses by combining some of the variables; a third is to drastically heighten the required level of significance. We have decided to use the strategy of combining variables, because it also requires a choice on theoretical grounds and nevertheless leaves the possiblity to test the effects of all defense mechanisms even if their effect is looked for only in a certain combination. The 10 original mechanisms of defense as scored according to the DMT manual (Kragh, 1969) were combined in the manner as outlined in Table 13.4. Some of these combinations are easy to defend, for example, the clustering of the two mechanisms of introjection and the two autoaggressive mechanisms, identification with the aggressor and turning against self. The combination of projection and regression seems doubtful, but here it can be argued that they are the most pathologic ones according to the DMT-coding system.

We decided to have three anxiety groups, with high, medium, and low scores (corresponding to the respective 33% of the distribution) and two median-split groups of high and low defense scores on the five combinations of defense mechanisms. For each of the basic experimental conditions, i.e., understimulation and overstimulation, this creates five (3 × 2) two-way analyses of variance with a repeated measurement factor for the different conditions necessary, with the normal condition identical in both understimulation and overstimulation. The design is represented schematically in Table 13.5.

By using orthogonal contrasts in a repeated measurement design, the significance of the difference between the three concrete conditions to be compared in the two basic conditions of understimulation and overstimulation can be controlled. The null hypothesis ($H_0$) was that neither defense mechanisms nor anxiety should show an effect on the dependent variable. The working hypothesis can be specified to an expected effect of defenses

TABLE 13.4. The combinations of the perceptual defense mechanisms as used for the data analysis.

| | Groups as used in the analyses of variance | |
|---|---|---|
| Defense categories | >MDN | <MDN |
| Repression<br>Denial | + | – |
| Isolation<br>Reaction formation | + | – |
| Identification with the aggressor<br>Turning against the self | + | – |
| Introjection of the opposite sex<br>Introjection of another object | + | – |
| Projection<br>Regression | + | – |

MDN, median.

TABLE 13.5. Schematic presentation of the design of the study.

| | | Anxiety level | Conditions with varying degrees of information load | | | | | |
|---|---|---|---|---|---|---|---|---|
| | | | Understimulation | | | Overstimulation | | |
| | | | Monotony | Normal | Satiation | Stress 1 | Normal | Stress 2 |
| Defense level | High | A+ | | | | | | |
| | | A0 | | Errors | | | made | |
| | | A− | | | | | | |
| | Low | A+ | | | | | | |
| | | A0 | | in the | | | computer task | |
| | | A− | | | | | | |

and anxiety in the sense that both anxiety and defense influence the performance negatively in both understimulation and overstimulation conditions. With respect to the defense mechanisms, our hypothesis favored the isolation–reaction formation combination, but the other combinations were deliberately not excluded from the statistical tests, signifying the expectation that an effect on the performance was not regarded as impossible. All tests were done by means of the BMDP (Biomedical Computer Programs, P-series) program series (W.D. Dixon et al., 1981).

## Results

### *Differentiation of the Conditions in the Computer-Simulation Task in Terms of Difficulty*

Figure 13.2. gives the means of the errors in the different conditions. To see if the performances can be regarded as different under the conditions,

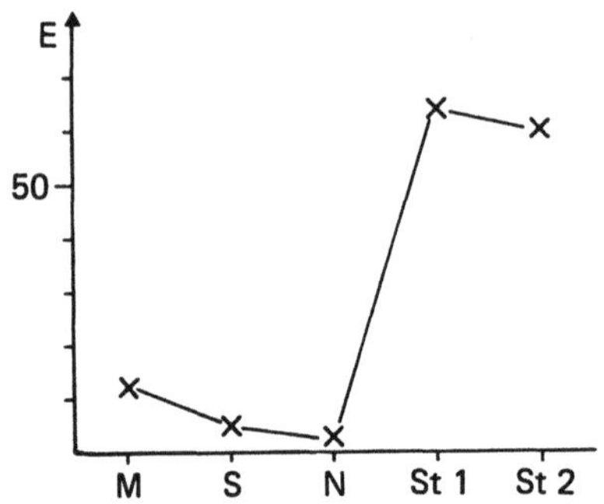


FIGURE 13.2. Means of the error percentage (E) in the different specific conditions (M, monotony; S, satiation; N, normal; St1, stress-level 1; St2, stress-level 2).

we calculated *t* tests for dependent variables between all conditions. Because we had 10 nonredundant tests, we set the level of significance at $p = 0.005$.

All comparisons were significant, which can be interpreted as a successful differentiation of the conditions in terms of the errors made. An obvious problem is the relation of the stress-1 and stress-2 condition. The common variance explained by the intercorrelations between the other conditions does not exceed 12%, while stress 1 and stress 2 show 69% common variance ($r = .83$). Moreover, stress 2, which was given after stress 1 elicited less errors than stress 1.

## *Effect of Anxiety and Defense in the Condition of Understimulation*

From the five possible analyses of variance, four could be calculated (for the defense combination identification with the aggressor-turning against self, the frequencies were too low). With the exception of a main effect of anxiety (which, of course, is the same in all four analyses), only one defense combination showed significant effects, that is, the isolation-reaction formation. The results of this analysis of variance are given in Table 13.6. The main effect of anxiety expressed itself by more errors in all conditions for the group with high anxiety. (The follow-up tests showed a significant ($p = .05$) difference between the upper group (A+) and the two other groups and no significant difference between the middle (A0) and the lower (A−) group.)

In Figure 13.3, the results are separately presented for the three anxiety groups. The most significant finding indicates in this case that subjects with high isolation-reaction formation combined with high anxiety made many more errors in the monotony situation. There was no difference between subjects with high and low defense in the A0 group, but in the group with low anxiety (A−), subjects with a low score on isolation-reaction

TABLE 13.6. Results of the analysis of variance with isolation-reaction formation for the condition *understimulation*.

| Effect | *df* | *F* | *p* |
|---|---|---|---|
| Anxiety | 2, 89 | 7.2 | <.01 |
| ir | 1, 89 | 1.1 | NS |
| Anxiety × ir | 2, 89 | 8.1 | <.001 |
| Repeated measures | 2, 178 | 24.2 | <.001 |
| Repeated measures × Anxiety | 4, 178 | 2.6 | NS |
| Repeated measures × ir | 2, 178 | 1.4 | NS |
| Repeated measures × Anxiety × ir | 4, 178 | 3.1 | <.05 |

ir, isolation-reaction formation.
*Note.* For testing the repeated measures effect and its interactions, the BMDP-program provided Greenhouse-Geisser probabilities.

formation had a slightly higher error score in the two understimulation conditions.

## *The Effects of Anxiety and Defense in the Condition of Overstimulation*

For the performance under the condition of overstimulation with the necessary exclusion of the defense combination identification with the aggressor-turning against self, we again calculated four (3 × 2) two-way analyses of variance. Compared to the condition of understimulation, the independent variables showed quite similar effects. We observed, however, no main effect of anxiety in this condition, but again, we observed an interaction of defense and anxiety for isolation-reaction formation among the different defense combinations (see Table 13.7).

TABLE 13.7. Results of the analysis of variance with isolation-reaction formation for the condition *overstimulation*.

| Effect | *df* | *F* | *p* |
|---|---|---|---|
| Anxiety | 2, 89 | 2.1 | NS |
| ir | 1, 89 | 2.1 | NS |
| Anxiety × ir | 2, 89 | 3.1 | <.05 |
| Repeated measures | 2, 178 | 468.2 | <.001 |
| Repeated measures × Anxiety | 4, 178 | 1.9 | NS |
| Repeated measures × ir | 2, 178 | 4.1 | <.05 |
| Repeated measures × Anxiety × ir | 4, 178 | 4.1 | <.01 |

ir, isolation-reaction formation.
*Note.* For testing the repeated measures effect and its interactions, the BMDP-program provided Greenhouse-Geisser probabilities.

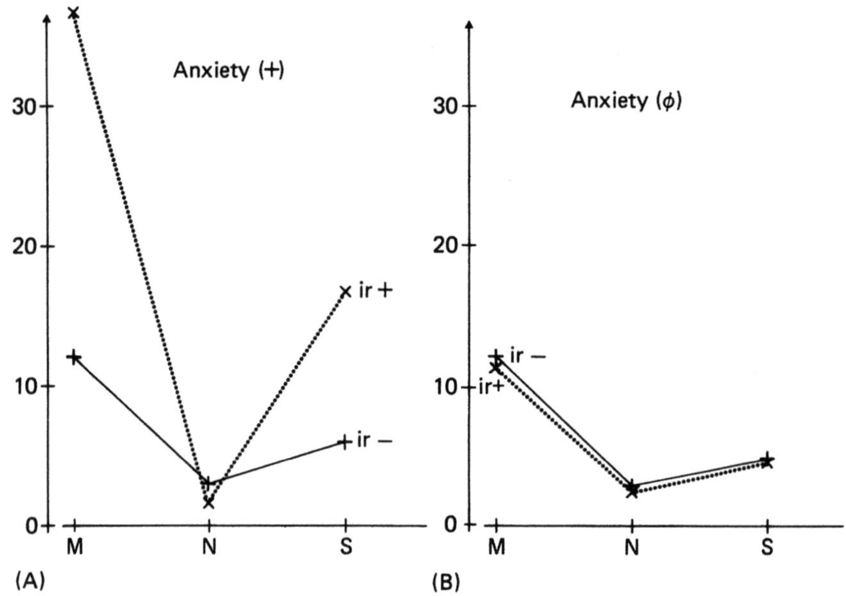


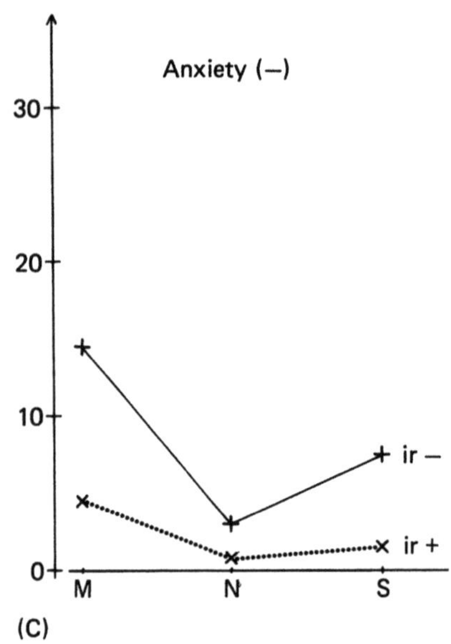


FIGURE 13.3. The effects of anxiety in interaction with defense on attention control in the condition of undersimulation. Part A gives the results for high anxiety (A+), part B for medium anxiety (A0), and part C for low anxiety (A−) (ir+, high scores on isolation-reaction formation; ir−, low scores; x-axes: M, monotony; N, normal; S, satiation; y-axes: percentage of possible errors).

The results are graphically presented in Figure 13.4. Subjects having scores above the median on isolation-reaction formation made more errors in the stress-1 and stress-2 situation if they belonged to the group with high or low anxiety. For subjects scoring high on anxiety and below the median

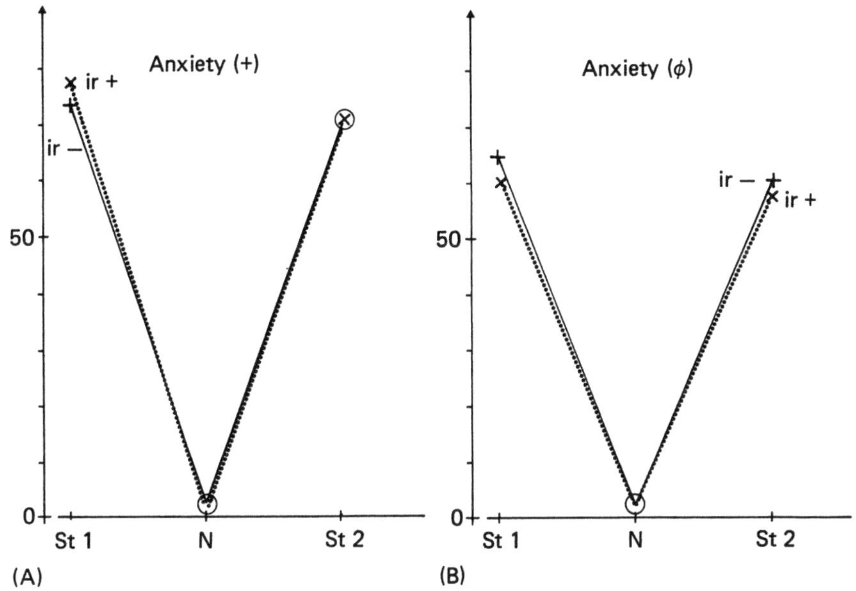


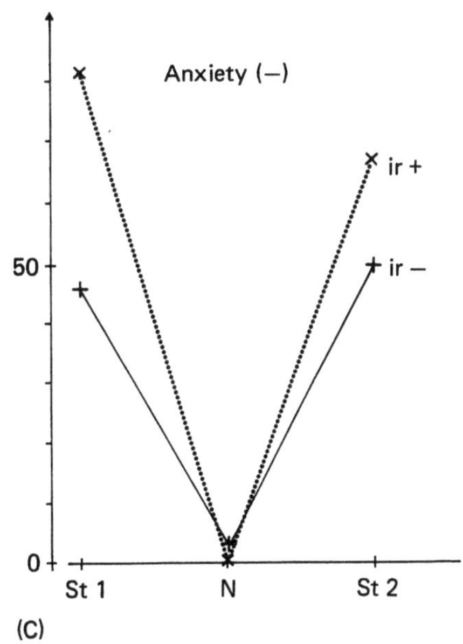


FIGURE 13.4. The effects of anxiety in interaction with defense on attention control in the condition of oversimulation. Part A gives the results for high anxiety (A+), part B for medium anxiety (A0), and part C for low anxiety (A−) (ir+, high scores on isolation-reaction formation; ir−, low scores; x-axes: St1, stress-level 1; N, normal; St2, stress-level 2; y-axes: percentage of possible errors).

on isolation-reaction formation, the performance was also hampered. Performance was significantly better for subjects scoring low on both anxiety and the isolation-reaction formation variable. The performance of the group with scores in the median range on the anxiety scale also showed medium scores on the dependent variable; statistically, they did not differ from the other groups. Also evident from Figure 13.5 is the result previously mentioned that the stress-2 situation did not elicit more errors than the stress-1 situation.

## Discussion

The different error rates for monotony and satiation in comparison to the normal situation on the one hand and stress 1 and stress 2 in comparison to the normal situation on the other can be seen as a clear indication that we succeeded to differentiate understimulation and overstimulation from a normal level of information load.

According to the experimental design, 10 two-way analyses of variance with a repeated measurement factor should have been calculated to test the effects of the independent variables on the attention control task. As a result of too low frequencies in one of the defense combinations, we could run only eight, from which two became significant. For both conditions, understimulation and overstimulation, a similar yet somewhat differing pattern appeared. The similarity results from the relevance of anxiety and isolation-reaction formation in both conditions. The specificity can be attributed to the general condition (e.g., the main effect of anxiety only for understimulation) as well as to the specific situations (e.g., the differences in performance for monotony and satiation). We stated in the formulation of the working hypothesis that in addition to anxiety, there would most probably be an effect from the combination of isolation-reaction formation on performance. This expectation was mostly based on previous results, mentioned in the introduction, and our experience with the DMT in regard to the frequency and distribution of the different defense categories. This also means that our favorite hypothesis was formed only partially on purely theoretical grounds. The theory of defense should, and actually does, make it possible to postulate the influence of other defense mechanisms. Thus, the results of our study can to some degree be regarded as a "method-effect." We know from comparisons between the DMT and the (Fragebogen zu Konflikt-bewältigungsstrategien [Conflict-Solving Strategy Inventory] (FKBS; Hentschel, Kießling, & Wiemers, in press), which is based on the same idea as the Defense Mechanism Inventory (DMI; Gleser & Ihilevich, 1969) and measures the same classes of defenses, that the correlation is pretty low between theoretically corresponding mechanisms of defense in both instruments (Hentschel, 1988). We also know that even the two percept-genetic techniques, DMT and MCT, having some of the same scoring categories, do not on the whole have much variance in common (Smith et al., 1980). To avoid broad verbal labels, as mentioned, it should be kept in mind that the effects that could be shown in the present study are related to specific instruments (i.e., the IAF and the DMT) and this implies a restriction for generalization but not a complete renounciation.

It is a well-documented fact that anxiety can have a disturbing effect on the output in a broad range of different tasks. In spite of a rather clear psychophysiological basis (Hall, 1980; Janke, 1986), the relationship between the physiological and the psychological representation still largely remains a puzzle, especially in regard to hypothetical psychophysiological patterns (Born, Lazarus-Mainka, & Stölting, 1980; Glanzmann & Fröhlich, 1986; Hentschel & Ternes, 1984; Johanson, Risberg, Silfveskiöld & Smith, 1986). Nevertheless, self-report anxiety inventories have a value of their own, and actually most of the results in anxiety research are probably based on such self-report inventories.

The DMT is a more specific test, as far as the method and its aim are concerned, and it is a well cross-validated instrument with reaction formation probably being one of the most relevant categories. Our results are similar to those obtained by Vaernes (1982), who in his experiment with divers, found deteriorating performance to be a correlate of reaction formation (in the DMT) and anxiety (in Taylors' 1953 Manifest Anxiety Scale), which thus could be used as an argument for a partial generalization. Although the results on the whole support the working hypothesis that both anxiety and defense influence the performance negatively, there is one remarkable exception for subjects having low scores on both anxiety and isolation–reaction formation. They show in the condition of understimulation a worse performance than those with low anxiety and a high level of defense. It is not so easy to develop a straightforward interpretation of this special result, but it seems as if some kind of internal filter is needed to keep up a certain level of motivation and performance. Nevertheless, the most clear-cut result for the understimulation condition is the deteriorating effect of both high anxiety and isolation–reaction formation, whereas for the condition of overstimulation, either of the two is detrimental.

In our experiment, the information load was varied for the different conditions and the dimension of attention control; thus, it became a central variable. In stress research, the control of the experimental effects is often restricted to overstimulation exclusively, whereas we have deliberately included the condition of understimulation. For shaping the latter condition, we sought different models than those usually used in stress research. Understimulation, seen as a specific condition of monotony, is usually implied in vigilance tasks using a signal detection design. In the most extreme form, it can also be found in sensory deprivation experiments, whereas the behavior effects of satiation were studied by Kurt Lewin (1935) and his co-workers (Karsten, 1928). Both variants of understimulation can occur while driving. Whereas monotony can easily be compared to driving on a desolate, straight long road, satiation could have a realistic counterpart in continuous stop-and-go traffic (especially in Europe, with a very low frequency of automatic transmissions). From self-experience in different driving situations, however, monotony seems to be the more frequent situation, which is also easier to trace.

Furthermore, in the computer simulation of the present study, the satiation condition seems to have been less error-inducing in general but nevertheless is a problematic situation for subjects having both high scores in anxiety and isolation-reaction formation.

Both stress loads evoked the hypothesized effect of heightening the number of errors for certain subgroups but without the expected differentiated effect between stress 1 and stress 2. We still think that stress-level 2 was more difficult than level 1, but a learning effect may have negated the greater difficulty because the stress-2 condition was presented after stress 1.

The background analogy for the design for our computer-simulation task was car-driving. In the research on accident prevention, a rather long and varying list of variables can be found. The accident-prone personality type has for a long time dominated the field as the main paradigm and was replaced by different variables contributing to a higher risk for accidents, such as aggressivity; competitive behavior; field dependence; extraversion; neuroticism; anxiety; depression; a general tendency to take high risks; alcohol and drug addiction; intelligence, particularly social intelligence; and also variables like the length of driving experience and sociodemographic variables (for a systematic overview of the literature see Kießling & Hentschel, 1989; see also Klebelsberg, 1982).

Although differing to some degree, on the whole, the portion of variance of the criterion (accidents) explained by these constructs is not very high (see Kießling & Hentschel, 1989). Attention regulation is to be found among the more promising predictor variables (Kahnemann, Ben-Ishai, & Cotan, 1973). One of the best predictors for accident-free driving, however, still seems to be the accumulated experience of driving. Critics of the approach of this research have argued that a number of problems are related to the criterion. The external conditions affecting the information load (e.g., weather, traffic density) and hence the internal state of the driver are usually ignored.

In our simulation experiment, we have tried to consider the internal state variables with the restriction that a direct measurement of the internal states of the subjects seemed impossible, but with the basic idea that the information load has, in interaction with stable personality traits, an effect on the states of a person and his performance.

We are aware of the fact that information load is not the only relevant input variable for car driving. Schlesinger (1980–1981) has reported that he could infer from the reports of some of his patients that their risk taking in driving, as well as his own, increased dangerously after the Guyana massacre and the assassination of the mayor of San Francisco. He has interpreted this remarkable observation as an attempt to prove one's own invulnerability, through a defensive derealization of the vulnerability of others actually encountered. This example can also exemplify the possibility that the source of the input can change. In this case, the input variable is to be found within the driver, the actual driving related information load from outside being of lesser importance. It can also exemplify the irrational part of our behavior, which in driving cannot be reduced meaningfully to purely rational, cognitive reactions. Both of the constructs chosen as predictors in the present experiment have a stronger weight on the affective-emotional side. We do not, of course, regard these as the only possible relevant variables in this context; quite a number of others have already been mentioned, but we think that it is all too seldom that affective-emotional variables are considered potential predictors for cognitive performances. In percept-genetic variables, there is always a mixture of affective and cognitive elements. The process of meaning assignment in percept-genesis is steered by cognitive mechanisms like the accumulation of experience, the elimination of irrelevant options, the rejection of inadequate constructions, and the eventual spontaneous generation of new interpretations (cf. Hentschel et al., 1986; Smith et al., 1980), but it always has an affective-emotional load; otherwise, it would not be possible to speak of meaning assignment.

The most basic assumption for percept-genesis, the correctness of which can be inferred from many studies, is that the process reflects enough personality-related variance. Objectively, the DMT series begins with a stimulus that is too short to be identified correctly and ends up with exposure times sufficient for identification by the majority of subjects. The evolvement of the correct "endgestalt" in between these two extremes with its relation to the personal history of the subject reveals diagnostically valuable information about internal structures that obviously are able to hamper or facilitate a reality-adequate perception in general.

The hypothesized anchorage of the percept-genetic approach in the biological theories of the functional circle and the gestalt-region theory has already been mentioned. Another possible link, which as far as we know has not yet been established, is to social representation theory (e.g., Moscovici, 1961). This theory could be of special value for the interpretation of broader socially meaningful contents of subjective perceptions, which in group-specific experience are shaped through the interaction with socially relevant others. These social representations are embedded in the individual learning history and can in turn determine adaptation to reality, including also social interactions.

One clear advantage of the percept-genetic approach is that it provides quantifiable variables that can be used as predictors for behavior in such different fields as psychopathology, intelligence, creativity, reactions to stress and as in our study, to situation-specific attention control.

The observed interaction of isolation-reaction formation with anxiety in our study shows some parallels to the results reported by Vaernes (1982) and seems interesting enough to be also controlled for in further experiments. In spite of the promising results of the present study, it remains an open question how close we have come with the analogy that has inspired the design of the attention-control task to reality, that is, how well our independent variables would predict the behavioral output of driving under real-life conditions. However, the link between the analogy of driving and the computer-simulation task is not an absolutely necessary one; the results can also be seen to stand in their own right, as a specific effect of anxiety and defense—as measured by the IAF and the percept-genetic DMT, respectively—on attention-control in situations of under-stimulation and overstimulation in a computer task.

## References


Becker, P. (1982). *Interaktions-Angst-Fragebogen (IAF)* [Interaction-Anxiety-Questionnaire, IAF]. Weinheim, Germany, Beltz Test.

Birbaumer, N. (1977). Angst als Forschungsgegenstand der experimentellen Psychologie [Anxiety as research topic in experimental psychology]. In N. Birbaumer (Ed.), *Psychophysiologie der Angst* [Psychophysiology of anxiety] (pp. 1–14). Munich: Urban & Schwarzenberg.

Born, C., Lazarus-Mainka, G., & Stölting, E. (1980). Die paradoxe Reaktion nichtängstlicher Personen [The paradoxical reaction of non-anxious persons]. *Zeitschrift Für Experimentelle und Angewandte Psychologie, 27*, 369–383.

Brunswik, E. (1955). Representative design and probabilistic theory in a functional psychology. *Psychological Review, 62*, 193–217.

Cattell, R.B., & Scheier, I.H. (1961). *The meaning and measurement of neuroticism and anxiety*. New York: Ronald.

Chance, M.R.A. (1976). Social attention: Society and mentality. In M.R.A. Chance & R.A. Larsen (Eds.), *The social structure of attention* (pp. 315–333). London: Wiley.

Cooper, L.A., & Regan, D.T. (1982). Attention, perception, and intelligence. In R.J. Sternberg (Ed.), *Handbook of human intelligence* (pp. 123–169). Cambridge, UK: Cambridge University Press.

Dixon, N.F. (1981). *Preconscious processing*. Chichester, UK: Wiley.

Dixon, N.F., Hentschel, U., & Smith, G.J.W. (1986). Subliminal perception and microgenesis in the context of personality research. In A. Angleitner, A. Furnham, & G. van Heck (Eds.), *Personality psychology in Europe: Vol. 2. Current trends and controversies* (pp. 239–255). Lisse, The Netherlands: Swets & Zeitlinger.

Dixon, W.D., Brown, M.B., Engleman, L., Frane, J.W., Hill, M.A., Jennrich, R.I., & Toporek, J.D. (Eds.). (1981). *BMDP statistical software 1981*. Los Angeles: University of California Press.

Draguns, J.G. (1984). Why microgenesis? An inquiry into the motivational sources of going beyond the information given. In G.J.W. Smith, W.D. Fröhlich, & U. Hentschel (Eds.), *From private to public reality* (pp. 5–16). Bonn: Bouvier.

Eriksen, C.W., & Pierce, J. (1968). Defense mechanisms. In E.F. Borgatta & W.W. Lambert (Eds.), *Handbook of personality theory and research* (pp. 1007–1040). Chicago: Rand McNally.

Eysenck, M.W. (1982). *Attention and arousal*. Berlin: Springer-Verlag.

Fleischman, E.A., & Hempel, W.E. (1956). Factorial analysis of complex psychomotor and related skills. *Journal of Applied Psychology*, *40*, 96–104.
Freud, A. (1946). *The Ego and the mechanisms of defense*. New York: International Universities Press.
Freud, S. (1949). The neuro-psychoses of defence. In J. Strachey (Ed. and Trans.), The *standard edition* of the complete psychological works of Sigmund Freud (Vol. 3, pp. 43–61). London: Hogarth Press. (Original work published 1894)
Freud, S. (1959). Inhibitions, symptoms and anxiety. In J. Strachey (Ed. and Trans.), The *standard edition* of the complete psychological works of Signund Freud (Vol. 20, pp. 77–172). London: Hogarth Press. (Original work published 1926)
Fröhlich, W.D. (1978). Stress, anxiety and the control of attention. In C.D. Spielberger & I.G. Sarason (Eds.), *Stress and anxiety* (Vol. 5, pp. 99–130). Washington DC: Hemisphere.
Fröhlich, W.D. (1983). Perspektiven der Angstforschung [Perspectives of anxiety research]. In H. Thomae (Ed.), *Enzyklopädie der Psychologie. Serie: Motivation und Emotion, Bd. 2: Psychologie der Motive* [Encyclopedia of psychology. Series: motivation and emotion, Vol. 2: Psychology of motives] (pp. 110–320). Göttingen, Germany: Hogrefe.
Glanzmann, P.G., & Fröhlich, W.D. (1986). Anxiety and covert changes of attention control. In U. Hentschel, G. Smith, & J.G. Draguns (Eds.), *The roots of perception* (pp. 381–400). Amsterdam: North-Holland.
Glass, A.L., Holyoak, K.J., & Santa, J.L. (1979). *Cognition*. Reading, MA: Addison-Wesley.
Gleser, G.C., & Ihilevich, D. (1969). An objective instrument for measuring defense mechanisms. *Journal of Consulting and Clinical Psychology*, *33*, 51–60.
Gray, J.A. (1971). *The psychology of fear and stress*. London: World University Library.
Hall, R.C.W. (1980). Anxiety. In R.C.W. Hall (Ed.), *Psychiatric presentation of medical illness* (pp. 13–35). Lancaster, England: MTP Press.
Heinrich, D., & Spielberger, C.D. (1982). Anxiety and complex learning. In H.W. Krohne & L. Laux (Eds.) *Achievement, stress and anxiety* (pp. 145–165). Washington, DC: Hemisphere.
Hentschel, U. (1984). Microgenesis and process description. In W.D. Fröhlich, G. Smith, J.G. Draguns, & U. Hentschel (Eds.), Psychological processes in cognition and personality (pp. 59–70). Washington, DC: Hemisphere.
Hentschel, U. (1988, June). *Empirical referents for the concept of defense*. Paper presented at the Fourth European Conference on Personality. Stockholm, Sweden.
Hentschel, U., Kießling, M. & Wiemers, M. (in press). *Fragebogen zu Konfliktbewältigungsstrategien* [Conflict solving strategy inventory]. Weinheim: Beltz Test.
Hentschel, U., & Kießling, M. (1990). Are defense mechanisms valid predictors of performance on cognitive tasks? In G. van Heck, S. Hampson, J. Reykowsky, & J. Zakrzewski (Eds.), *Personality psychology in Europe: Vol. 3. Foundations, models, and inquiries* (pp. 203–223). Lisse, The Netherlands: Swets & Zeitlinger.
Hentschel, U., & Schneider, U. (1986). Psychodynamic personality correlates of creativity. In U. Hentschel, G.J.W. Smith, & J.G. Draguns (Eds.), *The roots of perception* (pp. 249–275). Amsterdam: North-Holland.

Hentschel, U., Smith, G.J.W., & Draguns, J.G. (1986). Subliminal perception, microgenesis and personality. In U. Hentschel, G.J.W. Smith, & J.G. Draguns (Eds.), *The roots of perception* (pp. 3–36). Amsterdam: North-Holland.

Hentschel, U., & Ternes, G. (1984). Moderating effects of trait anxiety on electordermal reactions in different learning conditions. *Psychological Reports, 54*, 803–809.

Hunt, E. (1980). Intelligence as an information processing concept. *Journal of British Psychology, 71*, 449–474.

James, W. (1890). *Principles of psychology*. New York: Holt.

Janke, W. (1986). Angst: Definition und somatische Grundlagen [Anxiety: definition and somatic basis]. In W. Janke & P. Netter (Eds.), *Angst und Psychopharmaka* [Anxiety and psychopharmacy] (pp. 19–42). Stuttgart, Germany: Kohlhammer.

Johanson, A.M., Risberg, J., Silfverskiöld, P., & Smith, G.J.W. (1986). Regional changes in cerebral blood flow during increased anxiety in patients with anxiety neurosis. In U. Hentschel, G.J.W. Smith, & J.G. Draguns (Eds.), *The roots of perception* (pp. 353–360). Amsterdam: North-Holland.

Kahnemann, D., Ben-Ishai, R., & Cotan, M. (1973). Relation of a test of attention to road accidents. Journal of Applied Psychology, *58*, 113–115.

Karsten, A. (1928). Psychische Sättigung [Psychic satiation] *Psychologische Forschung, 10*, 142–254.

Kießling, M., & Hentschel, U. (1989). *Literaturrecherche: Persönlichkeitsvariablen als Prädiktoren für das Verhalten im Strassenverkehr* [Review: Personality variables as predictors for traffic behavior]. Report for the Daimler-Benz Research Unit in West-Berlin, University of Mainz. Unpublished manuscript.

Klebelsberg, D. (1982). *Verkehrspsychologie* [Traffic-psychology]. Berlin: Springer-Verlag.

Kragh, U. (1955). *The actual-genetic model of perception-personality*. Lund, Sweden: Gleerup.

Kragh, U. (1969). *Manual till DMT—Defense Mechanism Test* [Manual for the DMT—Defense Mechanism Test]. Stockholm: Skandinaviska Testförlaget.

Kragh, U. (1970a). The Defense Mechanism Test (DMT) as a method for diagnosis and personnel selection. In U. Kragh & G.J.W. Smith (Eds.), *Percept-genetic analysis* (pp. 179–189). Lund, Sweden: Gleerup.

Kragh, U. (1970b). Defensive organisation in percept-genesis. In U. Kragh & G. Smith (Eds.), *Percept-genetic analysis* (pp. 105–118). Lund, Sweden: Gleerup.

Kragh, U. (1985). *Manual for the Defense Mechanism Test (DMT)*. Stockholm: Persona.

Kreitler, S., & Kreitler, H. (1984). Meaning assignment in perception. In W.D. Frölich, G.J.W. Smith, J.G. Draguns, & U. Hentschel (Eds.), *Psychological processes in cognition and personality* (pp. 173–191). Washington, DC: Hemisphere.

Lewin, K. (1935). *A dynamic theory of personality Selected papers New York: McGraw Hill.*

Linschoten, J. (1959). Aktualgenese und heuristisches Prinzip [Microgenesis and the principle of heuristics]. *Zeitschrift für experimentelle und angewandte Psychologie, 6*, 449–473.

Meldman, M.J. (1970). *Diseases of attention and perception*. Oxford: Pergamon Press.

Moscovici, S. (1961). *La psychanalyse, son image et son public*. Étude sur la représentation sociale de la psychanalyse [The psychoanalysis, its image and its public. A study on the social representation of psychoanalysis]. Paris: Presses Universitaires de France.

Murray, H.A. (1938). *Explorations in personality*. New York: Oxford University Press.

Neuman, T. (1967). Personlighet och anpassning till militärflygning (II). Försvarsmekanismer som stabila personlighetsstrukturer: Två studier över DMT-seriers reliabilitet. [Personality and adaptation to military flying (II). Defense mechanisms as stable personality structures: Two studies on the reliability of the DMT-series] *MPI-rappórt No. 52*.

Neuman, T. (1978). Dimensionering och validering av perceptgenesens förvarsmekanismer. En hierarkisk analys mot pilotens stressbeteende [Structure and validity of perceptgenetic defense mechanisms. A hierarchical analysis of the behavior of pilots under stress]. *FOA rapport* (No. 55020-H6). Stockholm: Fösvarets forskningsanstalt.

Pribram, K.H. (1981). The brain as the locus of cognitive controls on action. In G. d'Ydewalle & W. Lens (Eds.), *Cognition in human motivation and learning* (pp. 141–157). Hillsdale, NJ: Lawrence Erlbaum.

Prinz, W. (1986). Looking at some New Look problems from an information processing point of view. In U. Hentschel, G.J.W. Smith, & J.G. Draguns (Eds.), *The roots of perception* (pp. 419–426). Amsterdam: North-Holland.

Rompe, K., & Heißing, B. (1985). Menschliches Fehlverhalten und technische Unfallursachen [Human errors and technical reasons for accidents]. In K. Rompe (Ed.), *Verkehrssicherheit und Wirksystem Fahrer-Fahrzeug-Umwelt* [Traffic safety and systems effects of driver-car-outside conditons] (pp. 115–138). Cologne, Germany: TÜV Rheinland.

Schlesinger, K. (1980–1981). On the creative process and the human capacity to construe. *International Journal of Psychoanalytic Psychotherapy, 8*, 483–500.

Smith, G.J.W., Fröhlich, W.D., & Hentschel, U. (Eds.). (1984). *From private to public reality*. Bonn: Bouvier.

Smith, G.J.W., Johnson, G., & Almgren, P.E. (1982). *MCT—Metakontrasttekniken* [MCT—Metacontrasttechnique]. Stockholm: Psykologiförlaget.

Smith, G.J.W., Kragh, U., & Hentschel, U. (1980). Perceptgenetische Vefahren: Historische und methodologische Übersicht [Perceptgenetic techniques: Historical and methodological overview]. In U. Hentschel & G. Smith (Eds.), *Experimentelle Persönlichkeitspsychologie* [Experimental personality psychology] (pp. 31–63). Wiesbaden, Germany: Akademische Verlagsge sellschaft.

Spielberger, C.D., Gorsuch, R.L, & Lushene, R.E. (1970). *Manual for the State–Trait Anxiety Inventory*. Palo Alto, CA: Consulting Psychologists Press.

Taylor, J.A. (1953). A personality scale of manifest anxiety. *Journal of Abnormal and Social Psychology, 48*, 285–290.

Uexküll, J. von (1921). *Umwelt und Innenwelt der Tiere* [Outer and inner world of animals]. Berlin: Springer-Verlag.

Vaernes, R. (1982). The Defense Mechanism Test predicts inadequate performance under stress. *Scandinavian Journal of Psychology, 23*, 37–43.

Vaillant, G.E. (1974). *Adaptation to life*. Boston: Little, Brown.

Weizsäcker, V. von (1947). *Der Gestaltkreis* [Gestalt region theory] (3rd ed.). Stuttgart, Germany: Thieme.

# 14
# Microgenetic Techniques of Personality Assessment

JURIS G. DRAGUNS

Following Sander (1928/1962) and Froehlich (1983), microgenesis[1] is the process of percept formation that occurs in consciousness and is observable in its entirety, from beginning to end. Of the several developmental progressions, for example, ontogenesis and phylogenesis, microgenesis is the only one that lends itself to observation throughout all of its stages. It is often brought about by artificially extending the perceptual process and obstructing the instantaneous recognition of the object presented. This objective is accomplished by some technique of stimulus impoverishment, most prominently exemplified by tachistoscopic presentation.

Sander (1928/1962), one of the pioneers of microgenetic investigation, reported three findings that are relevant to personality research and assessment. First, microgenesis proceeds in a noncontinuous and irregular manner. Instead of constructing a percept gradually, in a piecemeal fashion, hunches are formed that outstrip the available evidence and are then modified, elaborated, or discarded. The process is easily divisible into qualitatively distinct stages. Second, there is a disproportionate amount

[1] In this Chapter as well as in much of the current English-language usage, microgenesis is employed as a generic term for all developmental progressions which occur over a short time span and are observable in their entirety. This definition corresponds to the meaning of the term *Aktualgenese* in German which was coined by Sander and was sometimes translated into English as actual genesis. Microgenesis was introduced into English usage by Werner (1948, 1956). The two terms are often regarded as equivalent. Some of the authorities on this subject, e.g., Graumann (1959), draw the distinction between Aktualgenese as a descriptive term and microgenesis as an explanatory concept, laden with the implications of micro-macro correspondence between various developmental progressions. To reiterate, the use of the term microgenesis in the present Chapter is free of these theoretical implications.

The third overlapping term in current use is perceptgenesis. It refers exclusively to the several perceptual techniques of clinical and personality assessment developed at Lund University. Several of these instruments will be described later in the Chapter.

of emotional participation, seemingly incongruous in such an apparently innocuous task. To borrow from contemporary vernacular, microgenesis acquires the characteristics of an encounter between the whole person and a gradually emergent stimulus. In this process, not only perception and cognition are implicated but affect as well. Third, the early investigators of microgenesis were quick to observe individual differences in several features of this progression. Specifically, some people started with details, others began with wholes, while there were also instances of persons proceeding integratively, by organizing specific components into supraordinate configurations.

The goal of the present Chapter is to bridge that gap between these early observations and the current state of microgenetic techniques and findings. In more specific terms, the question may be asked, Has an accumulation of results emerged that is actually or potentially useful for the practical tasks of personality assessment? In other words, what, if anything, can microgenetic methods of inquiry contribute to the three major tasks of personality assessment (Draguns, 1975)? These three tasks are the identification of individual differences among people in responding to identical situations and stimuli, the stability of individual responses despite variations in time and context, and the personally characteristic organization of such responses.

By way of a preliminary response to these questions, let us admit that the current role of microgenetic techniques in personality assessment is not prominent. The microgenetic model of personality assessment is overshadowed by the two principal approaches to personality assessment: projective techniques and self-report inventories. What remains to be communicated is the personality-relevant yield of microgenetic research in two areas. First, there are relatively numerous, but brief, forays into personality psychology by means of a variety of techniques. The most that can be said about these ventures is that they are promising. This promise, however, remains to be fulfilled. Second, there are the results of a systematic research effort built on an explicit conceptual foundation and pursued consistently and vigorously over the past years. Reference is made here to the techniques developed and the results obtained by researchers at Lund University in Sweden. Their work has been described and reviewed in a number of sources (Hentschel & Smith, 1980; Kragh & Smith, 1970; Smith & Westerlundh, 1980), and it is also featured in several Chapters of this volume. Nonetheless, in as much as the Lund research team has made the major contribution to the integration of microgenesis and personality, the latter part of this Chapter will be devoted to it.

# Early Formulations and Findings: Three Pioneers of Microgenesis

## *Sander's Contribution*

Three major contributors to psychological research and theory co-discovered microgenesis. Sander (1928/1962) has already been mentioned. As an experimental psychologist and Wundt's youngest co-worker and assistant, Sander was interested in empirically studying the emergence of percepts. This interest was embedded in a theoretical framework that was holistic and developmental. Unlike the proponents of the much better known Berlin school of Gestalt psychology, the adherents of holistic developmental psychology (*Genetische Ganzheitspsychologie*) went beyond perception in their emphasis on the primacy of holistic experience. Krueger (1928), the originator of this school of thought, posited the inextricable unity of perception, cognition, motivation, conation, and affect in determining human behavior and experience. In particular, he emphasized the primacy of feeling from which the other, developmentally later, psychological functions eventually emerge.

The implications based on this theoretical framework for microgenesis are twofold. First, the eventual recognition of gradually emerging stimuli would proceed from the affectively colored experience of global reactions. By and large, Sander and his co-workers (e.g., Hausmann, 1935; Wohlfahrt, 1932) confirmed these expectations. In passing, it may be interjected that it may be inexact to speak of expectations and hypotheses. As Sander (1928/1962) relates it, he and his collaborators almost stumbled on the features of the early stages of microgenesis, with their globality and affective involvement. Nonetheless, the prominence accorded to these two types of experience in Sander's theory made it easier for him to focus on these phenomena. Second, Sander was quick to recognize two qualitatively distinct types of microgenesis: *hologenetic* (German: *hologen*, from the Greek, based on or arising from wholes) and *merogenetic* (German: *merogen*, from the Greek, based on or arising from parts) (Froehlich, 1984). Of interest in the context of this Chapter, Sander reported that the type of microgenesis experienced was based on the characteristics of the stimulus but also on the personality of the individual.

In his definitive review of the experimental results of Gestalt psychology, Sander (1928/1962) devoted a section to the incidental observations and serendipitous discoveries of the expression of personality characteristics in the microgenetic process. Then and later, he expressed the conviction that the whole- and detail-oriented types of microgenesis offer a variety of clues to the functioning of individuals in a wide variety of situations, on the basis of the assumption of stylistic consistency as embodied in the much newer notions of cognitive or personal style, such as field dependence and field independence (Witkin, Dyk, Faterson, Goodenough, & Karp, 1962). In fact, close parallels are discernible between the characteristics of field dependent persons as described by Witkin et al. and the global and undifferentiated mode of responding attributed to the holistic type by Sander (1928/1962). As far as the detail-oriented or, possibly, the field-independent person is concerned, his features, as expressed in the course of microgenesis, were not discovered until somewhat later, when the integrative type was described (Schmidt-Durban, 1939). These persons are capable of fitting components into supraordinate stimuli and, conversely, can extract details from complex wholes. Beyond the identification of these three types, personality-oriented research on microgenesis progressed little, although systematic verification of the existence of these three types, subject to the state of statistical data analysis at the time, was provided (Schmidt-Durban, 1939). Further advances, however, remained stymied for two reasons: the rudimentary state of statistical techniques of analysis, which has already been alluded to, and the nondynamic and general formulation of personality variables within the conceptual framework, which Sander and his co-workers had espoused. In other words, their theory did not go beyond the identification of personality dimensions and left open the questions of their origins, interrelationships, and consequences. Thus, all that remains of these pioneering formulations is the expectation that personality style is revealed in the microgenetic progression, and a few illustrative and corroborating findings in support of this link.

## *Werner's Contribution*

The other key figure in the demonstration of microgenetic phenomena and in their theoretical explication is Heinz Werner, an Austrian-born psychologist. He embarked on his career as an experimental psychologist in Germany. On Hitler's rise to power, Werner emigrated and became a prominent developmental theorist in the United States. He is best remembered for proposing the orthogenetic principle (Werner, 1948, 1957), according to which all development proceeds from global, undifferentiated experience through fragmentation into discrete detail to hierarchic integration of components into organized wholes. Werner regarded microgenesis as a developmental progression that abided by this general principle.[2]

[2] There is an implicit disagreement on this subject between the two pioneers of microgenesis, Sander and Werner. Sander, as indicated elsewhere in this chapter, differentiated two types of microgenesis, proceeding from wholes and details, respectively. Werner emphasized the uniformity of all delevopmental progres-

Morevoer, it had the advantage unshared by any other developmental experience of being open to observation throughout the entire process, as has already been pointed out. As a theorist, Werner was much more concerned with general rather than differential psychology. Nonetheless, he made an important if controversial contribution to microgenesis as an avenue of individually oriented investigation and, potentially, applied clinical assessment. In providing a developmental formulation of aphasia, he suggested that the abortive attempts at finding the right word, so characteristic of this disorder, be constructed as arrests at an early stage of microgenesis (Werner, 1956). This proposal was compatible with the conceptualizations of deficits in a variety of neuropsychological disorders, including aphasia, by the German psychiatrist Klaus Conrad (1947) and the Belgian psychologist André Ombredane (1951). The effect of these three converging formulations was to transform microgenesis from the description of a phenomenon to an explanatory concept. This development has sparked debate (Flavell & Draguns, 1957; de Koningh, 1967; Graumann, 1959; Linschoten, 1959), which has not died down to this day. In the context of this Chapter, it is not necessary to focus on this controversy. It is, however, important to note that Werner's, Conrad's, and Ombredane's ideas, contested though they are, opened the door to the use of microgenetic techniques in clinical settings for the purpose of diagnostic differentiation.

## Gemelli's Contribution

In contrast to the preceding two figures, for whom microgenesis was central in their conceptual scheme, Agostino Gemelli, a prominent Italian psychologist, contributed a number of important ideas and findings about microgenesis rather casually and never followed up on these innovative formulations. If Sander's and Werner's contributions to describing and explaining microgenesis were focused on its developmental and affective aspects, Gemelli (1928) emphasized a succession of cognitive operations in microgenesis. Of these he distinguished three: organization of sensory data, incorporation of meaning based on the person's experience and knowledge, and the final naming of the object. This formulation anticipates Bruner's (1957b) hypothesis theory, which holds that our experiences and expectations co-determine the content of our percepts together with the physical features of the stimuli. It can be regarded as the remote antecedent of modern microgenetic approaches to personality assessment, which conceive the various responses occuring before the veridical identification of the stimulus as reflections of enduring personality tendencies, for example, defenses.

---

sions. In any case, Lesswing (1973) was unable to corroborate empirically Werner's expectation that microgenesis invariably starts with the perception of amorphous wholes, thereby indirectly providing support for Sander's position.

## Microgenesis and Projective Techniques: Similarities and Differences

Microgenetic approaches have some obvious points of contact with projective techniques. What differentiates these two modes of presenting ambiguous stimuli remains less readily apparent. In Frank's (1939, p. 389) influential formulation, projective techniques are characterized by "a field with relatively little structure and cultural patterning, so that the personality can project upon that plastic field his way of seeing life, his meanings, significance, patterns, and especially his feelings."

What projective and microgenetic assessment techniques have in common is that the stimuli can easily be structured in a multiplicity of ways. In both kinds of techniques, the person is invited "to go beyond the information given" (Bruner, 1957a), to complete the incomplete and to express one's personality characteristics while ostensibly doing something else (Draguns, 1985). The purpose of capturing the elusive emerging stimulus at the first opportunity in a microgenetic progression is subtly different in purpose. What the person is asked to do is to establish what the incomplete, only partially revealed stimulus *really* is. Thus, as Jenkin (1957) has recognized, the attempts to impose meaning upon the stimuli are more attuned to reality and are less of a springboard for the expression of fantasy as compared with the responses to Rorschach inkblots and Thematic Apperception Test (TAT) pictures. The balance is tipped toward a more stimulus-based and realistic appraisal. Moreover, in contrast to the typical projective technique, a microgenetic stimulus is shown as part of a series that typically proceeds from maximal ambiguity to optimal clarity. In both cases, several competing response tendencies come to the surface. In microgenesis, however, there is a more general conflict between reality-oriented and fantasy-expressive tendencies. A subject might ask, "Shall I at all times concentrate on what this picture will eventually become, or shall I allow a free reign to my fantasies and simply say what it reminds me of?" In microgenesis, these two questions would exercise a pull into two opposite directions. On the presentation of a discrete projective stimulus, complementary answers would appear more likely.

## A Survey of Available Techniques

This section is devoted to the description of various potentially useful options for microgenetic personality assessment. While they greatly vary in content and format, they provide for the serial presentation of the stimulus under gradually improving conditions of viewing. Microgenesis typically spans the range between the absolute and differential thresholds (Draguns, 1984, 1986). It starts then with a detectable but not yet identifiable stimulus and ends whenever the stimulus is correctly named or identified. The range between these two points is artificially extended by devices that restrict a person's viewing time, for example, tachistoscopes, or otherwise interfere with instantaneous recognition, for example, by reducing contrast or illumination, photographic blurring, other forms of physical distortion, or omission of various components of the stimuli. Thus basic to the mode of these stimuli is serial presentation from maximal ambiguity through several graduations to optimal clarity.

### Sander's Techniques for the Study of Microgenesis

Sander (1928/1962) not only emphasized the role of personality in microgenesis in his writings, but he also pioneered the development of microgenetic techniques that would be useful for the demonstration of individual differences. To this end, he constructed a series of pictures composed initially of a few unconnected, seemingly random lines. In successive trials, additional features were provided, and in the end, the figure of a female farm worker ("peasant woman") was instantly recognizable. It is by means of this series that Sander and other German investigators of microgenesis discovered the detail-oriented and holistically-oriented "types" of microgenesis. Sander's (1928/1962) classic account contains several suggestions for the development of techniques for the exploration of individual differences in microgenesis. None of them, according to my knowledge, has been systematically investigated. An example, limited in its application to the musically trained, is playing a melody, stopping it short of completion, and having the subject provide the ending. The holistic and analytic types performed very differently on this task, with the former experiencing a distinct advantage in bringing the melody to a harmonious conclusion.

## *The Rorschach as a Microgenetic Test: Inkblots Presented Tachistoscopically*

As every Rorschach user knows, responses to the inkblots alternate. Wholes give way to details and vice versa. Could this succession be construed in microgenetic terms? Meyerhoff (1950) attempted to do just that and to assimilate the Rorschach response sequence to a microgenetic progression. The difficulty with this proposal is that the various inkblot responses appear stable and "final" from both the subject's and the external observer's point of view. No reduction in subjective uncertainty is experienced between the first and the last Rorschach response. Thus, the parallels between imposing meaning on inkblots and genuine microgenetic progressions appear tenuous. Perhaps for this reason, Meyerhoff's ideas have failed to produce resonance.

Independent of this formulation, a small number of investigators have experimented with the tachistoscopic presentation of Rorschach cards. The earliest study of this kind was by Stein (1949), who exposed the Rorschach cards at .01, .10, 1.0, and 10 s. With 27 normal subjects, he was able to establish a number of statistically significant trends. The number of wholes (W) decreased at higher levels; the reverse was true of details (D). Human movement (M) occurred in increasing numbers at the longer exposures, but inanimate movement (m) was concentrated at the early levels of presentation, perhaps, as an expression of tension, which is often reported to accompany the early stages of microgenesis. Not surprisingly, human and animal details (Hd and Ad) were predominantly found toward the end of the microgenetic sequence, while color responses (FC, CF, C) exhibited no clear trend across the four exposure speeds. Beyond these statistical findings, Stein provided several detailed case studies that illustrated the clinical utility of tachistoscopic inkblot presentation. In Stein's words:

> Tachistoscopic presentation of Rorschach cards was suggested as a possible technique for use in a variety of clinical and research situations where a complete diagnosis of the personality is necessary; for differential diagnosis, as a screening device, for the prediction of behavior in Social groups, and in evaluating a patients' progress in psychotherapy. Such applications, however, mush await the replication of the experiment discussed here with a large number and wide variety of subjects. (1949, p. 413)

To this day, however, such a replication has not been done. A few small steps toward investigating the value of the tachistoscopic Rorschach presentation have been taken. Phillips and Framo (1954) reported the results of the two doctoral dissertations by Framo and Freed, who investigated the effect of timed exposure on normal and schizophrenic subjects, respectively. The subjects were divided into four groups, each of which was shown Rorschach cards at only one exposure level. Nonetheless, the results shed some light on the normal process of microgenesis and on its peculiarities in schizophrenia. As expected, there was an abundance of W and a paucity of M at short exposures. The responses of normals changed more from short to long presentations while supposedly primitive responses were characteristic of schizophrenics at all exposures. Horiuchi (1961) in Japan limited herself to an intensive study of two tachistoscopically presented Rorschach cards, III and VI. She compared normals, schizophrenics, and neurotics and was able to demonstrate the effect of psychopathology on the perceptual process. Schizophrenics and neurotics produced a greater number of indefinite responses at longer exposure levels, even though for all three groups, Ws were predominant at early exposure levels. M and shading (Fc) characterized late exposures, although the latter category appeared earlier in normals than in schizophrenics. Animal (A) and plant (Pl) were the two most frequent content categories at all exposure levels. Horiuchi concluded that there were characteristic perceptual processes for each of the three groups. In light of these promising findings, it is regrettable that the study of the tachistoscopic Rorschach has not progressed beyond the first few isolated and tentative steps. Its few investigators recommend it as an avenue of bypassing defenses, although this potential has been illustrated only at the case level.

## *Microgenesis in Diagnostic Differentiation: The Picture Recognition Test*

Brengelmann (1953) used two objects, a pair of glasses and a sculpture of a human head and shoulders, both presented tachistoscopically, to study any differences between normal, neurotic, and psychotic subjects in the perceptual process. This preliminary study yielded significant results; the two groups of patients lagged behind normal controls in the recognition of the two objects. Even sharper differentiation was obtained with the spatial or three-dimensional perception of these stimuli. On the basis of these findings, Pinillos and Brengelmann (1953) developed the Picture Recognition Test (PRT), by means of which they were again able to differentiate psychotics from normals. The recognition scores of neurotics fell between the other two groups and were significantly different from those of normals but not psychotics. The PRT consists of 15 photographs of common objects, such as a tooth brush, a fountain pen, and an ashtray, which were presented at increasing exposure speeds from .01 s to 1 min. A total of 11 exposures were used. An incidental finding of this study was that pictures presented from an unusual perspective proved especially useful for group differentiation. Other constructors of microgenetic measures made similar observations. Conversely, highly familiar objects whose shapes constitute good gestalten resist distortion and disintegration even under unfavorable conditions of presentation and tend to be recognized early in the perceptual process. Independently of these observation, Froehlich (1964, 1984) emphasized the role of incongruity in extending and individualizing microgenesis. Objects that are distinctly out of place (e.g., a road sign in an office), retard the recognition of the entire stimulus and bring into play individualized reactions rooted, presumably, in personal experience and adaptation.

## *Tachistoscopic Techniques and Personality Dimensions*

In contrast to diagnostically oriented work, the tachistoscopic exploration of personality variables has been characterized by scatter and heterogeneity. Moreover, few positive results have been obtained. On the basis of the information presented earlier in this Chapter, there appears to be a high probability of a relationship between field dependence and a holistic style in responding to serial tachistoscopic presentation of pictorial stimuli. Yet Schiller's (1970) attempt to demonstrate such a link ended in failure. On a more ambitious plane, Lastowski (1984) attempted to link temperament variables, as measured by the Cattell 16 Personality Factor Questionnaire (Cattell, Eber, & Tatsuoka, 1972) and a checklist of her own devising with the speed of veridical recognition of emotionally arousing and neutral stimuli in tachistoscopically presented progressions. Few significant relationships emerged; they must be considered tentative until they are replicated. Negative findings clearly predominated. Yet Lastowski also observed a wide range and great variety of individual differences in coping with these stimuli. The difference between the recognition thresholds for emotional and neutral stimuli was highly significant. Moreover, qualitative observations yielded a panorama of suggestive but inconclusive findings. As Lastowski (1984, pp. 99–100) put it:

> When the data are examined qualitatively, however, individual differences are noted not only in the speed of recognition but in the styles of reporting what was seen. With respect to speed of recognition or number of trials necessary to achieve veridical perception, several groups stood out. First, there were those who very quickly perceived and accurately described the stimuli—many as early as Trial 1. For most of these subjects it was not possible to observe the entire microgenetic sequence. There was the opposite set of subjects, who took a long time to describe the stimuli accurately, many of whom at the end of the maximum number of trials still had not achieved veridical recognition. Patterns of differential responding to emotionally valent versus neutral stimuli were also observed. A small group of subjects appeared to be perceptually vigilant for emotionally valent stimuli. Some of these subjects took a relatively long time to come to grips with nonthreatening stimuli, as if they were less important to figure out than the emotional ones. Other subjects appeared to have no differential responding and took equally long or short times to achieve recognition. The majority of subjects, however, gave the appearance of perceptually defending against emotionally valent stimuli in that it took them proportionately longer to achieve veridical perception of the threatening stimuli. Still other subjects appeared to be vigilant as well as defensive in that very early they had the correct impression of an emotionally valent stimulus but then lost it (some to the extent of describing a totally different scene). Several trials later these subjects went back to their initial impressions.

The preceding description provides a rich slice of the "raw material" of microgenesis as it appears on the presentation of personally relevant and complex stimuli. The challenge is to tie to the variables that loom large in present-day personality psychology, and this challenge has not yet been met.

## *Blurred Pictures: Another Approach to Microgenesis*

Voigt (1956a) in Germany and Zucchi (1960) in Italy independently developed sets of pictures in which recognition was impeded not by the speed of presentation, but by different degrees of blur, produced by moving the objective of a camera progressively out of focus. Voigt's (1956a) technique was designed as a general psychodiagnostic test for which its author devised a rather complicated scoring system. It incorporated such indicators as the stage at which attribution of meaning occurred, the number of qualitatively different answers across the presentations, as well as formulae for process value and process descriptions. As these proposed scores have so far seen very little application, the specific ways of deriving them need not detain us here. In addition to describing his proposed measure, Voigt (1956b) provided a report on the application of this technique in a study on individual differences in response to fatigue. Several types of fatigue experiences were reflected in the process of responding to blurred pictures, including attempts to overcompensate for fatigue, which, however, tended to remain unsuccessful in that they required more time for response attainment or entailed a reduction of response quality. Nothing has appeared since these two reports, and the promise of Voigt's proposed measure remains unrealized.

Zucchi's (1960) approach was quite different. His subjects were young children, and his goals were to achieve a maximum degree of obstruction of veridical recognition while keeping the stimulus easily noticeable. These twin objectives were accomplished by combining a constant speed of presentation, at .03 s, with progressive blurring of the pictures. Zucchi's study was, for the most part, concerned with age differences. Thus, his results are not germane to the topic of this chapter. However, his method of extending the perceptual process is applicable for a variety of personality-related purposes.

Draguns (1962, 1963) used the principle of blurring for the purpose of developing several series of pictures. Unlike Voigt's (1956a) and Zucchi's (1960), his stimuli consisted of photographic prints that could be used indefinitely in an identical manner. They were also presented to the subjects for a finite, but ample, period of time. In a study with acute and chronic schizophrenics, he found that members of both groups differed from normal subjects in attempting to impose meaning on blurred stimuli prematurely. In the process, they committed significantly more errors than the normal controls did. Actually, there was a pronounced trend toward bimodality in the schizophrenic data; while the majority overestimated the amount of information available, a minority tended toward the other extreme and withheld responses past the point at which normal subjects were able to impose meaning on the picture. Cashdan (1966) confirmed both of these tenderncies in a study that aimed at establishing the microgenetic features associated with delusion formation. Ebner and Ritzler (1969) extended these findings in a more naturalistic study of the emergence and alternation of meaningful responses to blurred pictures. Worthy of mention is the research by Draguns and Multari (1961), who in a study of grade-school children, related the appearance of first meaningful responses to age. In line with Werner's (1948, 1957) comparative developmental theory, younger children were found to be quicker to venture such responses than older ones. A parallel is apparent between the microgenetic response styles of the majority of schizophrenics and those of younger children. The number of studies using blurred pictures is small, but they have produced convergent findings, especially in relation to schizophrenia. Information use in this disorder is disrupted, and efficient and realistic responding under conditions of uncertainty is impaired.

### *Conclusions*

A variety of techniques have been described. None of them, however, have been investigated systematically on extensively enough to qualify as tests with established psychometric properties, that is, adequate data on their reliability and validity. Thus, they provide a variety of choices for interested researchers. It is premature, however, to recommend any of them for individual-centered personality assessment. The situation is quite different with the percept-genetic methods, which will be introduced in the following section.

## Percept-Genesis as an Avenue of Exploring Personality

### *Theoretical Foundations*

For approximately the last 40 years, a cluster of process-oriented techniques have been developed and investigated by a team of researchers centered at Lund University in Sweden. These methods are collectively referred to as percept-genetic. They consititute so far the only set of interrelated microgenetic approaches that have been studied systematically and continuously over several decades. Moreover, the focus of these research approaches has been on the process-oriented investigations of personality variables. The Lund researchers, more than any other group of investigators, have taken seriously the idea of microgenesis constituting, if not the "road royal", then at least a major avenue for exploring personality. In the present section, the concept of percept-genesis as formulated by the Lund research group will be presented and discussed. This information will serve as an introduction for the appraisal of the current state of knowledge and the potential contribution of the several innovative techniques of personality assessment that have as yet not been widely adopted and applied outside of the locus of its origin.

Hentschel and Smith (1980) introduced percept-genesis as a special case of microgenesis. The research conducted by the Lund investigators is restricted exclusively to visual investigation. Auditory and tactile techniques, which have played a marginal role in the development of microgenesis (Bohm, 1959; Flavell & Draguns, 1957; Graumann, 1959), have so far not been within the scope of Lund investigators' concern. Theoretically, percept-genesis rests on the controversial assumption, upheld by some and rejected by other investigators of microgenesis, that all perception constitutes a process. In everyday commerce with the environment, the preparatory phases of perceptual activity are shortended and even collapsed as a result of massive experience and extensive familiarity with the objects in our environment. Smith, Kragh, and Hentschel (1980) pinpoint four principles that are basic for the understanding of the process of constructing reality in a perceptual act: (1) accumulation of information across the stages or phases of this process; (2) spontaneous emergence of new impressions; (3) an increasing number of leads that are eliminated as irrelevant or misleading for the development of a percept; (4) the disqualification of several stylistic and structural approaches to percept formation that are germane to the early and "primitive" phases of this process but that obstruct the attainment of the veridical percept in its terminal phases.

> It may be apposite to compare these principles of percept-genesis (especially those of accumulation of experience and disqualification) with the assumptions about development in epigenetic theories: Although the preceding stages are invariably incorporated into the successive ones, a new level of regulation and organization appears in each new phase. (Smith, Kragh, & Hentschel, 1980, p. 38)[3]

On another plane, Kragh and Smith (1970) describe the percept-genetic progression as follows. In the initial phases of the perceptual process, the person's reaction to the emerging stimulus is affective, global, and personal. External and internal sources of this experience are poorly and inadequately differentiated. As information is added in serial representation, these personal and affective components are gradually screened out. The perceptual operations become more focal as they are purified of their marginal components. Another facet of this process is stabilization; at the beginning of percept-genesis, a sense of lability prevails as the initial impressions are laden with multiple potentialities. The distance between the perceiver and the object to be perceived is minimal. As the image becomes clearer, it is, figuratively speaking, separated from the person and "objectified." In Kragh's and Smith's terminology, transformation occurs from a "stimulus-distal" to a "stimulus-proximal" mode of perceiving. To put it differently, the perceiver experiences a transition from an essentially physiognomic mode of perception to a reality-adapted and object-oriented one. In the process, the percept becomes stabilized and resistant to change.

Over and above these specific features, the percept-genetic model rests on two general assumptions. First, perception is conidered an event over time (Smith, 1957). Second, the unity of perception and personality is explicitly asserted. This unity comes to the fore in the perceptual progressions uncontaminated by the stabilization and automatization that make

[3] Translated from the German by the author.

much of everyday perception instantaneous and veridical. Percept-genesis then becomes a vehicle for the investigation of personality and for its assessment in practical situations and in dealing with specific individuals.

Three kinds of conceptualization and research have coalesced in making the emergence of the percept-genetic process possible. One of its conceptual bases is the classic demonstration of perceptual defense (Bruner & Postman, 1949) in the form of an elevated recognition threshold for emotionally arousing verbal stimuli. This study, however, did not provide the opportunity for the subjects to exhibit a variety of defenses in the face of a threatening stimulus. Rather, in terms of the conventional classification of defense mechanisms (Freud, 1946; Fenichel, 1945; Sjöbäck, 1973), the operations of the study compelled their resorting to denial as the only possible mode of defense under those circumstances. The Lund researchers, however, constructed more complex and realistic representations of perceptual threat and solicited more open-ended responses to them. In this manner, the entire gamut of defenses as described by the psychoanalysts comes into play. The second basis from which the percept-genetic model rises is the classic microgenetic research and theory, as presented in the earlier portions of this chapter. The third component is derived from traditional Freudian psychoanalytic theory, from which the percept-genetic researchers have borrowed the concepts of conflict, threat, anxiety, and defense. The result of integrating these three principles of formulations and findings is a number of percept-genetic tests and techniques, which will be described in the following section.

## *The Defense Mechanism Test*

The Defense Mechanism Test (DMT) was developed by Kragh (1955) who experimented with the tachistoscopic presentation of TAT-type stimuli. Gradually, on the basis of theoretical percept-genetic considerations, a format of stimuli was developed, which remains constant to this day. In each picture, two figures are presented. The hero is placed in foreground and is of the same gender as the subject. In the background, an angry and threatening figure of the opposite or the same sex is presented. The picture then connotes a psychodynamically significant threat, for example, of the Oedipal nature. The hero is the potential victim of the threatening figure. Thus, a vicarious situation of conflict-arousal is created; the person is asked to cope under conditions of decreasing ambiguity as the stimulus is presented 22 times by means of a specially constructed tachistoscope at increasing exposure speeds from 5 to 2000 ms. Because the gist of the test task lies in the discovery of the stimulus, it is not advisable at this point to provide a detailed description of the several pictures included in the test nor to illustrate this chapter with the reproductions of these stimuli.

The subject is instructed to report what he sees. The subject is admonished to be sensitive to his or her impressions and to report them spontaneously, as they occur. Because of the importance of the spatial placement of the figures perceived, verbal responses are supplemented by schematic drawings.

Defenses are operationally defined as the deformations or distortions of the stimulus figures or other features of the picture before their correct recognition. Over the years, Kragh and his associates (e.g., Westerlundh, 1976) have provided definitions and scoring rules for all of the major mechanisms of defense. Space limitations preclude the full inclusion of this information in the present chapter. Suffice it to say that repression, for example, is scored when the hero and/or the peripheral person "have a quality of rigidity or inanimateness or of being masked, or are animals" (Kragh, 1985, p. IV-5). Isolation is deemed to occur when the hero and the threat figure "are separated from each other in the field, parts of the configuration are excluded or 'whitened'; parts of the P-phase sequence are excluded." (Kragh, 1985, p. IV-5). Reaction formation is indicated when "the threat is turned into its opposite" (Kragh, 1985, p. IV-5).

### Psychometric Properties

The current test manual (Kragh, 1985) provides extensive data on interrater reliability, which appear to be psychometrically satisfactory. Test-retest reliability coefficients also are reported, on relatively small members of subjects, over periods of 1 and 5 years, respectively. All of the scores are statistically significant, and the Spearman *rho* remains .53 even after 5 years.

The appraisal of DMTs validity is more complicated. The test was never validated in a conventional manner on a representative and/or random sample of the population of Sweden, where it was developed. It should be recognized, however, that such normative data would be irrelevant to the test's rationale. At best, they would be of marginal empirical interest in providing information on the empirical distribution of the various defenses, something that apparently never has been done with any measure on any population. The thrust of the DMT is directed elsewhere, specifically, toward the demonstration of the correspondence of the defense mechanisms as revealed in the percept-genetic progression and as they occur in "real life." The validation of the DMT against these criteria has accrued in the form of a mosaic of findings obtained over more than 35 years. It can be summarized under five headings: mental health indicators, personality correlates, practical applications, systematic case studies, and investigations of the micro–macro correspondence between percept-genetic sequences and biographical events.

#### *Mental Health*

Psychoanalytic theory (e.g., Fenichel, 1945; Sjöbäck, 1973) posits that defense mechanisms are differentially associated with diagnostic entities.

Obsessive–compulsives should rely on isolation while hysterics would favor repression. Nilsson (1983) was able to demonstrate these relationships with clinical groups of reliably diagnosed patients in the preceding two categories. Kragh's (1955) findings on obsessive–compulsive neurotics showed a paucity of prerecognition responses in this group. These patients tended to operate in an "all-or-none" fashion and avoid offering a succession of responses in the early and intermediate stages of perceptgenesis. Anxiety tends to be reflected on the DMT in the form of reactivity to blackness and darkness (Kragh, 1985). In general, psychological impairment goes hand in hand with the predominance of scorable defense responses; less adequately functioning individuals exhibit more defensiveness. Primitive defenses indicative of an early developmental level, such as regression and denial, occur in a parallel way in the DMT protocols and real-life manifestations (Kragh, 1985). They are also similar to the genetically early anxiety-reduction mechanism observed with somewhat different percept-genetic techniques in children (Smith & Danielsson, 1977).

Conversely, individuals successfully engaged in stressful and dangerous activities (e.g., junior Danish naval officers trained as attack divers), typically exhibit less reliance on defenses, sometimes virtually appearing "defenseless" in the face of threatening stimuli (Kragh, 1962). Such people tend to look danger in the eye without flinching and have less of a habit or need of distorting or denying the threatening aspects of reality when they are confronted with them. In general, the composite findings on the DMT in clinical groups of subjects substantiate the diagnostically differential usefulness of this test. More important, these results corroborate the presence of those defense mechanisms in various diagnostic groups that are expected on the basis of clinical experience and psychodynamic theory. Also, the negative relationship between the adequacy of adaptive resources and defensiveness has in general been upheld in DMT research. To be sure, the groups investigated were sometimes small and many varieties of psychopathology have not yet been studied by means of the DMT. In particular, there is as yet a paucity of research with depressed and schizophrenic patients, although the few unpublished reports cited in the test manual (Kragh, 1985) confirm clinically based expectations on the prevalence of various mechanisms in these two conditions.

### *Personality-Oriented Research*

In addition to studies of clinical populations, a considerable amount of work has been done on the antecedents and correlates of various defensive operations in normal populations. Sharma (1977) tested the predictive validity of the DMT against the ratings of defensive functioning by psychotherapists after 6 months of intensive therapy. In this study, the DMT was found to be capable of predicting such mechanisms as turning against self, projection, identification with the aggressor, "polymorphous identification," and regression. Johnson (1970) found that high isolation scores were associated with a low rate of recalling dreams. In a major experimental study, Westerlundh (1976) was able to predict successfully the emergence of the mechanisms of reaction formation, isolation, introaggression, and identification with a female role on the DMT. Of further interest is Westerlundh's finding that the effect of mild aggressive arousal produced only nonsignificant effects in the form of the appearance of these defenses. When, however, intense anger was provoked, the defenses appeared as predicted.

A number of easily interpretable defensive distortions were documented in delinquent adolescents (Kragh & Kroon, 1966): At late stages of percept-genesis, these subjects reported less aggression than did controls while they relied on repression, isolation, and reaction formation. Aggression by father figures toward younger males ("sons") was often misperceived, and boys were distorted into girls when they were subject to paternal aggression. In intensely religious subjects, a distinct minority in the contemporary Swedish population (Kragh & Johnson, 1962), prominence of turning against self and disruption and distortion of the father relationship appeared as the salient findings.

Gitzinger (1988) was able to report positive findings in a group of psychosomatic and neurotic patients whose DMT scores were correlated with expert ratings and with two German paper-and-pencil personality inventories. Isolation, introjection, and repression were found to be the mechanisms characteristic of this group. In general, defense scores correlated positively with raters' judgments. Fewer such correlations were obtained with the two personality tests, and the coefficients tended to be lower. Diagnoses, both at the symptom and the personality level, shared relatively little variance with the DMT. In the early portion of percept-genesis, primary-process mechanisms, such as reaction formation, projection, denial, and regression were predominant. Defenses associated with the secondary process, such as isolation and introjection, were distributed over the entire sequence of presentation. These findings, however, are complicated by the tendency for isolation to appear at the intermediate points in the series, where presumably the transition from primary to secondary process takes place. Gitzinger (1988, p. 273) concluded that "the DMT is a highly informative procedure for the assessment of preconscious defense mechanisms."[4] Collectively, this sampling of relevant results highlights the potential of the DMT for bringing to the surface psychodynamic characteristics that fit in with the subjects' biographical experience and their characteristic behaviors, values, and attitudes.

---

[4] Translated from the German by the author.

*Practical Applications*

Much of Kragh's early research was done within the context of military psychology. He was able to demonstrate the usefulness of the DMT, especially in the selection of pilots. Over the years, this research has been pursued by Neuman (1978). The basic finding was that the defensive structure of successful pilot candidates differed from that of unsuccessful ones. The initial criterion was the failure to complete successfully the pilot-training program. Follow-up data are now available on flight accidents (Neuman, 1978). Again, significant differentiation of accident-free military pilots has been achieved. Neuman has developed a rather elaborate scheme, which takes into account the nature of the defense and the phase at which this defense appears, to which different weights are assigned. To simplify, the presence of genetically early, "primitive" defenses, such as denial, is associated with maladaptive, stressful, and emergency conditions. More elaborate, developmentally mature defenses under similar circumstances are conducive to adaptive responses under these kinds of exceptional circumstances. The various signs of unsatisfactory flight performance on the DMT are now being used for pilot selection not only in the Swedish air force but in several other Scandinavian air forces as well. They have also been applied in selecting airline pilots, and their use has spread beyond Scandinavia. Moreover, data (Kragh, 1985) are available to show that the usefulness of the DMT is not limited to pilot selection but extends to other activities that require quick and exact performance under stress. The defensive structure of accident-free drivers, for example, differs from that of their accident-prone counterparts (Kragh, 1985). The DMT performance of naval attack drivers has already been mentioned earlier in this chapter. The theoretical import of all of these findings lies in demonstrating the parallel between handling intrapsychic stress on the DMT and reality stress in a variety of situations that require quick, complex, and exact performance under conditions of emotional arousal and danger.

*Case Studies*

Kragh has pioneered the use of detailed, quantified, and predictive case studies for the demonstration of similarities between life-history events and DMT responses. In his view, this approach constitutes an integral component of DMT validation. In one such study, Kragh (1986) formulated 38 predictive statements, 26 of which were confirmed while only 7 were rejected in light of the available autobiographic data, and 5 remained undecided. Beyond the demonstration of a qualitative correspondence between the two sources of biographic information, Kragh was able to pinpoint chronologically the occurrence of various events. As an example, the subject's response to the fourth and fifth presentations of a DMT picture was as follows: "This boy is wearing garters and a white shirt with black stripes. An old lady with grey hair and a knot" (Kragh, 1986, p. 149). Kragh formulated the following five falsifiable inferences about the subject at 5 years of age: "You were in the habit of wearing trousers with garters; Grandmother still exerted great influence on you; You were a goodlooking boy in your opinion; You were nicely dressed; Your grandmother was an authoritarian person" (Kragh, 1986, p. 149). The subject accepted four of these statements as true and was uncertain only about his grandmother still exerting great influence on him at that age. This illustration introduces what is probably the most far-reaching and arguable aspect of Kragh's formulations: his postulate of micro–macro correspondence between DMT sequences and the chronology of life events. It is to this subject that the next section is devoted.

### *Micro–Macro Correspondence*

Werner (1948, 1957), it may be recalled, posited formal correspondence in the sequence of developmental progressions of all durations and types. Kragh and Smith (1970) went considerably further in predicting parallels between percept-genesis and ontogenesis in the content of experiences reported. The following statement summarizes their position:

> The assumption of a sequential correspondence involves that experiences are actualized, in the present "micro-process," in the same order at they appeared in the "macro-process" of life. The initial stages of the perceptual process should be described in terms of a "global" stirring up or "priming" of infantile experiences and infantile modes of perceptual organization, not as a conscious regression to childhood. The more differentiated, "isolated," and veridical subsequent stages of the process again, would actualize successively more mature sections of the ontogenesis. (Kragh & Smith, 1970, p. 38)

In systematic studies, this principle was tested (Kragh, 1955) by comparing adult subjects who had lost their fathers with those who had not experienced such a loss. Six hypotheses were formulated and confirmed. Of central interest for the validation of the principle of micro-macro correspondence was the demonstration that the percept-genesis of a father–son picture required more exposures before correct recognition in the group who had experienced the loss of father by comparison with controls. The "fatherless" subjects also reported a less distinct perception of the father figure during percept-genesis. In both groups, the older man's reported age increased from the early to the late stages of percept-genesis. Other studies of the correspondence between DMT and life sequences (e.g., Smith & Kragh, 1955) have also produced positive results. Thus, the daring and, to many readers of this volume, implausible proposition of micro–macro correspondence has proved to be heuristically useful. The skeptics are faced with the challenge of more parsimoniously explaining the results obtained without the recourse to this principle; its proponents are stimulated to develop increasingly definitive and crucial demonstrations of such parallels.

### Other Percept-Genetic Techniques

The amount of detailed information on the DMT presented here may serve as a prototype for the introduction of the other percept-genetic techniques of personality assessment. They share with the DMT its assumptions and rationale. Quite often, they have been studied by means of the same methods and validated against similar criteria. For all of these reasons, a more succinct presentation appears justified.

#### *The Meta-Contrast Technique*

The origin of the Meta-Contrast Technique (MCT) procedure goes back to a study by Smith and Henriksson (1955), in which a subliminally presented stimulus was superimposed on a supraliminal one. The expected effect on the supraliminal stimulus was substantiated in this study. More surprisingly, Smith and Henriksson observed substantial individual differences in the susceptibility to the initially subliminal stimulus, which they were able to relate tentatively to the defense mechanism of isolation. The procedure and the results of this study served as the foundation for the MCT in which, however, more personally relevant and affectively arousing subliminal stimuli were substituted. Early in the program of these studies, the Lund University research group (Nyman & Smith, 1961; Smith & Johnson, 1962; Smith & Nyman, 1961); correlated the effects of the incidental stimulus with a number of abnormal behavior patterns. Obsessive–compulsive patients, for example, were little influenced by the subtle changes brought about by the subliminal stimulus. Other groups, characterized by paranoid symptoms, were drastically affected by such stimuli. Socially anxious persons also exhibited hypersensitivity to incidental situation, albeit in a different way. Subsequent clinical observations and experimental studies reflected the operation of such defenses as denial, projection, and operation while coming to grips with near-threshold emotionally disruptive stimulation.

Smith and Johnson (1962, 1963) documented the extent and limits of various somatic and psychological therapies on the perceptual responses to MCT. The nature of such defenses as repression and isolation changed little during therapy; but expressions of depression and manifestations of psychosis were much reduced in light of MCT indicators. A relatively benign, as opposed to clearly paranoid, projection was demonstrated to decline substantially.

More recent work on the MCT focused on the comparison of adaptive and defensive strategies of children and adolescents. (Smith & Danielsson, 1977, 1982) The development from preschool age to adolescence in handling perceptual threat can be described as a progression from open flight to symbolic and perceptual tactics (Smith & Danielsson, 1977). On the MCT, the reaction of the youngest children was in the form of closing the eyes and leaving the room. This primitive strategy was replaced by the vicarious manifestations of the same mechanism, that is, denial, in the form of attributing these characteristics to the constantly and supraliminally presented figure. Thus, even within the scope of the same mechanism, important transformations took place. The changes that took place ontogenetically were roughly similar to those that were observable in the course of percept-genesis, from early to late exposures. Older children and adolescents exhibited in their initial reactions some of the mechanisms that were characteristic of the younger subjects throughout the percept-genetic sequence. Similarly, a clinical sample of children, most of whom had severe anxiety problems, manifested disruption and primitivization of response to covert perceptual threat in a manner that made their responses resemble those of young normal children and/or the reactions to the early stages of the MCT. Moreover, the defensive strategies of children were found to be related to Piagetian measures of developmental level (Piaget & Inhelder, 1941); by and large, cognitively mature children, with age level held constant, displayed more sophisticated and complex defensive operations and eschewed responding to anxiety by means of open and direct flight.

Smith, Sjöholm, and Nielzen (1976) focused on the MCT responses of patients with anxiety, phobic, and obsessive–compulsive symptoms and identified the characteristic defenses associated with these clinical states. Obsessive–compulsives tended toward isolation as their preferred defense mechanism. Anxiety responses were characteristic of the three clinical groups. Repression appeared mainly in the responses of subjects with hysteroid tendencies. Mechanisms appearing late in the series showed the greatest amount of correspondence with clinical symptoms. Repression was characteristic of anxiety patients, yet negatively related to the intensity of anxiety symptoms. Thus, the accumulated findings on the MCT, of which the foregoing results constitute a haphazard and nonrandom sample, strongly point to its clinical utility and relevance. They also suggest that the MCT is a promising technique for the developmental assessment of cognitive and perceptual maturity of mechanisms used to reduce covert and incidental threat.

### *Color–Word Technique*

The Stroop Color-Word Test (CWT) is well known as an auxiliary technique used in neuropsychology and also as a tool for the investigation of cognitive style (Jensen & Rohwer, 1966). The percept-genetic investigators have put it to a new use by going beyond the total time and error scores on this measure and recording the process of responses to the various portions of this measure. Seemingly, this technique has little in common with such typical percept-genetic procedures as the DMT and MCT. No new response is attained, and no meaning is discovered in the course of this progression. It shares, however, with the other percept-genetic measures the property of serial presentation. On the response side, it provides the opportunity of observing the stabilization and automatization that are the basic hallmarks of percept-genesis. The serial CWT was applied by Nyman and Smith (1961) in groups of ambulatory clinic patients and normal controls. This research was preceded by that of Smith and Nyman (1959), who studied a broader range of psychiatric patients, including psychotic and hospitalized. In both projects, diagnostically distinct patterns of responding were observed. The dissociative, anxiety, and obsessive–compulsive styles stood out especially well and were described by Nyman and Smith (1961, p. 27) as follows:

(1) One group was characterized by primary dissociative patterns of adaptation and included patients diagnosed as primitive or hysteroid. This adaptive style has been described as reflecting flexible but inconsistent controls, i.e., an incoherently organized way of behaving.
(2) The common style of another group was primary cumulation or recurring adaptive lag. Thus patients had difficulties in handling new adaptive requirements without resorting to previous, inadequate sets. This style has been proved to be typical of subjects with symptoms of anxiety coupled with averting defenses against insight and corresponded here, more specifically, to symptoms of manifest anxiety in patients with compulsive or phobic defense mechanisms.
(3) A third category contained only obsessive–compulsive subjects and differed above all from the group of phobics or anxiety hysterics by an adaptive strategy stamped by initial stupor and a quick subsequent adjustment to a time level which was then but little affected by subsequent new attempts.

Nyman and Smith (1961), however, also reported that the relationship between defenses and cognitive styles, as measured by the MCT and CWT respectively, was complex. This observation constituted the point of departure for a major research project by Hentschel (1980), who attempted to specify the terms of this relationship. This study included some percept-genetic methods but went beyond them to encompass a variety of relevant measures. Of interest in the present context are the findings that the serial CWT significantly differentiated normal and clinical groups and that good performance on interference tasks exemplified by, but not limited to, the serial CWT was positively correlated with the defense mechanism of isolation. Thus, the relatively simple, innocuous, and impersonal task of reading color names from a list printed in incongruous hues has demonstrated its utility in both psychodiagnostic and personological contexts.

### *Visual Aftereffects*

Most psychologists are familiar with visual afterimages. They can be easily produced by, for example, turning off a television set, closing one's eyes, and looking at a blank wall (Smith, Hentschel, & Andersson, 1980). As

Smith et al. (1980) demonstrate, the phenomenon cannot be explained on a purely physiological basis. Specifically, visual aftereffects (VAE) are influenced by psychoactive drugs; they can be conditioned; and they can be provoked by an imaginary stimulus. Above all, they exhibit fluctuations across the course of stimulus presentation, and they produce individual differences in the size, brightness, and color of afterimages (AI) experienced. These parameters have been put to use in the development of standardized methods of producing afterimages, which have been employed at Lund University for over 40 years (Smith, 1949). As described by Smith and Danielsson (1982), the apparatus consists of a semitransparent Plexiglass screen that can be moved along two horizontal bars. The stimulus is projected from behind the screen and is viewed through an eyepiece. The illumination of the room is kept low. The stimulus is a red oval figure with two eyes and a down-turned "sad" face schematically drawn in black. The subject is instructed to focus on the nose. A total of 16 trials constitute a complete series for presentation with adults. With children, the number of trials is limited to 10. The subjects are asked to rate the stimulus in brightness, on a scale from 1 to 10. The reported color of the AI and its size are also noted.

Over the years, a great many personality-relevant results have been produced with this method and with a closely related technique in which the aftereffect of a spiral is investigated. These results are summarized by Andersson, Nilsson, Ruuth, and Smith (1972) and by Smith, Hentschel, and Andersson (1980). The pattern of the results obtained is analogous to the findings with the other three percept-genetic techniques; they pertain to diagnostic differentiation, assessment of the developmental level, and diagnosis of defense and anxiety (Anderson et al., 1972; Andersson & Weikert, 1974; Smith, & Danielsson, 1982; Smith, Ruuth, Franzen, & Sjöholm, 1972; Smith, Sjöholm, & Nielzen, 1976). In all of these areas, positive results have been obtained, and many of them have been cross-validated. The scoring system for VAE is rather complicated and cannot be effectively presented in the limited space available. Anxiety, for example, is expressed through the darkening of the AIs. Schizophrenia is often indicated through what Smith et al. (1972) called *intermittent regression*, that is, reverting to earlier and developmentally lower scores in size, intensity, color, and content. The characteristic pattern of responses in depression was termed *depressive retardation*, expressed in the form of perseverative and stereotyped responses. One problem with the VAE technique is that its relationship with personality dimensions and diagnostic categories is not readily apparent on a common-sense basis. There is also no ready-made theory to account for the individual differences and the personality and psychopathological correlates discovered by the Lund University researchers. To fill this gap, Andersson (1984) formulated an elaborate and sophisticated dialectic scheme based on Piagetian and psychodynamic concepts. With this development, future results with the VAE can be predicted and not just explained post hoc.

## *Preliminary Appraisal*

An impressive amount of clinically relevant data has been amassed by means of the percept-genetic techniques. Yet these procedures have spread relatively little from their point of origin and remain completely unknown to the typical working clinician in the United States or outside Scandinavia. Perhaps the last few decades have not been propitious for the introduction and adoption not only of a set of new techniques but of a different and unfamiliar format of assessment. Yet the techniques developed by the Lund University investigations appear to merit scrutiny by applied psychologists, in clinical and other settings, throughout the world. Gradually, a very impressive body of findings has come into being that not only has the potential for doing the job of conventional personality assessment as performed by projective techniques and paper-and-pencil measures but that holds the promise of venturing into new areas of personality assessment as well. The direct scoring of defenses is one such feature. More centrally, however, the explicit introduction of the notion of time as a variable of personality holds promise, and the results recapitulated here indicate that this promise has to a large extent already been realized. The outer edge of time-oriented personality assessment is the daring and controversial hypothesis that percept-genetic progressions recapitulate life history. Certainly, it is premature to say at this point that this principle has been sufficiently substantiated to make clinical biographical inferences on the basis of percept-genetic information. It is, however, a far-reaching principle that deserves to be taken seriously and to be investigated rigorously by its proponents and skeptics alike. On the individual plane, the appearance of potentially useful biographic information in a percept-genetic sequence should neither be dismissed nor credulously accepted. At this point, the appropriate status of such bits of data is that of leads or hypotheses to be pursued and eventually accepted or dismissed on the strength of other available sources of information.

As yet, the yield of percept-genetic research has come, with few exceptions, from one source. It is a tribute to the Lund researchers that they have been able to accumulate a coherent pattern of findings on the basis of process-oriented techniques. This has been accomplished by the congruence of research methods and conceptual framework. As a result, a high rate of confirmatory and positive findings has been obtained. However, the percept-genetic procedures have not yet endured the massive onslaught of skeptical and, indeed, hostile scrutiny that has been lavished on both the projective techniques and the personality questionnaires. An inevitable by-product of the probable internationalization of the percept-genetic approach will be the mushrooming of research on these techniques in a variety of contexts and from a multiplicity of perspectives. This salutory development will establish the limits of usefulness and validity of the several percept-genetic measures which, as of now, have not been tapped.

## Conclusions

A brief survey has been provided of the attempts going back over 60 years of integrating research techniques of microgenetic investigation with the objectives and concerns of personality assessment. With the exception of the percept-genetic approach, recapitulated in the preceding portion of this chapter, no concerted effort has been expended on any one technique or method of personality appraisal. The result is a number of leads of varying degrees of promise but no firm factual foundation from which to proceed. The pattern of results, however, seems to support the expectation on which these microgenetic ventures into personality assessment rest; namely, that personality characteristics are revealed through varying the span between the absolute and differential thresholds in which the stimulus can be structured in a variety of ways. In addition to this expectation, which the personality-oriented proponents of microgenesis share with the users of projective techniques, is the opportunity to observe in the course of microgenesis the person's characteristic modes of coping with uncertainty, filling gaps in the available evidence, and transcending the information given. These are tasks that are ubiquitous, essential, and indeed, existential. Microgenesis provides a window on how these tasks are tackled; its potential for elucidating these operations in their individuality and richness remains to be realized.

## *References*

Alvarez Villar, A., & Narros Martin, G. (1958). La percepción visual en las diversas entidades nosologicas psiquiatricas. *Revista de Psicológia General y Aplicada*, *13*, 739–766.

Andersson, A.L. (1984). Toward a dialectical conception of the percept-genetic approach to perception personality. In W.D. Froehlich, G. Smith, J.G. Draguns, & U. Hentschel (Eds.), *Psychological processes in cognition and personality* (pp. 125–134). Washington, DC: Hemisphere.

Andersson, A.L., Nilsson, A., Ruuth, E., & Smith, G. (1972). *Visual aftereffects and the individual adaptive system*. Lund, Sweden: Gleerup.

Andersson, A.L., & Weikert, C. (1974). Adult defensive organization as related to adaptive regulation of spiral aftereffect duration. *Social Behavior and Personality*, *2*, 56–75.

Bohm, W. (1959). Methodische Möglichkeiten der experimentellen Wahrnehmungserschwerung bei der auditiven Aktualgenese. *Zeitschrift für Experimentelle und Angewandte Psychologie*, *6*, 474–495.

Brengelmann, J.C. (1953). Der visuelle Objekterkennungstest. *Zeitschrift für Experimentelle und Angewandte Psychologie, 6*, 422–452.

Bruner, J.S. (1957a). Going beyond the information given. In J.S. Bruner, E. Brunswik, L. Festinger, F. Heider, K.F. Münzinger, C.E. Osgood, & D. Rapaport (Eds.), *Contemporary approaches to cognition* (pp. 41–69). Cambridge, MA: Harvard University Press.

Bruner, J.S. (1957b) On perceptual readiness. *Psychological Review, 64*, 156–170.

Bruner, J.S., & Postman, L. (1949). Perception, cognition, and behavior. *Journal of Personality, 18*, 14–31.

Cashdan, S. (1966). Delusional thinking and the induction process in schizophrenia. *Journal of Consulting Psychology, 30*, 207–212.

Cattell, R.B., Eber, H.W., & Tatsuoka, M.M. (1972). *The 16 Personality Factor Questionnaire handbood*. Champaign, IL: Institute for Personality and Abilities Testing.

Conrad, K. (1947). Über den Begriff der Vorgestalt und seine Bedeutung für die Hirnpathologie. *Nervenarzt, 19*, 315–323.

Costa Molinari, J.M., Rom Font, J., Malga Montserrat, A., & Ponzo, W. (1964). Tipificaci6n de nuestra t6cnica taquistosc6pica. *Revista de Psicol6gia General y Aplicada, 19*, 577–585.

de Koningh, H.L. (1967). Over de Vorgestalt theorie van Conrad: Een psychologische evaluatie. *Nederlands Tiidschrift voor de Psychologie, 22*, 98–129.

Draguns, J.G. (1962). *Schizophrenic responses to cognitive and perceptual ambiguity*. Unpublished doctoral dissertation, University of Rochester, Rochester, New York.

Draguns, J.G. (1963). Responses to cognitive and perceptual ambiguity in chronic and acute schizophrenics. *Journal of Abnormal and Social Psychology, 66*, 24–30.

Draguns, J.G. (1975). *Personality assessment*. New York: General Learning Corporation.

Draguns, J.G. (1984). Microgenesis by any other name. In W.D. Froehlich, G. Smith, J.G. Draguns, & U. Hentschel (Eds.), *Psychological processes in cognition and personality* (pp. 3–17). Washington: Hemisphere.

Draguns, J.G. (1985). Projective techniques. In W. Kuiper & J. Kuiper (Eds.), *Encyclopedia of social science*. London: Methuen.

Draguns, J.G. (1986). Subliminal perception as the first stage of perception: Can personality be revealed so early in the sequence? In G. Smith, U. Hentschel, & J.G. Draguns (Eds.), *The roots of perception* (pp. 331–349). Amsterdam: Elsevier.

Draguns, J.G., & Multari, G. (1961). Recognition of perceptually ambiguous stimuli in grade school children. *Child Development, 32*, 541–550.

Ebner, E., & Ritzler, B. (1969). Perceptual recognition in chronic and acute schizophrenics. *Journal of Consulting and Clinical Psychology, 33*, 200–206.

Fenichel, O. (1945). *The psychoanalytic theory of neurosis*. New York: Norton.

Flavell, J.H., & Draguns, J.G. (1957). A microgenetic approach to perception and thought. *Psychological Bulletin, 54*, 197–217.

Frank, L.K. (1939). Projective methods for the study of personality. *Journal of Psychology, 8*, 389–413.

Freud, A. (1946). *The ego and the mechanisms of defense*. New York: International Universities Press.

Froehlich, W.D. (1964). *Unstimmigkeit, Erwartung und Kompromiss*. Unpublished dissertation, University of Bonn.

Froehlich, W.D. (1983). *Wörterbuch der Psychologie* (7th ed.). Munich: Deutscher Taschenbuchverlag.

Froehlich, W.D. (1984). Microgenesis and information processing. In W.D. Froehlich, G. Smith, J.G. Draguns, & U. Hentschel (Eds.), *Psychological processes in cognition and personality* (pp. 19–52). Washington, DC: Hemisphere.

Gemelli, A. (1928). Contributo allo studio della percezione: IV. Il comparire e lo scomparire delle forme. *Contributi del Laboratorio di Psicologia e Biologia. Università Cattolica del Sacro Cuore*, *3*, 385–436.

Gitzinger, I. (1988). *Operationalisierung von Abwehrmechanismen*. Unpublished diploma thesis. University of Freiburg, Germany.

Graumann, C.F. (1959). Aktualgenese, die deskriptiven Grundlagen und theoretische Wandlungen des aktualgenetischen Forschungsansatzes. *Zeitschrift für Experimentelle und Angewandte Psychologie*, *6*, 473–499.

Hausmann, G. (1935). Zur Aktualgenese räumlicher Gestalten. *Archiv für die gesamte Psychologie*, *93*, 289–334.

Hauss, K. (1966). Zur Frage des Nachweises subjektiver Gestaltungstendenzen im optischen Wahrnehmungsprozess mit Hilfe des Bilderkennungstests von Pinillos und Brengelmann. *Psychiatria et Neurologia*, *149*, 36–48.

Hauss, K. (1970). *Emotionalität und Wahrnehmung*. Göttingen, Germany: Hogrefe.

Hentschel, U. (1980). Kontrollprinzipien und Neurosenformen. In U. Hentschel & G. Smith (Eds.), *Experimentelle Persönlichkeitspsychologie: Die Wahrnehmung als Zugang zu diagnostischen Problemen* (pp. 227–321). Wiesbaden: Akademische Verlagsgesellschaft.

Hentschel, U., & Smith, G. (Eds.). (1980). *Experimentelle Persönlichkeitspsychologie: Die Wahrnehmung als Zugang zu diagnostischen Problemen*. Wiesbaden, Germany: Akademische Verlagsgesellschaft.

Horiuchi, H. (1961). A study of the perceptual process of Rorschach cards by tachistoscopie method on movement and shading responses. *Journal of Personality Assessment*, *25*, 44–53.

Jenkin, N. (1957). Affective processes in perception. *Psychological Bulletin*, *54*, 100–127.

Jensen, A.R., & Rohwer, W.D., Jr. (1966). The Stroop Color-Word Test: A review. *Acta Psychologica*, *24*, 398–408.

Johnson, M. (1970). Dream reports related to percept-genetic defensive organization in the DMT. In U. Kragh & G. Smith (Eds.), *Percept-genetic analysis* (pp. 206–214). Lund, Sweden: Gleerup.

Kragh, U. (1955). *The actual-genetic model of perception-personality*. Lund, Sweden: Gleerup.

Kragh, U. (1962). Prediction of success by Danish attack divers by the Defense Mechanism Test. *Perceptual and Motor Skills*, *15*, 103–106.

Kragh, U. (1985). *DMT manual*. Stockholm: Persona.

Kragh, U. (1986). Life panorama under the microscope: A paradigmatic case study. In U. Hentschel, G. Smith, & J.G. Draguns (Eds.), *The roots of perception* (pp. 145–160). Amsterdam: Elsevier.

Kragh, U., & Johnson, M. (1962). An experimental study of the religious personality by means of subliminal techniques. *Psychological Research Bulletin, Lund University*, *2*(9).

Kragh, U., & Kroon, T. (1966). An analysis of aggression and identification in young offenders by the study of perceptual development. *Human Development*, *9*, 209–221.

Kragh, U., & Smith G. (Eds.). (1970). *Percept-genetic analysis*. Lund, Sweden: Gleerup.

Krueger, F. (1928). The essence of feeling. *The Wittenberg Symposium: Feelings and emotions*. Worcester, MA: Clark University Press.

Lastowski, F.A., (1984). Individual differences and microgenesis. In W.D. Froehlich, G. Smith, J.G. Draguns, & U. Hentschel (Eds.), *Psychological processes in cognition and personality* (pp. 95–106). Washington, DC: Hemisphere.

Lesswing, N.J. (1973). *Perceptual microgenesis: A descriptive inquiry*. Unpublished master's thesis, The Pennsylvania State University.

Linschoten, J. (1959). Aktualgenese und heuristisches Prinzip. *Zeitschrift für Experimentelle und Angewandte Psychologie*, *6*, 449–473.

McKeever, W.F. (1986). Tachistoscopie methods in neuropsychology. In H.J. Hannay (Ed.), *Experimental techniques in human neuropsychology* (pp. 167–211). New York: Oxford University Press.

Meyerhoff, H. (1950). Der Rorschach-Test als aktualgenetischer Versuch. *Psychiatrie, Neurologie, Medizinische Psychologie*, *2*, 373–378.

Neuman, T. (1978). Dimensionering och validering av perceptgenesens forsvarsmekanismer. En hierarisk analys mot pilotens stressbeteende. *FAO-rapport* nr. C55020-H6.

Nilsson, A. (1983). Application of a percept-genetic approach to separation and Oedipal conflict problems in primitive hysteria and obsessive–compulsive neurosis. *Archiv für Psychologie*, *82*, 178–188.

Nyman, G.E., & Smith, G. (1961). Experimental differentation of clinical syndromes within a sample of young neurotics. *Acta Psychiatrica et Neurologica Scandinavia*, *37*, 14–31.

Ombredane, A. (1951). *Aphasie et l'élaboration de la pensée explicite*. Paris: Presses Universitaires de France.

Phillips, L., & Framo, J. (1954). Developmental theory applied to normal and psychopathological perception. *Journal of Personality*, *22*, 464–474.

Piaget, J., & Inhelder, B. (1941). *Le développement des quantités chez l'enfant*. Neuchatel, Switzerland: Delachaux & Niestlé.

Pinillos, J., & Brengelmann, J.C. (1953). Bilderkennung als Persönlichkeitstest. *Zeitschrift für Experimentelle und Angewandte Psychologie*, *1*, 480–500.

Sander, F. (1928/1962). Experimentelle Ergebnisse der Gestaltpsychologie. In F. Sander & H. Volkelt (Eds.), *Ganzheitspsychologie* (pp. 73–112). Munich: Beck. (Original work published 1928)

Schiller, M. (1970). Feldabhängigkeit, Unstimmigkeit, Kompromiss. Unpublished doctoral dissertation. University of Bonn.

Schmidt-Durban, W. (1939). Experimentelle Untersuchungen zur Typologie der Wahrnehmung. *Neue Psychologische Studien*, *15*(2), 1–87.

Sharma, V.H.P. (1977). *Application of a percept-genetic test in a clinical setting.*

Unpublished manuscript, Psykologiska Institutionen, Lunds Universiteit, Lund, Sweden.
Sjöbäck, H. (1973). *The psychoanalytic theory of defensive processes*. Lund, Sweden: Gleerup.
Smith, G. (1949). *Psychological studies of twin differences*. Lund, Sweden: Gleerup.
Smith, G. (1957). Visual perception: An event over time. *Psychological Review*, *64*, 306–313.
Smith, G., & Danielsson, A. (1977). From open flight to symbolic and perceptual tactics. *Scripta Minora Regiae Societatis Humanorum Litteratorum Lundensis*, *3* (entire issue).
Smith, G., & Danielsson, A. (1982). *Anxiety and defensive strategies in childhood and adolesence*. New York: Interational Universities Press.
Smith, G., & Henriksson, M. (1955). The effect of an established percept on a perceptual process beyond awareness. *Acta Psychologica*, *11*, 346–355.
Smith, G., Hentschel, U., & Andersson, A. (1980). Physiologische und psychologische Annahmen und Methodologie. In G. Smith & U. Hentschel (Eds.), *Experimentelle Personlichkeitspsychologie* (pp. 135–160). Wiesbaden, Germany: Akademiscae Verlagsanstalt.
Smith, G., & Johnson, M. (1962). The influence of psychiatric treatment upon the process of reality construction. *Journal of Consulting Psychology*, *26*, 520–526.
Smith, G., & Johnson, M. (1963). Esperimental prediction of the long-term effect of psychiatric therapy. *Journal of Consulting Psychology*, *27*, 373.
Smith, G., & Kragh, U. (1955). Do micro-genetic sequences reflect life history? *Acta Psychologia*, *11*, 504–512.
Smith, G., Kragh, U., & Hentschel, U. (1980). Historische und methodologische Ubersicht. In U. Hentschel & G. Smith (Eds.), *Experimentelle Persönlichkeitspsychologie: Die Wahrnehmung als Zugang zu diagnostischen Problemen* (pp. 31–63). Wiesbaden, Germany: Akademische Verlagsanstalt.
Smith, G., & Nyman, G.E. (1959). Psychopathologic behavior in a serial experiment. Investigations of neurotic, psychotic, and normal subjects. *Lunds Universitets Arsskrift, N.F. Avd. 2.*, *56*(5).
Smith, G., & Nyman, G.E. (1961). A serial tachistoscopic experiment and its clinical application. *Acta Psychologica*, *18*, 67–84.
Smith, G., Ruuth, E., Franzen, G., & Sjöholm, L. (1972). Intermittent regressions in a serial afterimage experiment as signs of schizophrenia. *Scandinavian Journal of Psychology*, *13*, 27–33.
Smith, G., Sjöholm, L., & Nielzen, S. (1976). Anxiety and defense against anxiety as reflected in perceptgenetic formations. *Journal of Personality Assessment*, *40*, 151–161.
Smith, G., & Westerlundh, B. (1980). Percept genesis: A process perspective on perception-personality. *Review of Personality and Social Psychology*, *1*, 94–124.
Spreen, O. (1957). Uber Tachistoskop-Versuche bei Normalen, Hirnverletzten und Neurotikern. *Psychologische Beiträge*, *3*, 80–93.
Stein, M.J. (1949). Personality factors involved in the temporal development of Rorschach responses. *Journal of Projective Technique*, *13*, 355–414.
Voigt, J. (1956a). Die Aktualgenese in der psychologischen Diagnostik. *Psychologische Beiträge*, *2*, 586–636.
Voigt, J. (1956b). Uber individuelle Varietäten der Ermüdung, *Zeitschrift für experimentelle und angewandte psychologie*, *4*, 274–306.

Werner, H. (1948). *Comparative psychology of mental development*. New York: International Universities Press.
Werner, H. (1956). Microgenesis and aphasia. *Journal of Abnormal and Social Psychology*, *52*, 347–353.
Werner, H. (1957). The concept of development from a comparative and organismic point of view. In D.B. Harris (Ed.), *The concept of development*. Minneapolis: University of Minnesota Press.
Westerlundh, B. (1976). *Aggression, anxiety, and defense*. Lund, Gleerup.
Witkin, H.A., Dyk, R.B., Faterson, H.F., Goodenough, D.P., & Karp, S.A. (1962). *Psychological differentiation*. New York: Wiley.
Zucchi, M. (1960). Ricerche tachistoscopiche sulla percezione ambigua del bambino. *Archivio di Psicologia, Neurologia e Psichiatria*, *21*, 183–208.

# Appendix:
## Selected References on Microgenesis


Arieti, S. (1962). The microgeny of thought and perception. *Archives of General Psychiatry*, *6*, 76–90.

Bachmann, T. (1987). Different trends in perceptual pattern microgenesis as a function of the spatial range of local brightness averaging. *Psychological Research*, *49*, 107–111.

Bachmann, T. (1989). Microgenesis as traced by the transient paired-forms paradigm. *Acta Psychologica*, *70*, 3–17.

Brown, J.W. (1972). *Aphasia, apraxia, and agnosia*. Springfield, IL: Charles C. Thomas.

Brown, J.W. (1977), *Mind, brain, and consciousness*. New York: Academic Press.

Brown, J. W. (1988). *The life of the mind*. Hillsdale, NJ: Lawrence Erlbaum.

Calis, G., Sterenborg, J., & Maarse, F. (1984). Initial microgenetic steps in single-glance face recognition. *Acta Psychologica*, *55*, 215–230.

Catán, L. (1986). The dynamic display of process: Historical development and contemporary uses of the microgenetic method. *Human Development*, *29*, 252–263.

Cegalis, J.A. (1984). On the role of conflict in microgenesis. In W. Froehlich, G. Smith, J. Draguns, & U. Hentschel (Eds.), *Psychological processes in cognition and personality* (pp. 107–121). Washington, DC: Hemisphere.

Conrad, K. (1947). Über den Begriff der Vorgestalt und seine Bedeutung für die Hirnpathologie. *Nervenarzt*, *18*, 289–293.

Dixon, N.F. (1971). *Subliminal perception: The nature of a controversy*. New York: McGraw-Hill.

Dixon, N.F. (1981). *Preconscious processing*. Chichester, UK: Wiley.

Draguns, J.G. (1983). Why microgenesis? An inquiry on the motivational sources of going beyond the information given. *Archives of Psychology*, *135*, 5–16.

Draguns, J.G. (1984). Microgenesis by any other name. . . . In W. Froehlich, G. Smith, J. Draguns, & U. Hentschel (Eds.), *Psychological processes in cognition and personality*. Washington, DC: Hemisphere.

Flavell, J.H., & Draguns, J.G. (1957). A microgenetic approach to perception and thought. *Psychological Bulletin*, *54*, 197–217.

Froehlich, W.D. (1984). Microgenesis as a functional approach to information processing through search. In W. Froehlich, G. Smith, J. Draguns, & U. Hentschel (Eds.), *Psychological processes in cognition and personality*. Washington, DC: Hemisphere.

Froehlich, W., Smith, G., Draguns, J., & Hentschel U. (Eds.). (1984). *Psychological processes in cogniton and personality*. Washington, DC: Hemisphere.
Goldberg, G. (1985). Supplementary motor area structure and function: Review and hypotheses. *Behavioral and Brain Sciences*, *8*, 567–616.
Goldberg, G. (1987). From intent to action. Evolution and function of the premotor systems of the frontal lobe. In E. Perecman (Ed.), *The frontal lobes revisited* (pp. 273–306). New York: IRBN Press.
Graumann, C.G. (1959). Aktualgenese: Die deskribptiven Grundlagen und theoretischen Wandlungen des aktualgenetischen Forschung sansatzes. *Zeitschrift fur experimentelle und angewandte Psychologie*, *6*, 410–448.
Hanlon, R.E., & Brown, J.W. (1989). Microgenesis: Historical review and current studies. In A. Ardila & F. Ostrosky-Solis (Eds.), *Brain organization of language and cognitive processes* (pp. 3–15). New York: Plenum Press.
Hanlon, R.E., Brown, J.W., & Gerstman, L. (1990). Enhancement of naming in nonfluent aphasia through gesture. *Brain and Language*, *38*, 298–314.
Hentschel, U., Smith, G., & Draguns, J.G. (Eds.). (1986). *The roots of perception*. Amsterdam: Elsevier North-Holland.
Hoffman, R., & Sledge, W. (1984). A microgenetic model of paragrammatisms produced by a schizophrenic speaker. *Brain and Language*, *21*, 147–173.
Kragh, U. (1955). *The actual-genetic model of perception-personality*. Lund, Sweden: Gleerup.
Kragh, U., & Smith, G.J.W. (1970). *Percept-genetic analysis*. Lund, Sweden: Gleerup.
Linschoten, J. (1959). Aktualgenese und heuristisches Prinzip. *Zeitschrift für experimentelle und angewandte Psychologie*, *6*, 449–473.
Pick, A. (1913). *Die agrammatischen Sprachstörungen*. Berlin: Springer-Verlag.
Pick, A. (1973). *Aphasia* (J.W. Brown, Trans.). Springfield, IL: Charles C. Thomas. (Original work published 1931)
Pötzl, O. (1960). The relationship between experimentally induced dream images and indirect vision. Monograph 7. *Psychological Issues*, *2*, 41–120. (original work published 1917)
Sander, F. (1962). Experimentelle Ergebnisse der Gestaltpsychologie. In F. Sander & H. Volkelt (Eds.), *Ganzheitspsychologie* (pp. 73–112). Munich: Beck. (Original work published 1928)
Schilder, P. (1951). On the development of thoughts. In D. Rapaport (Ed.), *Organization and pathology of thought* (pp. 497–518). New York: Columbia University Press.
Sergent, J. (1986). Microgenesis of face perception. In H.D. Ellis, M.A. Jeeves, F. Newcombe, & A. Young (Eds.), *Aspects of face processing*. Dordrecht, The Netherlands: Martinus Nijhoff.
Smith, G.J.W. (1957). Visual perception: An event over time. *Psychological Review*, *64*, 306–313.
Smith, G.J.W. (1984). Stabilization and automatization of peceptual activity over time. In W. Froehlich, G. Smith, J. Draguns, & U. Hentschel (Eds.), *Psychological processes in cognition and personality* (pp. 135–142). Washington, DC: Hemisphere.
Smith, G.J.W., & Danielsson, A. (1982). *Anxiety and defensive strategies in childhood and adolescence. Psychological Issues, Monograph 53*. New York: International Universities Press.

Smith, G.J.W., Johnson, G., & Almgren, P.E. (1989). *MCT—The meta-contrast technique*. Stockholm: Psykologiforlaget.

Smith, G.J.W., & Westerlundh, B. (1980). Perceptgenesis: A process perspective on perception-personality. *Review of Personality and Social Psychology*, *1*, 94–124.

Werner, H. (1948). *Comparative psychology of mental development*. New York: International Universities Press.

Werner, H. (1956). Microgenesis and aphasia. *Journal of Abnormal Social Psychology*, *52*, 347–353.

Werner, H. (1957). The concept of development from a comparative and organismic point of view. In D.B. Harris (Ed.), *The concept of development: An issue in the study of human behavior* (pp. 125–148) Minneapolis: University of Minnesota Press.

Westerlundh, B. (1976). *Aggression, anxiety and defense*. Lund, Sweden: Gleerup.

Yakovlev, P. (1948). Motility, behavior and the brain. *Journal of Nervous and Mental Disease*, *107*, 313–335.

# Index

MIX
Papier aus verantwortungsvollen Quellen
Paper from responsible sources
FSC® C105338

If you have any concerns about our products,
you can contact us on
**ProductSafety@springernature.com**

In case Publisher is established outside the EU,
the EU authorized representative is:
**Springer Nature Customer Service Center GmbH**
**Europaplatz 3, 69115 Heidelberg, Germany**

Printed by Libri Plureos GmbH
in Hamburg, Germany